SPANISH
TERMINOLOGY
for the Dental Team

Terminología En Español
para el Equipo Dental

SPANISH TERMINOLOGY
for the Dental Team

Terminología En Español para el Equipo Dental

THIRD EDITION

Amber Lovatos, RDH, BSDH
Public Health Dental Hygienist
The Latina RDH
Spring, Texas

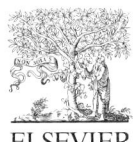

ELSEVIER

Elsevier
3251 Riverport Lane
St. Louis, Missouri 63043

SPANISH TERMINOLOGY FOR THE DENTAL
TEAM, THIRD EDITION

ISBN: 978-0-443-11482-3

Notice

Practitioners and researchers must always rely on their own experience and
knowledge in evaluating and using any information, methods, compounds or
experiments described herein. Because of rapid advances in the medical sciences, in
particular, independent verification of diagnoses and drug dosages should be made.
To the fullest extent of the law, no responsibility is assumed by Elsevier, authors,
editors or contributors for any injury and/or damage to persons or property as a
matter of products liability, negligence or otherwise, or from any use or operation of
any methods, products, instructions, or ideas contained in the material herein.

Previous editions copyrighted 2011 and 2004.

Senior Content Strategist: Kelly Skelton
Senior Content Development Specialist: Vasowati Shome
Publishing Services Manager: Deepthi Unni
Senior Project Manager: Beula Christopher
Designer: Margaret Reid

Printed in India

Last digit is the print number: 9 8 7 6 5 4 3 2 1

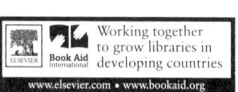

Reviewers

Margaret J. Fehrenbach, RDH, MS
Director, Dental Hygiene Educational Consulting
Oral Biology Technical Writer and Webinar Presenter
Past Adjunct Faculty
Dental Hygiene Program, Seattle Central College
Seattle, Washington

Natalie Stephanie Cruz, CMI-Spanish
Certified Medical Interpreter
UNC-Chapel Hill Adams School of Dentistry
Chapel Hill, North Carolina

How to Use This Book

Hispanic is a term used to identify people from Spanish-speaking countries, particularly those from Latin America and Spain. The largest Hispanic populations in the United States reside in Arizona, California, Colorado, Florida, New Mexico, New York, and Texas. Because it is not possible to detail every conceivable vocabulary preference, this book uses a universally accepted dialect. However, you will probably encounter some Spanish words unfamiliar to your area. It is important to recognize that different dialects exist not only between countries but also within regions of the same country. However, no particular version of Spanish is more correct than another.

ORGANIZATION

This book is organized into three parts and follows a logical sequence of how a practitioner would interact with a patient from initial greeting to specialty appointments.

The book addresses the use of the formal "you" (usted) in situations among adults and the appropriate use of the informal "you" (tú) in situations in which adults are addressing children.

In cases where two or more words or phrases are appropriate, each is separated by a slash (/).

In this example, the word translator or interpreter can be used to complete the sentence:

I need a (translator/interpreter)—wait a minute.

Necesito un (traductor/intérprete)—espere un minuto.

In cases where several words or phrases are appropriate, choices have been placed into boxes. These choices may pertain to more than one sentence in the section. In this example, any of the choices in the box may be correct.

What is the relationship of the subscriber to you? (Box 2.1)

Throughout the text, boxes containing helpful information relating to a topic will appear for readers to reference. (Box 11.2)

Box 2.1
People who may carry insurance for a dental patient

- Husband
- Wife
- Father
- Mother
- Self

Box 11.12
Flossing steps

- Break off about a foot and a half of floss and wind most of it around one of your middle fingers.
- Wind the remaining floss around the same finger of the opposite hand so that it will take up the floss as it becomes dirty.
- After winding the floss, hold the floss tightly between your thumbs and forefingers.
- Guide the floss between the contacts of your teeth using a gentle motion.
- Curve the floss into a "C" shape against one tooth and gently slide it into the space between the gum and the tooth.
- Hold the floss tightly against the tooth and gently rub the side of the tooth with up-and-down motions.
- Floss each tooth thoroughly with a clean section of floss.

RESOURCES

We have included audio resources that you may find helpful as you learn to communication in Spanish. The enhanced ebook version, included with every new print purchase, features audio pronunciation of phrases in English and Spanish. The access information is on the inside front cover.

Inside the book, we have included helpful information about the use of accents, verbs, nouns, and adjectives within the Spanish language. A pronunciation guide is also included. At the back of the book, an extensive English-to-Spanish glossary is provided for quick reference. The glossary is divided into categories, such as dental terms, numbers, and months of the year. An alphabetical Spanish-to-English listing of each of the vocabulary words and a list of informal expressions used in conversation are also provided.

Contents

Contenido

Appendix B and Informal Expressions are available in the eBook at ebooks.health.elsevier.com. See inside cover for access details.

PART I
Anatomy

PARTE I
Anatomía (Audio 1.0)

Capítulo 1
Anatomía Oral (Audio 1.1)

DENTAL AND ORAL ANATOMIC TERMINOLOGY (SEE FIGS. 1.1–1.3)
TERMINOLOGÍA ANATÓMICA DENTAL Y ORAL (VEA LAS FIGURAS 1.1–1.3) (AUDIO 1.2)

Alveolar Bone
El hueso alveolar (Audio 1.3)

Blood
La sangre (Audio 1.4)

Blood vessels
Los vasos sanguíneos (Audio 1.5)

Bone
El hueso (Audio 1.6)

Buccal vestibule
El vestíbulo bucal (Audio 1.7)

Central incisor(s)
El(Los) incisivo(s) central(es) (Audio 1.8)

Cementum
El cemento (Audio 1.9)

Crown
La corona (Audio 1.10)

Cuspid(s)/canine(s)
El(Los) canino(s) /colmillo(s) (Audio 1.11)

Deciduous teeth (milk teeth)/primary teeth
Los dientes de leche/los dientes primarios (Audio 1.12)

Dentin
La dentina (Audio 1.13)

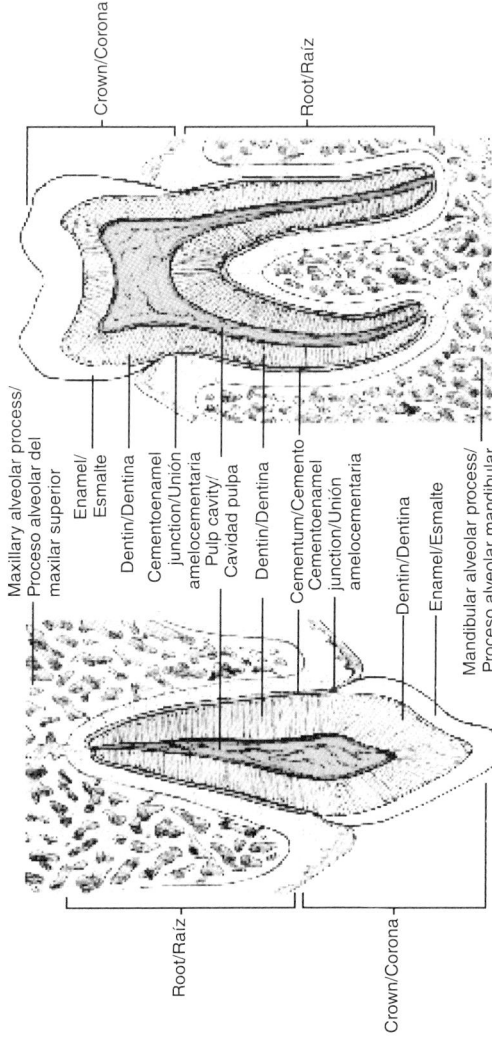

Crown/Corona

Root/Raíz

Maxillary alveolar process/ Proceso alveolar del maxilar superior

Enamel/ Esmalte

Dentin/Dentina

Cementoenamel junction/Unión amelocementaria

Pulp cavity/ Cavidad pulpa

Dentin/Dentina

Cementum/Cemento

Cementoenamel junction/Unión amelocementaria

Dentin/Dentina

Enamel/Esmalte

Mandibular alveolar process/ Proceso alveolar mandibular

Root/Raíz

Crown/Corona

Fig. 1.1 Diagram of the tooth. Diagrama de un diente. *(From Bath-Balogh M, Fehrenbach M): Illustrated dental embryology, histology and anatomy, ed 2. Philadelphia, 2006, Saunders.)*

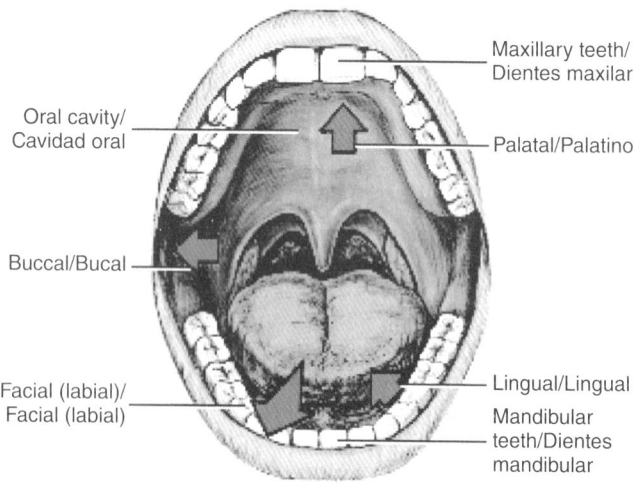

Fig. 1.2 Diagram of an oral cavity. Diagrama de una cavidad bucal. *(From Bath-Balogh M, Fehrenbach MJ: Illustrated dental embryology, histology and anatomy, ed 2. Philadelphia, 2006, Saunders.)*

Enamel
El esmalte (Audio 1.14)

Floor of the mouth
El piso (suelo) de la boca (Audio 1.15)

Frenum/frenulum
El frenillo (Audio 1.16)

Gingiva/gum(s)
La Gingiva/la(s) encía(s) (Audio 1.17)

Hard palate
El Paladar duro (Audio 1.18)

Incisor(s)
El(Los) incisivo(s) (Audio 1.19)

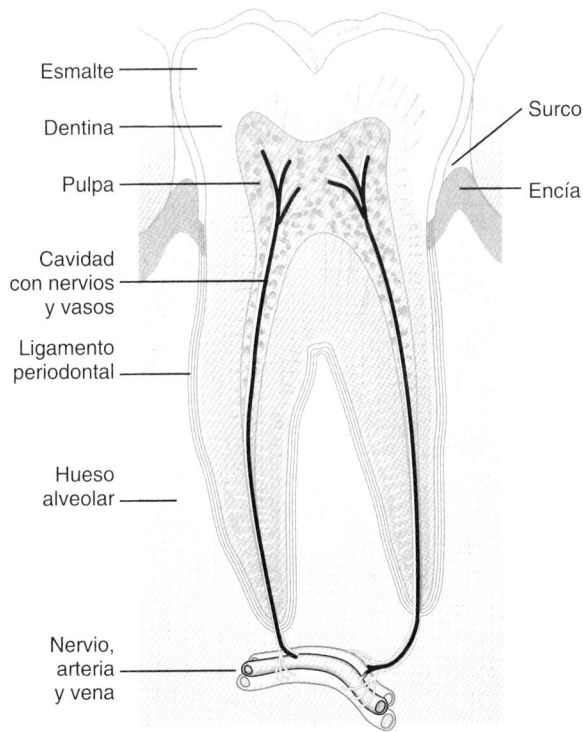

Fig. 1.3 Tooth anatomy. Anatomia del diente. *(From Raymond, K: Krause.*
Mahan's Food & the Nutrition Care Process, 15e., *2021 Elsevier.)*

Lateral incisor
El incisivo lateral (Audio 1.20)

Lip(s)
El(Los) labio(s) (Audio 1.21)

Lower left/right first premolar
El primer premolar inferior izquierdo/derecho (Audio 1.22)

Mandible/jaw
La mandíbula/la quijada (Audio 1.23)

Mandibular lateral incisors
Los incisivos laterales inferiores (Audio 1.24)

Mandibular tooth
El diente de la mandíbula/El diente mandibular (Audio 1.25)

Maxilla
El maxilar (Audio 1.26)

Maxillary central incisors
Los incisivos centrales superiores (Audio 1.27)

Maxillary/mandibular cuspid
El (canino/colmillo) superior/inferior (Audio 1.28)

Molar(s)
La(Las) muela(s)/El(Los) molar(es) (Audio 1.29)

Nerve
El nervio (Audio 1.30)

Oral cavity
La cavidad bucal/la cavidad oral (Audio 1.31)

Oral mucosa
La mucosa oral (Audio 1.32)

Oropharynx
La orofaringe (Audio 1.33)

Palate
El paladar (Audio 1.34)

Papilla
La papilla (Audio 1.35)

Periodontal ligament
El ligamento periodontal (Audio 1.36)

Pharynx
La faringe (Audio 1.37)

Premolar(s)/bicuspid(s)
El(Los) premolar(es) (Audio 1.38)

Pulp
La pulpa (Audio 1.39)

Pulp canal (root canal) *(anatomy not procedure)*
La cavidad con nervios y vasos (Audio 1.40)

Pulp cavity
La cavidad pulpar (Audio 1.41)

Pulp chamber
La cámara pulpar (Audio 1.42)

Root/tooth root
La raíz/raíz del diente (Audio 1.43)

Root canal *(anatomy)*
El canal de la raíz/el conducto radicular (Audio 1.44)

Saliva
La saliva (Audio 1.45)

Salivary gland(s)
La(Las) glándula(s) salival(es) (Audio 1.46)

Soft palate
El paladar blando (Audio 1.47)

Sulcus
El surco gingival (Audio 1.48)

Tongue
La lengua (Audio 1.49)

Tonsils
Las amígdalas/Las anginas (Audio 1.50)

Tooth/teeth
El diente/Los dientes (Audio 1.51)

Upper left/right first/second/third molar
El primer/segundo/tercer molar superior izquierdo/derecho
(Audio 1.52)

Uvula
La úvula (Audio 1.53)

Wisdom tooth/wisdom teeth
La(s) muela(s) de(l) juicio/La muela cordal/Las cordales (Audio 1.54)

Chapter 2
Head and Neck Anatomy

Capítulo 2
Anatomía de Cabeza y Cuello (Audio 2.1)

ANATOMIC TERMINOLOGY OF THE HEAD AND NECK (SEE FIGS. 2.1 AND 2.2)
TERMINOLOGÍA ANATÓMICA DE LA CABEZA Y EL CUELLO (VEA LAS FIGS. 2.1 Y 2.2) (AUDIO 2.2)

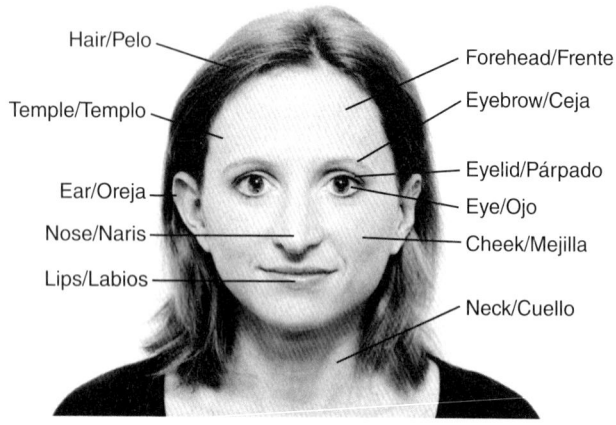

Fig. 2.1 Frontal view of the face. Vista frontal de la cara.

Artery (arteries)
La(Las) arteria(s) (Audio 2.3)

Blood vessels
Los vasos sanguíneos (Audio 2.4)

Buccal fat pad
La almohadilla grasa bucal (Audio 2.5)

Cheek(s)
La(Las) mejilla(s)/(el/los) cachete(s) (Audio 2.6)

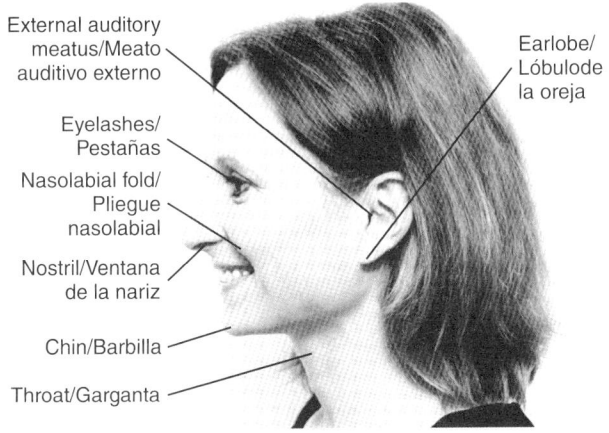

External auditory meatus/Meato auditivo externo

Eyelashes/Pestañas

Nasolabial fold/Pliegue nasolabial

Nostril/Ventana de la nariz

Chin/Barbilla

Throat/Garganta

Earlobe/Lóbulo de la oreja

Fig. 2.2 Lateral view of the face. Vista lateral de la cara.

Cheek bone/zygoma
El hueso (de la/del) (mejilla/cachet)/cigomático/hueso malar (Audio 2.7)

Chin
La barbilla (Audio 2.8)

Ear/ears
La(Las) oreja(s) (Audio 2.9)

Eardrum (tympanic membrane)
El tímpano (Audio 2.10)

Esophagus
El esófago (Audio 2.11)

Eustachian tube(s)
La(Las) trompa(s) de eustaquio (Audio 2.12)

Eye(s)
El(Los) ojo(s) (Audio 2.13)

Eyebrow(s)
La(Las) ceja(s) (Audio 2.14)

Eyelash(es)
La(Las) pestaña(s) (Audio 2.15)

Forehead
La frente (Audio 2.16)

Hair
El pelo (Audio 2.17)

Head
La cabeza (Audio 2.18)

Larynx
La laringe (Audio 2.19)

Lip(s)
El(Los) labio(s) (Audio 2.20)

Lymph node(s)
El(Los) ganglio(s) linfático(s) (Audio 2.21)

Lymphatics
Los linfáticos (Audio 2.22)

Mandible
La mandíbula (Audio 2.23)

Maxilla
El maxilar (Audio 2.24)

Minor salivary glands
Las glándulas salivales menores (Audio 2.25)

Mouth
La boca (Audio 2.26)

Muscle(s)
El(Los) músculo(s) (Audio 2.27)

Muscles of mastication
Los músculos de la masticación/músculos masticadores (Audio 2.28)

Neck
El cuello (Audio 2.29)

Nerve
El nervio (Audio 2.30)

Nerve canal (anatomy)
El canal del nervio/conducto radicular (Audio 2.31)

Nose
La nariz (Audio 2.32)

Nostril
La ventana de la nariz (Audio 2.33)

Oral cavity
La cavidad oral (Audio 2.34)

Parathyroid glands
Las glándulas paratiroides (Audio 2.35)

Parotid gland(s)
La(Las) glándula(s) parótida(s) (Audio 2.36)

Pharynx
La faringe (Audio 2.37)

Scalp
El cuero cabelludo (Audio 2.38)

Sinus
Los senos nasales (Audio 2.39)

Sublingual gland(s)
La glándula sublingual/Las glandulas sublinguales (Audio 2.40)

Submandibular gland
La glándula submandibular (Audio 2.41)

Throat
La garganta (Audio 2.42)

Thyroid gland
La glándula tiroides (Audio 2.43)

Trachea
La tráquea (Audio 2.44)

Vein(s)
La(Las) vena(s) (Audio 2.45)

Chapter 3
General Anatomy

Capítulo 3
Anatomía General (Audio 3.1)

GENERAL ANATOMIC TERMINOLOGY (SEE FIGS. 3.1 AND 3.2)
TERMINOLOGÍA ANATÓMICA GENERAL VEA LAS FIGS. 3.1 Y 3.2) (AUDIO 3.2)

Abdomen
El abdomen (Audio 3.3)

Adrenal gland(s)
La(Las) glándula(s) suprarrenal(es) (Audio 3.4)

Ankle(s)
El(Los) tobillo(s) (Audio 3.5)

Anus
El ano (Audio 3.6)

Aorta
La aorta (Audio 3.7)

Arm(s)
El(Los) brazos) (Audio 3.8)

Back
La espalda (Audio 3.9)

Brain
El cerebro (Audio 3.10)

Breast(s)
El(Los) seno(s)/El(Los) pecho(s) (Audio 3.11)

Buttocks/rear end
Las nalgas/El trasero (Audio 3.12)

Calf muscle(s)/gastrocnemius
La(Las) pantorrilla(s)/gastrocnemio (Audio 3.13)

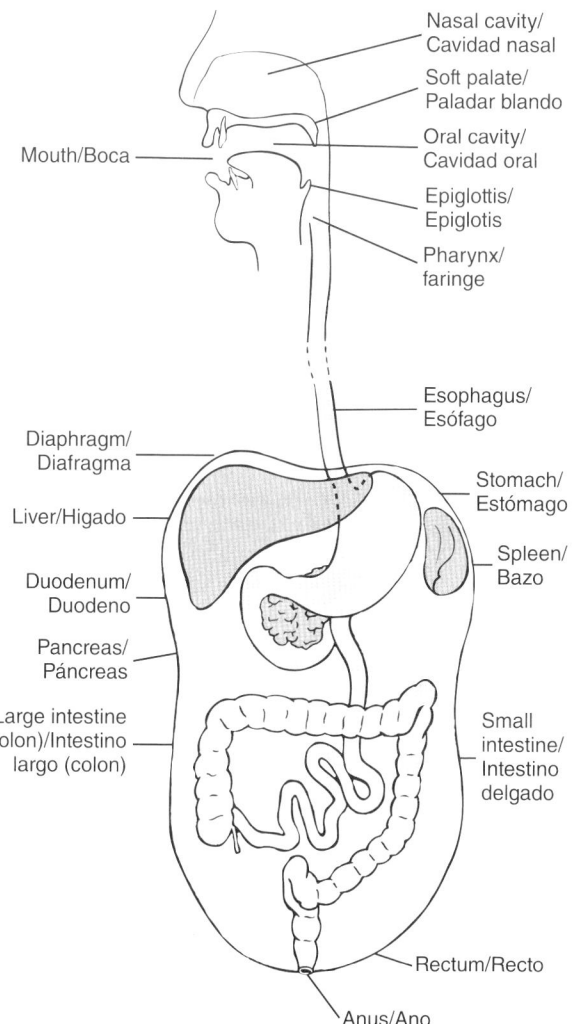

Fig. 3.1 Diagram of A, the head, B, the neck, and C, the torso (with internal organs). Diagrama de A, la cabeza, B, el cuello y C, el torso (con órganos internos). *(From Liebgott B: The Anatomical Basis of Dentistry, ed 3. Mosby, St. Louis, 2010.)*

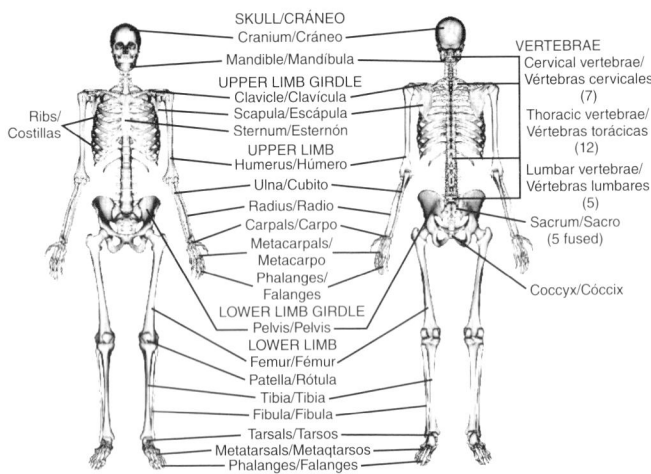

Fig. 3.2 Diagram of the skeleton. Diagrama del esqueleto. *(From Liebgott B: The Anatomical Basis of Dentistry, ed 3. Mosby, St. Louis, 2010.)*

Carpal bones
Los huesos del carpo (Audio 3.14)

Cervical vertebra (cervical vertebrae)
La(Las) vértebra(s) cervical(es) (Audio 3.15)

Chest
El pecho (Audio 3.16)

Clavicle
La clavicula (Audio 3.17)

Coronary arteries
Las arterias coronarias (Audio 3.18)

Cranial nerves
Los nervios craneales/pares craneales (Audio 3.19)

Diaphragm
El diafragma (Audio 3.20)

Elbow(s)
El(Los) codo(s) (Audio 3.21)

Fallopian tube(s)
La(Las) trompa(s) de falopio (Audio 3.22)

Femur
El femur (Audio 3.23)

Femoral artery
La arteria femoral (Audio 3.24)

Finger(s)
El(Los) dedo(s) (Audio 3.25)

Fingernail(s)
La(s) uña(s) (Audio 3.26)

Forearm(s)
El(Los) antebrazo(s) (Audio 3.27)

Foot/feet
El pie/Los pies (Audio 3.28)

Gallbladder
La vesícula biliar (Audio 3.29)

Groin
La ingle (Audio 3.30)

Hand(s)
El(Las) mano(s) (Audio 3.31)

Head
La cabeza (Audio 3.32)

Heart
El corazón (Audio 3.33)

Heel
El calcañar/talón (Audio 3.34)

Hips
Las caderas (Audio 3.35)

Intestines
Los intestinos (Audio 3.36)

Joints
Los articuláciones (Audio 3.37)

Kidney(s)
El(Los) riñón(es) (Audio 3.38)

Knee(s)
La(Las) rodilla(s)(Audio 3.39)

Kneecap/patella
La rótula (patela) (Audio 3.40)

Knuckles
Los nudillos (Audio 3.41)

Leg(s)
La(Las) pierna(s) (Audio 3.42)

Ligament
El ligamento (Audio 3.43)

Liver
El hígado (Audio 3.44)

Lungs
Los pulmónes (Audio 3.45)

Nipple(s)
El(Los) pezón(es) (Audio 3.46)

Ovaries
El(Los) ovario(s) (Audio 3.47)

Palm(s)
La(Las) palma(s) (Audio 3.48)

Pancreas
El páncreas (Audio 3.49)

Pectoralis muscles
Los músculos pectorales (Audio 3.50)

Pelvis
La pelvis (Audio 3.51)

Penis
El pene (Audio 3.52)

Prostate gland
La glándula de la próstata (Audio 3.53)

Rectum
El recto (Audio 3.54)

Ribs
Las costillas (Audio 3.55)

Rotator cuff
El manguito de los rotadores/ manguito rotador (Audio 3.56)

Sacrum
El sacro (Audio 3.57)

Scapula
La escápula (Audio 3.58)

Sciatic nerve
El nervio ciático (Audio 3.59)

Shin
La espinilla (Audio 3.60)

Shoulder(s)
El(Los) hombro(s) (Audio 3.61)

Skin
La piel (Audio 3.62)

Sole
La planta (Audio 3.63)

Spinal cord
La médula espinal (Audio 3.64)

Spine
El espinazo (Audio 3.65)

Sternum
El esternón (Audio 3.66)

Stomach
El estómago (Audio 3.67)

Tendon(s)
El(Los) tendón(es) (Audio 3.68)

Testicle(s)
El(Los) testículo(s) (Audio 3.69)

Thigh(s)
El(Los) muslo(s) (Audio 3.70)

Thoracic vertebrae
La vértebra torácica (Audio 3.71)

Thumb(s)
El(Los) pulgar(es) (Audio 3.72)

Toe(s)
El(Los) dedo(s) del pie (Audio 3.73)

Toenails
La(Las) uña(s) de los pies (Audio 3.74)

Torso
El torso (Audio 3.75)

Ureter(s)
El(Los) uréter(es) (Audio 3.76)

Urethra
La uretra (Audio 3.77)

Urinary bladder/bladder
La vejiga urinaria/vejiga (Audio 3.78)

Uterus
El útero (Audio 3.79)

Vagina
La vagina (Audio 3.80)

Vertebrae
Las vértebras (Audio 3.81)

Vertebral disc
El disco vertebral/disco intervertebral (Audio 3.82)

Waist
La cintura (Audio 3.83)

Wrist(s)
La(Las) muñeca(s) (Audio 3.84)

PART II
Dental Terminology

PARTE II
Terminología Dental (Audio 4.0)

Chapter 4
Emergencies in the Dental Office (Audio 4.1)

Capítulo 4
Emergencias en el Consultorio Dental (Audio 4.2)

MEDICAL EMERGENCIES
EMERGENCIAS MÉDICAS (AUDIO 4.3)

Don't swallow. We will help remove it from your mouth.
No trague. Le ayudaremos a removerlo de su boca. (Audio 4.4)
Are you not feeling well? Tell me how you feel. (See Box 4.1)
¿No se está sintiendo bien? Dígame cómo se siente. (Vea el Cuadro 4.1) (Audio 4.5)

Are you feeling _____? (See Box 4.1)
¿Se siente _____? (Vea el Cuadro 4.1) (Audio 4.6)

_____, (Name) has this happened to you before at the dentist?
¿_____, (Nombre) le ha pasado esto antes en el dentista? (Audio 4.7)

Is there someone we should call?
¿Hay alguien a quien deberíamos llamar? (Audio 4.8)

You have (fainted/had a seizure).
Usted (se desmayó/tuvo una convulsión). (Audio 4.9)

Turn your head this way to vomit.
Volte la cabeza a este lado para vomitar. (Audio 4.10)

I will call the dentist in since you are not feeling well.
Voy a llamar al dentista ya que usted no se está sintiendo bien. (Audio 4.11)

We will reschedule your appointment since you are not feeling well today.
Vamos a volver a programar su cita ya que no se siente bien hoy.
Reprogramaremos su cita ya que no se siente bien. (Audio 4.12)

The dentist will be in charge.
El/La dentista va a estar a cargo. (Audio 4.13)

Box 4.1
Descriptions of how a patient feels (Audio 4.136)

- Cold and clammy (Audio 4.137)
- Cold (Audio 4.138)
- Disoriented (Audio 4.139)
- Dizzy (Audio 4.140)
- Hot (Audio 4.141)
- Light-headed (Audio 4.142)
- Nauseated (Audio 4.143)
- Stomachache (Audio 4.144)
- Sleepy/drowsy (Audio 4.145)
- Sweaty (Audio 4.146)
- Tired (Audio 4.147)

Cuadro 4.1
Descripciones de cómo se siente el paciente (Audio 4.136)

- Frío(a) y húmedo(a) (Audio 4.137)
- Frío(a) (Audio 4.138)
- Desorientado(a) (Audio 4.139)
- Mareado(a) (Audio 4.140)
- Caliente (Audio 4.141)
- Mareado(a) (Audio 4.142)
- Con náuseas (Audio 4.143)
- Dolor de estómago (Audio 4.144)
- Soñoliento(a)/somnoliento(a)/con sueno (Audio 4.145)
- Sudoroso(a) (Audio 4.146)
- Cansado(a) (Audio 4.147)

Remain calm; we are here for you.
Manténgase calmado(a); estamos aquí para usted. (Audio 4.14)

To keep from fainting, please remain calm and keep lying down.
Para evitar que se desmaye, por favor permanezca calmado(a) y quédese acostado(a). (Audio 4.15)

Call (911/medical assistance).
Llame (al 911/asistencia médica). (Audio 4.16)

We have called (911/medical assistance).
Hemos llamado (al 911/a asistencia médica). (Audio 4.17)

Medical assistance will soon be here.
La asistencia médica estará aquí pronto. (Audio 4.18)

We will stay with you until emergency help gets here.
Nos quedaremos con usted hasta que llegue la ayuda de emergencia. (Audio 4.19)

We will be taking your (blood pressure/pulse).
Le tomaremos (la/el) (presión arterial/pulso). (Audio 4.20)

Bring in the oxygen for this patient.
Trae el oxígeno para este paciente. (Audio 4.21)

(We are/I am) going to take your blood pressure.
(Le vamos/le voy) a tomar su presion. (Audio 4.22)

We will be placing you on oxygen.
Le vamos a administrar oxígeno. (Audio 4.23)

Here's the oxygen mask.
Aquí está la máscara de oxígeno. (Audio 4.24)

Breathe normally with the oxygen.
Respire normalmente con el oxígeno. (Audio 4.25)

Do you need your medications?
¿ Necesita sus medicamentos? (Audio 4.26)

Use your inhaler for your asthma attack.
Use su inhalador para su ataque de asma. (Audio 4.27)

Use your pills for your heart pain.
Use sus pastillas para el dolor del corazón. (Audio 4.28)

Are you having trouble breathing?
¿Está teniendo problemas para respirar? (Audio 4.29)

Slow down your breathing.
Respire más despacio. (Audio 4.30)

Are you having trouble swallowing?
¿Está teniendo problemas para tragar/pasar saliva? (Audio 4.31)

Is your skin itchy?
¿Tiene picazón en la piel? (Audio 4.32)

Do you feel heart palpations?
Está sintiendo palpaciones del corazon? (Audio 4.33)

Do you have any crushing pain in your chest?
Tiene dolor opresivo en el pecho? (Audio 4.34)

Is there shooting pain up your arm?
¿Tiene un dolor punzante en el brazo? (Audio 4.35)

Is there a change in your vision?

¿Hay algún cambio en su visión? (Audio 4.36)

We will be injecting you with medicine for your allergy attack.

Le inyectaremos medicamento para su ataque de alergia. (Audio 4.37)

(Eat/drink) this (sugar/orange juice) to help with your low blood sugar.

(Come/Bebe) (esta azúcar/este jugo de naranja) para ayudarle con su nivel bajo de azucar. (Audio 4.38)

We will be helping _____ (name) to breathe.

Le estaremos ayudando a _____ (nombre) a respirar. (Audio 4.39)

_____; (name) has gone into (cardiac arrest/ unconsciousness).

_____; (nombre) ha entrado en (un paro cardíaco/una pérdida de conocimiento). (Audio 4.40)

We will be performing cardiopulmonary resuscitation (CPR) on _____ (name).

Estaremos adminstrando los (primeros auxilios/reanimación cardiopulmonar) (RCP) a _____(nombre). (Audio 4.41)

We will be using the automated external defibrillator (AED) on _____ (name).

Estaremos usando el desfibrilador externo automatizado (DEA) en _____ (nombre). (Audio 4.42)

Stand back during the use of the automated external defibrillator.

Retroceda durante el uso del desfibrilador externo automatizado. (Audio 4.43)

DENTAL EMERGENCIES
EMERGENCIAS DENTALES (AUDIO 4.44)

Do you have a toothache?

¿Tiene dolor de dientes? (Audio 4.45)

Do your molars hurt?

¿Le duelen las muelas? (Audio 4.46)

Does your (tooth/jaw/TMJ joint) hurt?
¿Le duele su (diente/(mandíbula/quijada)/articulación temporomandibular)? (Audio 4.47)

Do your gums hurt?
¿Le duelen las encías? (Audio 4.48)

Are you in pain?
¿Tiene dolor? (Audio 4.49)

Is it a (sharp/deep/throbbing) pain?
¿Es un dolor (agudo/profundo/punzante)? (Audio 4.50)

Does it hurt you at night?
¿Le duele por la noche? (Audio 4.51)

Does it hurt when you are lying down?
¿Le duele cuando está acostado(a)? (Audio 4.52)

Is it worse during the day or night?
¿Es peor durante el día o la noche? (Audio 4.53)

Does it hurt when you get up in the morning?
¿Le duele cuando se levanta en la mañana? (Audio 4.54)

Does it hurt when you open wide?
¿Le duele cuando abre grande/completamente? (Audio 4.55)

Does the pain get better or worse when you (lie down/sit up)?
¿El dolor mejora o empeora cuando se (acuesta/sienta)? (Audio 4.56)

How long have you been in pain?
¿Cuánto tiempo lleva con dolor? (Audio 4.57)

Where does it hurt?
¿Dónde le duele? (Audio 4.58)

Please point to where you have the pain.
Por favor, señale dónde tiene el dolor. (Audio 4.59)

When did the pain start?
¿Cuándo comenzó el dolor? (Audio 4.60)

How many days ago?
¿Hace cuántos días? (Audio 4.61)

Did you have an accident?
Ha tenido algún accidente? (Audio 4.62)

Did you fall?
¿Usted se cayó? (Audio 4.63)

Were you hit in the face?
Se golpeó en la cara? (Audio 4.64)

You are bleeding.
Está sangrando. (Audio 4.65)

You are swollen.
Está hinchado(a). (Audio 4.66)

You have a cut on your _____. (See Box 4.2)
Tiene una cortada en su(s) _____. (Vea el Cuadro 4.2) (Audio 4.67)

We need to place some stitches to close the cut.
Necesitamos poner unas puntadas para cerrar la cortadura/cortada.
Necesitamos poner unos puntos para cerrar la cortadura/cortada.
(Audio 4.68)

Are you taking any medication for the pain?
¿Está tomando algún medicamento para el dolor? (Audio 4.69)

Is it working?
¿Está funcionando? (Audio 4.70)

Box 4.2
Parts of the mouth
that may be cut
(Audio 4.148)

- Cheek (Audio 4.149)
- Gums/gingiva (Audio 4.150)
- Lip (Audio 4.151)
- Roof of the mouth
  (Audio 4.152)
- Tongue (Audio 4.153)

Cuadro 4.2
Partes de la boca que
pueden estar cortadas
(Audio 4.148)

- Cachete/Mejilla (Audio 4.149)
- Encías (Audio 4.150)
- Labio (Audio 4.151)
- Cielo de la boca/techo de la
  boca (Audio 4.152)
- Lengua (Audio 4.153)

What medication are you taking?
¿Qué medicamentos está tomando? (Audio 4.71)

How often do you take the medication?
¿Con qué frecuencia toma el medicamento? (Audio 4.72)

How long have you been taking the medication?
¿Cuánto tiempo ha estado tomando el medicamento? (Audio 4.73)

Does anything make the pain worse?
¿Hay algo que empeora el dolor? (Audio 4.74)

Are any of your teeth sensitive to _____? (See Box 4.3)
¿Tiene dientes sensible (al/a lo) _____? (Vea el Cuadro 4.3)
(Audio 4.75)

Does it hurt when you bite (hard/soft) things?
¿Le duele cuando muerde cosas (duras/suaves)? (Audio 4.76)

Have you ever had a pain like this before?
¿Ha tenido un dolor como este antes? (Audio 4.77)

Does the tooth feel hot?
¿Se siente caliente el diente? (Audio 4.78)

Do you have (bleeding/swelling/pus)?
¿Tiene (sangrado/ hinchazón/ pus)? (Audio 4.79)

Box 4.3
Things that teeth can be sensitive to (Audio 4.154)

- Air (Audio 4.155)
- Biting (Audio 4.156)
- Cold (Audio 4.157)
- Drinking (Audio 4.158)
- Heat (Audio 4.159
- Sweets (Audio 4.160)

Cuadro 4.3
Cosas a las que pueden ser sensibles los dientes (Audio 4.161)

- Aire (Audio 4.155)
- Morder (Audio 4.156)
- Frío (Audio 4.157)
- Beber (Audio 4.158)
- Caliente (Audio 4.159)
- Dulce (Audio 4.60)

Does it hurt deep in the bone or where the tooth and gum meet?
¿Le duele en lo profundo del hueso o donde se une el diente con la encía? (Audio 4.80)

This tooth cannot be saved.
No podemos salvar este diente. (Audio 4.81)

Would you like to try to save this tooth?
¿Le gustaría tratar de salvar este diente? (Audio 4.82)

Does your tooth feel loose?
¿Se siente flojo su diente? (Audio 4.83)

Does more than one tooth hurt?
¿Le duele más de un diente? (Audio 4.84)

Does the pain extend to the top and bottom jaws?
¿El dolor se extiende hacia las quijadas de arriba y abajo? (Audio 4.85)

I am going to tap on your teeth slightly. Let me know if any tooth hurts.
Voy a darle golpecitos en los dientes. Hágame saber si algún diente le duele. (Audio 4.86)

Does it hurt when I press here?
¿Le duele cuándo presiono aquí? (Audio 4.87)

Which tooth hurts more, this one or this one?
¿Cuál diente le duele más, éste o éste? (Audio 4.88)

Does the tooth feel sharp?
¿Su diente se siente afilado? (Audio 4.89)

Is it cutting your tongue?
¿Le está cortando la lengua?? (Audio 4.90)

Please bite down slowly.
Por favor muerda lentamente. (Audio 4.91)

Please tap your teeth together.
Por favor, golpee sus dientes juntos. (Audio 4.92)

Bite normally.
Muerda normalmente. (Audio 4.93)

Bite with your back teeth.
Muerda con sus dientes posteriores. (Audio 4.94)

Please slowly bite down on this firmly. If it hurts, then stop biting immediately.
Por favor, muerda esto lentamente y firmemente. Si le duele, entonces deje de morder inmediatamente. (Audio 4.95)

Would you like me to take care of this problem now?
¿Le gustaría que me encargue de este problema ahora? (Audio 4.96)

Would you like me to give you medication/(a prescription) to relieve the pain?
¿Le gustaría que le diera medicamentos/(una receta) para aliviar el dolor? (Audio 4.97)

I want to give you medication to relieve the pain. Here is a prescription.
Quiero darle medicamento para aliviar el dolor. Aquí tiene una receta. (Audio 4.98)

Take the medicine every _____ hours.
Tome el medicamento cada _____ horas. (Audio 4.99)

This pain medication has a narcotic in it. Do not drink alcohol or drive or operate machinery if you take it.
Este medicamento para el dolor contiene un narcótico. No beba alcohol ni maneje o opere maquinaria si lo toma. (Audio 4.100)

This medication does not have a narcotic in it.
Este medicamento no contiene ningún narcótico. (Audio 4.101)

Does it hurt when you open and close your mouth?
¿Le duele cuando abre y cierra la boca? (Audio 4.102)

Does it hurt here?
¿Le duele aquí? (Audio 4.103)

We need to take a radiograph of this (area/tooth).
Necesitamos tomar una radiografía de (esta área/este diente). (Audio 4.104)

I will know more about your problem when I see the radiograph.
Voy a saber más sobre su problema cuando vea la radiografía. (Audio 4.105)

I can see on the radiograph that you have _____. (See Box 4.4)

Puedo ver en la radiografía que usted tiene _____.
(Vea el Cuadro 4.4) (Audio 4.106)

From this radiograph, I do not see anything wrong with your tooth.

En esta radiografía, no veo nada malo con su diente. (Audio 4.107)

Box 4.4 Problems that can be detected on a radiograph (Audio 4.162)	**Cuadro 4.4 Problemas que pueden ser detectados en una radiografía**
• An abscess (Audio 4.163)	• Un absceso (Audio 4.163)
• A cracked tooth (Audio 4.164)	• Un diente fracturado (Audio 4.164)
• A cyst (Audio 4.165)	• Un quiste (Audio 4.165)
• Decay (Audio 4.166)	• Descomposición (Picado) (Audio 4.166)
• A fractured jaw (Audio 4.167)	• Una mandíbula fracturada (Audio 4.167)
• A fractured tooth (Audio 4.168)	• Un diente fracturado (Audio 4.168)
• A gum infection (Audio 4.169)	• Una infección de encía (Audio 4.169)
• An impacted tooth (Audio 4.170)	• Un diente retenido (Audio 4.170)
• An infection (Audio 4.171)	• Una infección (Audio 4.171)
• A tumor (Audio 4.172)	• Un tumor (Audio 4.172)
• Bone fracture (Audio 4.173)	• Una fractura de hueso (Audio 4.173)
• Bone spur (Audio 4.174)	• Un espolón de hueso (Audio 4.174)
• Caries/cavities (Audio 4.175)	• Caries (Audio 4.175)
• Dry socket (Audio 4.176)	• Un alveolo seco (Audio 4.176)

Have you had treatment on this tooth recently?
¿Has recibido tratamiento en este diente recientemente?
(Audio 4.108)

If this tooth is extracted you should fill the space with a(n) (implant/bridge/partial denture) in the near future.
Si este diente es extraído, usted debe llenar el espacio con (un implante/un puente/una dentadura parcial) en un futuro no muy lejano. (Audio 4.109)

This procedure will stop the pain, but the treatment is not finished.
Este procedimiento detendrá el dolor, pero el tratamiento no se ha terminado. (Audio 4.110)

You need to come back in _____ days to have the treatment finished.
Usted necesita regresar en _____; días para terminar el tratamiento. (Audio 4.111)

You should return for a full exam.
Usted debe regresar para un examen completo. (Audio 4.112)

During the full exam, I can see if there are any other problems with your teeth.
Durante el examen completo, podré ver si hay otros problemas con sus dientes. (Audio 4.113)

DENTAL TRAUMA (AVULSED TOOTH)
TRAUMATISMO DENTAL (DIENTE AVULSIONADO) (AUDIO 4.114)

When was the accident?
¿Cuándo fue el accidente? (Audio 4.115)

Where was the accident?
¿Dónde fue el accidente? (Audio 4.116)

Where did you find the tooth?
¿Dónde encontró el diente? (Audio 4.117)

What did you do with the tooth?
¿Qué hizo con el diente? (Audio 4.118)

Do you have the tooth?
Tiene usted el diente? (Audio 4.119)

We need to take a radiograph of the area.
Necesitamos tomar una radiografía del área. (Audio 4.120)

We will reimplant the tooth.
Vamos a reimplantar el diente. (Audio 4.121)

We will stabilize the tooth with a splint.
Estabilizaremos el diente con una férula. (Audio 4.122)

The area will be very sore.
El área estará muy adolorida. (Audio 4.123)

The tooth will need to have a root canal treatment.
El diente necesitará un tratamiento de (endodoncia/conducto).
(Audio 4.124)

We need to see you again in _____ days.
Necesitaremos verl(o/a) otra vez en _____días. (Audio 4.125)

What happened that caused the tooth to come out?
¿Qué pasó que provocó que se saliera el diente? (Audio 4.126)

Did you reimplant the tooth?
¿Reimplantaste el diente? (Audio 4.127)

Did you soak the tooth in milk/liquid?
¿Remojaste el diente en leche/líquido? (Audio 4.128)

How did you store the tooth?
¿Cómo guardaste el diente? (Audio 4.129)

Did you clean the tooth?
¿Limpiaste el diente? (Audio 4.130)

We cannot reimplant the tooth.
No podemos reimplantar el diente. (Audio 4.131)

If a tooth comes out, do not clean it but put it in milk.
Si se sale un diente, no lo limpie sino póngalo en leche. (Audio 4.132)

If a tooth comes out, do not clean it but reimplant it.
Si se cae un diente, no lo limpie pero vuelva a implantarlo.
(Audio 4.133)

If the tooth is dirty, rinse it with salt water, do not scrub, and reimplant it.
Si el diente está sucio, enjuáguelo con agua salada, no frote y vuelva a implantarlo. (Audio 4.134)

If a tooth falls out, call us immediately.
Si se cae un diente, llámanos inmediatamente. (Audio 4.135)

Chapter 5
Dental Examination/Patient Assessment and Treatment Planning

Capítulo 5

Examen Dental/La Evaluación del Paciente y la Planificación del Tratamiento (Audio 5.1)

THE DENTAL EXAMINATION
EL EXAMEN DENTAL (AUDIO 5.2)

General Phrases
Frases Generales (Audio 5.3)

Please open your mouth.
Por favor, abra la boca. (Audio 5.4)

Are you happy with your smile?
¿Está usted contento(a) con su sonrisa? (Audio 5.5)

Do your teeth work well for you?
¿Funcionan bien sus dientes? (Audio 5.6)

Do you have any problems with your speech?
¿Tiene algún problema con su habla? (Audio 5.7)

Are you happy with the (color/shape) of your teeth?
¿Está contento(a) con (el color/la forma) de sus dientes? (Audio 5.8)

Is there anything you would like to change about your teeth?
¿Hay algo que le gustaría cambiar de sus dientes? (Audio 5.9)

Are you happy with your dental work?
¿Está contento(a) con su trabajo dental? (Audio 5.10)

Today I will give you a complete oral exam.
Hoy le haré un examen oral completo. (Audio 5.11)

We examine your teeth on your first visit.
Examinaremos sus dientes en su primera visita. (Audio 5.12)

33

We will reexamine your teeth each visit.
Reexaminaremos sus dientes cada visita. (Audio 5.13)

Are you comfortable while I examine your teeth?
¿Está cómodo(a) mientras le examino los dientes? (Audio 5.14)

Let me know if you are uncomfortable while I examine your teeth.
Hágame saber si está incómodo(a) mientras le examino los dientes. (Audio 5.15)

I will be using a (dental instrument/camera) to examine your teeth.
Usaré (un instrumento dental/una cámara) para examinarle los dientes. (Audio 5.16)

I will be gentle when examining your teeth.
Seré cuidadoso(a) mientras le examino los dientes. (Audio 5.17)

We will chart your fillings, (cavities/caries), tooth position, and bite.
Registraremos sus (rellenos/empastes), caries, posicion de sus dientes, y su mordida. (Audio 5.18)

I will examine your fillings to see if there is any decay around them.
Examinaré sus (calzas/empastes/rellenos) para ver si hay caries a su alrededor. (Audio 5.19)

I will examine your bite.
Examinaré su mordida. (Audio 5.20)

I will use this colored tape to check your bite.
Usaré esta cinta de color para examinar su mordida. (Audio 5.21)

We will also check the radiographs.
Revisaremos las radiografías también. (Audio 5.22)

Has any treatment been suggested for that tooth?
¿Se le ha sugerido algún tratamiento para ese diente? (Audio 5.23)

Has this tooth had (an abscess/a gum boil)?
¿Este diente ha tenido un (absceso/flemón)? (Audio 5.24)

Have you had a root canal on this tooth?
¿Ha tenido (una endodoncia/un tratamiento de conducto radicular) en este diente? (Audio 5.25)

(When/Why) did you have that tooth extracted?
¿(Cuándo/Por qué) fue extraído ese diente? (Audio 5.26)

Your dental chart will be stored in our computer.
Su expediente dental será guardado en nuestra computadora. (Audio 5.27)

Here's a (mirror/camera). Let's look at your teeth.
Aquí tiene (un espejo/una cámara). Veamos sus dientes. (Audio 5.28)

I want to check the position of your tongue when you swallow.
Quiero revisar la posición de su lengua cuando pase saliva. (Audio 5.29)

I will need to hold your lips apart to check your swallowing.
Necesitaré separar sus labios para revisar cómo traga. (Audio 5.30)

Put your teeth together.
Junte los dientes. (Audio 5.31)

Swallow/Pass your saliva.
Trague/pase su saliva. (Audio 5.32)

INTRAORAL ASSESSMENT
EVALUACIÓN INTRAORAL (AUDIO 5.33)

Hello, I am Doctor _____, your dentist.
Hola, soy el Doctor (M)/la Doctora (F) _____, su dentista/ odontologo(a). (Audio 5.34)

I will be performing an assessment on you today.
Hoy le estaré haciendo una evaluación. (Audio 5.35)

I will be planning your dental hygiene treatment based on my assessment.
Planificaré su tratamiento de higiene dental de acuerdo a mi evaluación. (Audio 5.36)

I will be (examining/palpating) your _____ in order to obtain some information about your health. (See Box 5.1)
Estaré (examinando/palpando) su _____ para obtener información sobre su salud. (Vea el Cuadro 5.1) (Audio 5.37)

For your protection, I will be wearing gloves while I (examine/palpate) your _____. (See Box 5.1)
Para su protección, usaré guantes mientras (examino/palpo) su _____. (Vea el Cuadro 5.1) (Audio 5.38)

With my fingers, I will be applying slight, temporary pressure in your mouth to examine it.
Aplicaré una presión leve y temporario en su boca con los dedos para examinarle. (Audio 5.39)

Box 5.1
Intraoral structures
(Audio 5.245)

- Cheek (Audio 5.246)
- Floor of the mouth (Audio 5.247)
- Gums/gingiva (Audio 5.248)
- Lip (Audio 5.249)
- Mouth (Audio 5.250)
- Mucosa (Audio 5.251)
- Ridge (Audio 5.252)
- Roof of the mouth (palate) (Audio 5.253)
- Salivary gland (Audio 5.254)
- Taste buds (Audio 5.255)
- Throat (pharynx) (Audio 5.256)
- Tongue (Audio 5.257)
- Tonsil (Audio 5.258)
- Uvula (Audio 5.259)

Cuadro 5.1
Estructuras intraorales
(Audio 5.245)

- Cachete/mejilla (Audio 5.246)
- Piso de la boca (Audio 5.247)
- Encías (Audio 5.248)
- Labio (Audio 5.249)
- Boca (Audio 5.250)
- Mucosa (Audio 5.251)
- Reborde (Audio 5.252)
- Cielo/techo de la boca (paladar) (Audio 5.253)
- Glándulas salivales (Audio 5.254)
- Papilas gustativas (Audio 5.255)
- Garganta (faringe) (Audio 5.256)
- Lengua (Audio 5.257)
- Amígdala/anginas (Audio 5.258)
- Úvula (Audio 5.259)

Are you comfortable while I examine your mouth?
¿Está cómodo(a) mientras examino su boca? (Audio 5.40)

Let me know if you are uncomfortable while I examine your mouth.
Hágame saber si está incómodo(a) mientras examino su boca. (Audio 5.41)

Remove your (appliance/denture/retainer).
Quítese su (aparato/dentadura/retenedor). (Audio 5.42)

(Open/Close) your mouth.
(Abre/Cierre) la boca. (Audio 5.43)

Partially open your mouth.
Abra la boca parcialmente. (Audio 5.44)

Close slightly.
Cierre poquito. (Audio 5.45)

Bend your head (forward/backward).
Incline la cabeza hacia (adelante/atrás). (Audio 5.46)

Turn your head to the (right/left).
Volte la cabeza hacia la (derecha/izquierda). (Audio 5.47)

Stick your tongue out.
Saque la lengua. (Audio 5.48)

Touch your tongue to the roof of your mouth.
Toque el (cielo/techo) de la boca con la lengua. (Audio 5.49)

I will need to hold your tongue to examine it.
Necesitaré sujetarle la lengua para examinarla. (Audio 5.50)

Move your jaw to the (right/left).
Mueva la quijada hacia (derecha/izquierda). (Audio 5.51)

Move your jaw (forward/backward).
Mueva la quijada hacia (adelante/atrás). (Audio 5.52)

Put your teeth together and bite down hard.
Junte los dientes y muerda fuertemente. (Audio 5.53)

Say "ah."
Diga "ah." (Audio 5.54)

Have your tonsils been (infected/removed)?
¿Ha tenido las amígdalas (infectadas/extraídas)? (Audio 5.55)

You have a chewing line in your cheek.
Usted tiene una línea de mordida en su cachete. (Audio 5.56)

Do you (bite/chew) your cheeks?
Se (muerde/mastica) los cachetes? (Audio 5.57)

Have you burned your mouth with hot food or drink recently?
¿Se ha quemado la boca con un alimento o bebida caliente recientemente? (Audio 5.58)

Do you feel any pain when I press here?
Siente dolor cuando presiono aquí? (Audio 5.59)

Do you feel pain when you do that?
Siente dolor cuando hace eso? (Audio 5.60)

Did you notice this?
¿Usted notó esto?(formal) ¿Notaste esto? (informal) (Audio 5.61)

Does this bother you?
¿Le molesta esto? (Audio 5.62)

How long have you had this?
¿Por cuánto tiempo ha tenido esto? (Audio 5.63)

Have you had (lip/mouth) cancer?
¿Ha tenido cáncer (del labio/de la boca)? (Audio 5.64)

Have you had trauma to your (face/teeth)?
¿Ha tenido algún trauma en su (cara/dientes)? (Audio 5.65)

Have you had treatment for this?
¿Ha tenido tratamiento para esto? (Audio 5.66)

I will be using this (brush/dye) and (light/rinse) to check your tissues.
Usaré este (cepillo/tinte) y (luz/enjuague) para examinar sus tejidos. (Audio 5.67)

DISCUSSION OF SOFT TISSUE FINDINGS
DISCUSIÓN DE LOS RESULTADOS EN EL TEJIDO
SUAVE (AUDIO 5.68)

Have you seen this____? (See Box 5.2)
¿Ha visto este/esta _____? (Vea el Cuadro 5.2) (Audio 5.69)

I found this _____ in your mouth. (See Box 5.2)
Encontré este/esta _____ en su boca. (Vea el Cuadro 5.2) (Audio 5.70)

You will need to have the _____ removed. (See Box 5.2)
Tendremos que extraer este/esta _____. (Vea el Cuadro 5.2)
(Audio 5.71)

An oral surgeon can do this for you.
Un(a) cirujano(a) oral puede hacer esto para usted. (Audio 5.72)

We can refer you to an oral surgeon.
Podemos referirlo(a) a un(a) cirujano(a) oral. (Audio 5.73)

STUDY MODEL IMPRESSIONS
IMPRESIONES DEL MODELO DE
ESTUDIO (AUDIO 5.74)

We are going to take an impression of your (teeth/mouth).
Vamos a tomar una impresión de (sus dientes/su boca). (Audio 5.75)

**A dental impression makes a negative copy of your (teeth/
mouth) using a (soft/pudding-like) material**.
Una impresión dental hace una copia negativa de (sus dientes/su
boca) usando un material blando. (Audio 5.76)

**Dental plaster is distributed into the impression to produce
a copy of your teeth**.
Se distribuye yeso dental en la impresión para producir una copia de
sus dientes. (Audio 5.77)

The material is soft now, but it will harden.
El material está blando ahora, pero se endurecerá. (Audio 5.78)

**We will then be able to remove it without damaging your
mouth**.
Entonces podremos quitarlo sin dañar su boca. (Audio 5.79)

Box 5.2
Common intraoral findings (Audio 5.260)

- Bleeding (hemorrhage) (Audio 5.261)
- Blister (vesicle) (Audio 5.262)
- Bruise (hematoma) (Audio 5.263)
- Burning (Audio 5.264)
- Change in color (Audio 5.265)
- Enlargement (Audio 5.266)
- Growth (Audio 5.267)
- Healing (Audio 5.268)
- Infection (Audio 5.269)
- Itching (Audio 5.270)
- Lesion (Audio 5.271)
- Numbness (paresthesia) (Audio 5.272)
- Patch (macule/papule/nodule) (Audio 5.273)
- Soreness (Audio 5.274)
- Tingling (Audio 5.275)
- Tumor (cancer) (Audio 5.276)
- Ulcer (Audio 5.277)

Cuadro 5.2
Hallazgos intraorales communes (Audio 5.260)

- Sangrado (hemorragia) (Audio 5.261)
- Ampolla (vesícula) (Audio 5.262)
- Magulladura/moretón (hematoma) (Audio 5.263)
- Quemadura (Audio 5.264)
- Cambio en color (Audio 5.265)
- Agrandamiento (Audio 5.266)
- Crecimiento (Audio 5.267)
- Curación (Audio 5.268)
- Infección (Audio 5.269)
- Picazón (Audio 5.270)
- Lesión (Audio 5.271)
- Adormecimiento (parestesia) (Audio 5.272)
- Parche (mácula/pápula/nódulo) (Audio 5.273)
- Dolor (Audio 5.274)
- Hormigueo (Audio 5.275)
- Tumor (cáncer) (Audio 5.276)
- Úlcera (Audio 5.277)

Let's try this dental tray to see if it fits.
Probemos esta bandeja dental para ver si le queda. (Audio 5.80)

I need to dry your mouth before the impression.
Necesito secarle la boca antes de tomar la impresión. (Audio 5.81)

I need to place some of the impression material on your teeth.
Necesito colocar un poco del material de impresión en sus dientes. (Audio 5.82)

Relax!
¡Relájese! (Audio 5.83)

Breathe through your nose.
Respire por la nariz. (Audio 5.84)

Are you comfortable with the impression?
¿Está cómodo(a) con la impresión? (Audio 5.85)

Let me know if you are not comfortable with the impression.
Hágame saber si está incómodo(a) con la impresión. (Audio 5.86)

Do you gag?
¿Le dan náuseas? (Audio 5.87)

We will use (nitrous oxide/topical spray) to help you with your gagging.
Usaremos (óxido nitroso/rocío tópico) para ayudarle con las náuseas. (Audio 5.88)

We need to take the impression again.
Necesitamos tomar la impresión nuevamente. (Audio 5.89)

Let's look at the plaster model made from the impression of your (mouth/teeth).
Veamos el modelo de yeso hecho de la impresión de (su boca/sus dientes). (Audio 5.90)

PHOTOGRAPHIC EXAMINATION
EXAMEN FOTOGRÁFICO (AUDIO 5.91)

We are going to take a picture of your _____. (See Box 5.3)
Vamos a tomar una foto de su(s) _____. (Vea el Cuadro 5.3) (Audio 5.92)

This camera takes a (picture/video) inside your mouth.
Esta cámara toma (una foto/un video) dentro de su boca. (Audio 5.93)

Your (picture/video) will be stored in our computer.
Su (foto/video) estará guardada(o) en nuestra computadora. (Audio 5.94)

Box 5.3
Common photos taken in the dental office (Audio 5.278)

- Face (Audio 5.279)
- Head (Audio 5.280)
- Lesion (Audio 5.281)
- Lips (Audio 5.282)
- Mouth (Audio 5.283)
- Profile (Audio 5.284)
- Smile (Audio 5.285)
- Tooth (teeth) (Audio 5.286)

Cuadro 5.3
Fotos comunes tomadas en la oficina del dentista (Audio 5.278)

- Cara (Audio 5.279)
- Cabeza (Audio 5.280)
- Lesión (Audio 5.281)
- Labios (Audio 5.282)
- Boca (Audio 5.283)
- Perfil (Audio 5.284)
- Sonrisa (Audio 5.285)
- Dental (dientes) (Audio 5.286)

EVALUATION OF THE TEETH AND RESTORATIONS
EVALUACIÓN DE LOS DIENTES Y LAS RESTAURACIONES (AUDIO 5.95)

Restorative Examination
Examen Restaurativo (Audio 5.96)

We will be examining your teeth for _____. (See Box 5.4)
Examinaremos sus dientes para _____. (Vea el Cuadro 5.4) (Audio 5.97)

Do you know what (caries are/a cavity is)?
¿Usted sabe lo que (son las caries/es una cavidad)? (Audio 5.98)

We have a new detection device that uses an extremely powerful light to check for (decay/caries/cavities).
Tenemos un nuevo aparato de detección que usa una luz extremadamente potente para averiguar si hay (descomposición/caries/cavidades). (Audio 5.99)

We will use an instrument called an explorer to look for (decay/caries/cavities) on all tooth surfaces.
Usaremos el instrumento llamado explorador para buscar (descomposición/caries/cavidades) en todas las superficies del diente. (Audio 5.100)

Box 5.4
Types of dental conditions commonly found at a restorative treatment appointment (Audio 5.287)

- Decay/caries/cavities (Audio 5.288)
- Attrition (Audio 5.289)
- Abrasion (Audio 5.290)
- Position (Audio 5.291)
- Staining (Audio 5.292)

Cuadro 5.4
Tipos de condiciones dentales encontradas comúnmente en una cita de tratamiento restaurativo (Audio 5.287)

- Descomposición/caries/cavidades (Audio 5.288)
- Desgaste (Audio 5.289)
- Abrasión (Audio 5.290)
- Posición (Audio 5.291)
- Manchas (Audio 5.292)

This is an explorer.
Esto es un explorador. (Audio 5.101)

When an explorer "sticks" in a crevice in your tooth, it means that we have found (decay/caries/a cavity) in your tooth.
Cuando el explorador se adhiere a la grieta de su diente, quiere decir que hemos encontrado una (descomposición/carie/cavidad) en su diente. (Audio 5.102)

Is this tooth sensitive to _____? (See Box 5.5)
¿Es este diente sensible al/a lo _____? (Vea el Cuadro 5.5) (Audio 5.103)

What type of pain are you having in this area? (See Box 5.6)
¿Qué tipo de dolor tiene en esta área? (Vea el Cuadro 5.6) (Audio 5.104)

Does it bother you when I do this?
¿Le incomoda cuando hago esto? (Audio 5.105)

Discussion of Findings
Discusión de los Resultados (Audio 5.106)

You have (caries/a cavity) in this tooth.
Usted tiene (caries/una cavidad) en este diente. (Audio 5.107)

Box 5.5
Things that teeth can be sensitive to (Audio 5.293)

- Air (Audio 5.294)
- Biting (Audio 5.295)
- Cold (Audio 5.296)
- Drinking (Audio 5.297)
- Heat (Audio 5.298)
- Sweets (Audio 5.299)

Cuadro 5.5
Cosas a las cuales los dientes pueden ser sensibles (Audio 5.293)

- Aire (Audio 5.294)
- Morder (Audio 5.295)
- Frío (Audio 5.296)
- Beber (Audio 5.297)
- Caliente (Audio 5.298)
- A lo dulce (Audio 5.299)

Box 5.6
Descriptions of pain (Audio 5.300)

- Intense (Audio 5.301)
- Spontaneous (Audio 5.302)
- Continuous (Audio 5.303)

Cuadro 5.6
Descripciones de dolor (Audio 5.300)

- Intenso (Audio 5.301)
- Espontáneo (Audio 5.302)
- Continuo (Audio 5.303)

This spot on the radiograph shows the location of the decay in your tooth.
Este punto en la radiografía muestra la localización de la descomposición en su diente. (Audio 5.108)

RESTORATIVE TREATMENT PLANNING
PLANIFICACIÓN DEL TRATAMIENTO RESTAURATIVO (AUDIO 5.109)

You need to have the decay removed and a filling put in place.
Es necesario remover la caries y colocar un (empaste/relleno). (Audio 5.110)

Box 5.7
Types of fillings
(Audio 5.304)

Cuadro 5.7
Tipos de empastes/
rellenos/calzas (Audio
5.304)

- Silver (Audio 5.305)
- White (Audio 5.306)
- Amalgam (Audio 5.307)
- Metal (Audio 5.308)
- Composite (Audio 5.309)
- Tooth colored (Audio 5.310)

- Bonded (Audio 5.311)
- Resin (Audio 5.312)

- Plata (Audio 5.305)
- Blanco (Audio 5.306)
- Amalgama (Audio 5.307)
- Metal (Audio 5.308)
- Compuesto(a) (Audio 5.309)
- Del color del diente
  (Audio 5.310)
- Consolidada (Audio 5.311)
- Resina (Audio 5.312)

We recommend _____ as the best filling material for this situation. (See Box 5.7)
Recomendamos el/la _____ como el mejor material de (empaste/relleno) para esta situación. (Vea el Cuadro 5.7) (Audio 5.111)

We will fill the tooth with _____. (See Box 5.7)
Llenaremos el diente con _____. (Vea el Cuadro 5.7) (Audio 5.112)

We will need to (anesthetize/numb/put to sleep) the tooth.
Necesitaremos (anestesiar/adormecer/dormir) el diente. (Audio 5.113)

We will be using anesthetic to do this.
Utilizaremos anestésico para hacer esto. (Audio 5.114)

We will then (anesthetize/numb/put to sleep) the tissue.
Necesitaremos (anestesiar/adormecer/dormir) el tejido. (Audio 5.115)

When we inject you, it may feel like a little mosquito bite.
Cuando le inyectamos, puede que lo sienta como una pequeña picadura de mosquito. (Audio 5.116)

DISCUSSION OF TOOTH-RELATED FINDINGS
DISCUSIÓN DE LOS RESULTADOS RELACIONADOS AL DIENTE (AUDIO 5.117)

This tooth is _____. (See Box 5.8)
Este diente está _____. (Vea el Cuadro 5.8) (Audio 5.118)

How long have you had _____? (See Box 5.8)
¿Por cuánto tiempo ha tenido _____? (Vea el Cuadro 5.8)
(Audio 5.119)

Box 5.8 **Common dental examination findings (Audio 5.313)**	**Cuadro 5.8** **Hallazgos comunes del examen dental (Audio 5.313)**
• Straightened (braces) (Audio 5.314)	• Enderezado (frenillos/frenos/brackets) (Audio 5.314)
• Bridge (Audio 5.315)	• Puente (Audio 5.315)
• Broken (Audio 5.316)	• Quebrado (Audio 5.316)
• Cap (crown) (Audio 5.317)	• Corona (Audio 5.317)
• Decayed (Audio 5.318)	• Descompuesto (Audio 5.318)
• Pulled (extracted) (extraction) (Audio 5.319)	• Sacado (extraído) (extracción) (Audio 5.319)
• Filling (restored) (restoration) (Audio 5.320)	• Relleno/empaste/calza/empastadura (restaurado) (restauración) (Audio 5.320)
• Implant (Audio 5.321)	• Implante (Audio 5.321)
• Lingual bar (Audio 5.322)	• Barra lingual (Audio 5.322)
• Root canal (Audio 5.323)	• Endodoncia/tratamiento de conducto (Audio 5.323)
• Sealant (Audio 5.324)	• Sellador/sellante dental (Audio 5.324)
• Sealed (Audio 5.325)	• Sellado (Audio 5.325)
• Space (Audio 5.326)	• Espacio (Audio 5.326)

This tooth needs to be _____. (See Box 5.8)
Este diente necesita ser _____. (Vea el Cuadro 5.8) (Audio 5.120)

We found _____ (cavities/caries).
Encontramos _____ (cavidades/caries). (Audio 5.121)

PATIENT ASSESSMENT AND TREATMENT PLANNING
LA EVALUACIÓN DEL PACIENTE Y LA PLANIFICACIÓN DEL TRATAMIENTO (AUDIO 5.122)

We will evaluate your oral health needs and present you with a treatment plan. Our treatment plans can be divided into four distinct phases: systemic, disease control, definitive, and maintenance.
Evaluaremos las necesidades de su salud oral y le presentaremos un plan de tratamiento. Nuestros planes de tratamiento pueden dividirse en cuatro fases: sistémica, control de enfermedad, definitiva, y mantenimiento. (Audio 5.123)

Note: Questions and statements in this chapter may pertain to more than one phase of treatment planning.
Nota: Las preguntas y declaraciones en este capítulo pueden ser apropiadas para más de una fase de la planificación de tratamiento. (Audio 5.124)

SYSTEMIC TREATMENT PHASE
FASE SISTÉMICA DEL TRATAMIENTO (AUDIO 5.125)

The systemic phase of treatment planning takes a holistic approach to your oral care.
La fase sistémica involucra un acercamiento holístico para su cuidado oral. (Audio 5.126)

The systemic phase takes into account your systemic health and the ways in which your oral conditions may be affecting it.
La fase sistémica toma en cuenta su salud sistémica y las maneras en que sus condiciones orales pueden estar afectándola. (Audio 5.127)

The systemic phase takes into account your oral health and the ways in which your systemic health may be affecting it. La fase sistémica toma en cuenta su salud oral y las maneras en que su salud sistémica puede estar afectándola. (Audio 5.128)

We have evidence that the inflammatory process infecting your gums may be at play in other systemic diseases of a similar nature, such as stroke, heart disease, and diabetes. Hay evidencia de que el proceso de inflamación infectando sus encías puede participar en otras enfermedades sistémicas de la misma naturaleza, como ataque cerebral, enfermedad cardíaca, y diabetes. (Audio 5.129)

How are you?
¿Cómo está usted? (Audio 5.130)

How do you feel today?
¿Cómo se siente hoy? (Audio 5.131)

Do you see a doctor regularly? How is your health?
¿Ve a su doctor(a) regularmente? ¿Cómo está su salud? (Audio 5.132)

Do you take any medication?
¿Toma algún medicamento? (Audio 5.133)

Did you take any medication today?
¿Tomó algún medicamento hoy? (Audio 5.134)

What medication do you take?
¿Qué medicamento toma? (Audio 5.135)

Do you have any bottles of the medication with you?
¿Tiene algunas botellas del medicamento con usted? (Audio 5.136)

Do you have high blood pressure?
¿Tiene la presión arterial alta? (Audio 5.137)

Do you have any heart problems?
¿Tiene alguna enfermedad del corazón? (Audio 5.138)

Do you take antidepressants?
¿Toma antidepresivos? (Audio 5.139)

Do you take blood thinners?
¿Toma anticoagulantes? (Audio 5.140)

Are you allergic to any medication?
¿Es alérgico(a) a algún medicamento? (Audio 5.141)

Do you have diabetes?
¿Tiene diabetes? (Audio 5.142)

Do you have a heart condition?
¿Tiene una condición cardíaca? (Audio 5.143)

Have you ever had a stroke?
¿Ha tenido alguna vez una (ataque cerebral/embolio)? (Audio 5.144)

Have you ever had a problem with novocaine or any dental local anesthetic?
¿Ha tenido alguna vez un problema con la novocaína o con algún anestésico local dental? (Audio 5.145)

Has a doctor ever told you that you need to take an antibiotic before seeing a dentist?
¿Algún(a) doctor(a) le ha dicho alguna vez que necesita tomar un antibiótico antes de ver al/a la dentista? (Audio 5.146)

What is your doctor's name and phone number?
¿Cuál es el nombre de su doctor(a) y su número de teléfono? (Audio 5.147)

Do you have a bleeding problem?
¿Tiene un problema de sangrado? (Audio 5.148)

Is there anything else related to your health that you would like to tell us?
¿Hay algo más relacionado a su salud que desea decirnos? (Audio 5.149)

Have you been in the hospital lately?
¿Ha estado en el hospital recientemente? (Audio 5.150)

When did you get out?
¿Cuándo salió? (Audio 5.151)

When were you admitted to the hospital?
Cuando lo(a) internaron en el hospital? (Audio 5.152)

Why were you admitted to the hospital?
¿Por qué fue internado(a) en el hospital? (Audio 5.153)

Medications you take can have an effect on your mouth.
Los medicamentos que usted toma pueden tener un efecto en su
boca. (Audio 5.154)

**(Physical/Systemic) problems that you have can affect your
mouth**.
Los problemas (físicos/sistémicos) que usted tiene pueden afectar su
boca. (Audio 5.155)

ACUTE TREATMENT PHASE
FASE DE TRATAMIENTO AGUDO (AUDIO 5.156)

**In the acute treatment phase, we focus on relieving your
immediate pain. During this phase, we also try to address
your other primary concerns, such as function or esthetics
(loss or fracture of front teeth)**.
En la fase de tratamiento agudo, nos centramos en el alivio del
dolor inmediato. Durante esta fase, también tratamos de responder
a otras preocupaciones primarias, como la función o la estética
(la pérdida o la fractura de los dientes delanteros). (Audio 5.157)

What is the reason for your visit today?
¿Cuál es el motivo de su visita hoy? (Audio 5.158)

What brings you to our office today?
¿Qué lo(a) trae a nuestra oficina hoy? (Audio 5.159)

Did you break a tooth?
¿Se quebró un diente? (Audio 5.160)

Did you lose a tooth?
¿Perdió un diente? (Audio 5.161)

Do you have a toothache?
¿Tiene dolor de dientes? (Audio 5.162)

**How would you rate your pain on a scale from zero
(no pain) to ten (most pain)?**
¿Cómo calificaría su dolor en una escala de cero (sin dolor) a diez
(mucho dolor)? (Audio 5.163)

Is your main concern pain?
¿Es su principal preocupación el dolor? (Audio 5.164)

Is your main concern esthetics?
¿Es su principal preocupación la estética? (Audio 5.165)

Can you eat?
¿Puede comer? (Audio 5.166)

Have you been able to sleep?
¿Ha podido dormir? (Audio 5.167)

What would you like for us to do for you today?
¿Qué quiere que hagamos hoy por usted? (Audio 5.168)

DISEASE CONTROL PHASE
FASE DE CONTROL DE LA ENFERMEDAD
(AUDIO 5.169)

In the disease control phase, we will focus on getting your (caries/periodontal disease) under control. We will also treat any other oral infections. At the end of the disease control phase, we will evaluate the treatment options for long-term solutions to your dental concerns. This phase typically involves simple fillings, initial periodontal therapy (cleaning), oral surgery (extractions), or endodontics (root canal therapy).
En la fase del control de la enfermedad, nos enfocaremos en dejar (sus caries/su enfermedad periodontal) bajo control. También trataremos cualquier infección oral. Al final de la fase del control de la enfermedad, evaluaremos las opciones de tratamiento para soluciones a largo plazo para sus preocupaciones dentales. Esta fase suele incluir (empastes/rellenos) simples, terapia periodontal inicial (limpieza), cirugía oral (extracciones), o endodoncia (terapia del canal radicular). (Audio 5.170)

You have _____ cavities.
Usted tiene _____ caries. (Audio 5.171)

You have _____ teeth that need treatment.
Usted tiene _____ dientes que necesitan tratamiento. (Audio 5.172)

You have _____ teeth that cannot be saved.
Usted tiene _____ dientes que no pueden ser salvados. (Audio 5.173)

You have _____ teeth with periodontal disease.
Usted tiene _____ dientes con enfermedad periodontal.
(Audio 5.174)

I suggest that we first take care of your gum problems and then do the fillings you need.
Le sugiero que primero nos encarguemos de sus problemas de las encías, y después hagamos los (empastes/rellenos) que necesita.
(Audio 5.175)

DEFINITIVE TREATMENT PHASE
FASE DE TRATAMIENTO DEFINITIVO (AUDIO 5.176)

The definitive phase of treatment includes all of the long-term solutions designed to provide maximal esthetics, phonetics, and function. We will let you know the type of dental restoration and (additional) periodontal (gum) therapy that you will need in order to achieve a healthy mouth. The treatment may involve orthodontia (braces) or elective oral surgery. It typically includes many forms of fixed or removable dental reconstruction. We will spell it out exactly for you.
La fase de tratamiento definitivo incluye todas las soluciones a largo plazo diseñadas para proveer máxima estética, fonética, y función. Le haremos saber qué tipo de tratamiento dentales de restauración periodontal (de encía y adicionales) usted necesitará para tener una boca saludable. El tratamiento puede incluir ortodoncia (frenillos/frenos) o cirugía dental electiva. Típicamente incluye muchas formas de reconstrucción dental fija o removible. Se lo explicaremos en detalle. (Audio 5.177)

I am going to refer you to a (periodontist/endodontist/oral surgeon).
Lo(a) voy a referire a un(a) (periodoncista/endodoncista/cirujano(a) oral). (Audio 5.178)

Are you interested in saving your teeth?
¿Está usted interesado(a) en salvar sus dientes? (Audio 5.179)

Your dental condition is (fair/good/excellent/poor).
Su condición dental es (regular/buena/excelente/mala). (Audio 5.180)

This would be a good option for you.
Esto sería una buena opción para usted. (Audio 5.181)

If you don't do this, you will probably have problems with this tooth (these teeth) in the future.
Si usted no hace esto, probablemente tendrá problemas con este diente (estos dientes) en el futuro. (Audio 5.182)

Orthodontics needs to be completed before the missing teeth are replaced.
Necesitamos terminar la ortodoncia antes de reemplazar los dientes que faltan. (Audio 5.183)

It is more efficient when all restorations in a quadrant are completed in one visit.
Es más eficiente cuando todas las restauraciones en un cuadrante se terminan en una visita. (Audio 5.184)

Fillings do not last forever.
Los empastes/rellenos no duran para siempre. (Audio 5.185)

The life of a filling depends on many factors out of the dentist's control.
La vida de una (empastadura/relleno/empaste/calza) depende de muchos factores fuera del control del dentista. (Audio 5.186)

Orthodontics cannot be started until all the decay has been removed.
No podemos iniciar los (frenos/frenillos/brackets) hasta que las caries hayan sido tratadas. (Audio 5.187)

MAINTENANCE TREATMENT PHASE
FASE DE MANTENIMIENTO DEL TRATAMIENTO
(AUDIO 5.188)

At the conclusion of your dental treatment, we will let you know exactly what steps you need to take in order to maintain a healthy mouth. Preventing future problems is our goal.
Al concluir su tratamiento dental, le haremos saber exactamente qué medidas necesita tomar para mantener una boca sana. La prevención de problemas futuros es nuestra meta. (Audio 5.189)

All the dental treatment you needed is now completed.
Todo el tratamiento dental que usted necesitabas ya está completo.
(Audio 5.190)

Do you have any questions?
¿Tiene preguntas? (Audio 5.191)

Remember to brush and floss every day.
Recuerde cepillarse y limpiar con hilo dental todos los días. (Audio
5.192)

**Don't forget to return to the office every _____ months to
have an exam and prophylaxis (cleaning)**.
No olvide volver a la consulta cada _____ meses para hacerle un
examen y una profilaxis (limpieza). (Audio 5.193)

**If you return regularly to the office for a checkup and a
cleaning, we can help you prevent future dental problems.
If dental problems start, they can be detected early and
treated easily**.
Si regresa regularmente a la consulta para un chequeo y una
limpieza, podemos ayudarle a prevenir problemas dentales futuros.
Si surgen problemas dentales, pueden ser detectados temprano y
tratarse fácilmente. (Audio 5.194)

Prevention of decay and gum disease is important.
Es importante prevenir las caries y la enfermedad de las encías.
(Audio 5.195)

**It is less expensive to prevent problems than to fix
problems**.
Es menos costoso prevenir los problemas que arreglarlos. (Audio
5.196)

Don't suck on hard candies or mints.
No chupe dulces o mentas duras. (Audio 5.197)

Don't smoke.
No fume. (Audio 5.198)

**Clean your (teeth/bridges/partials/dentures) as you have
been instructed**.
Limpie sus (dientes/puentes/dentaduras parciales/dentaduras) como
le han enseñado. (Audio 5.199)

It has been a pleasure helping you obtain great dental health.
Ha sido un placer ayudarle a obtener una excelente salud dental. (Audio 5.200)

Smile big.
Sonría grande. (Audio 5.201)

If you were pleased with our service, we would appreciate it if you would tell your friends and relatives about us.
Si estuvo satisfecho con nuestro servicio, le agradeceríamos que le contara a sus amigos y familiares sobre nosotros. (Audio 5.202)

COMMON PATIENT QUESTIONS AND RESPONSES
PREGUNTAS Y RESPUESTAS COMUNES DE PACIENTES (AUDIO 5.203)

Patient Questions
Preguntas de Pacientes (Audio 5.204)

Can this tooth be _____? (See Box 5.9)
¿Este diente puede ser _____? (Vea el Cuadro 5.9) (Audio 5.205)

How many teeth need to be _____? (See Box 5.9)
¿Cuántos dientes necesitan ser _____? (Vea el Cuadro 5.9) (Audio 5.206)

What are you going to do?
¿Qué va a hacer usted? (Audio 5.207)

Will it hurt?
¿Dolerá? (Audio 5.208)

Can you numb me?
¿Me puede adormecer? (Audio 5.209)

Do I have to be numbed?
¿Necesito ser adormecido(a)? (Audio 5.210)

Are you going to give me a shot?
¿Me va a dar una inyección? (Audio 5.211)

**Box 5.9
Common
procedures that
patients inquire about
(Audio 5.327)**

- Capped (crowned)
  (Audio 5.328)
- Pulled (extracted)
  (Audio 5.329)
- Filled (restored)
  (Audio 5.330)
- Lost (Audio 5.331)
- Root canal
  (Audio 5.332)
- Saved (Audio 5.333)

**Cuadro 5.9
Procedimientos
comunes sobre los que
los pacientes preguntan
(Audio 5.327)**

- Coronado(s)
  (Audio 5.328)
- Extraído(s)
  (Audio 5.329)
- Empastado(s) (restaurado(s))
  (Audio 5.330)
- Perdido(s) (Audio 5.331)
- Endodoncia/tratamiento de
  conducto (Audio 5.332)
- Salvado(s) (Audio 5.333)

Can I have gas?
¿Me va adiminstrar gas? (Audio 5.212)

Will I be able to drive home?
¿Podré manejar a mi hogar? (Audio 5.213)

Do I have to come back?
¿Tengo que regresar? (Audio 5.214)

How much will it cost?
¿Cuánto va a costar? (Audio 5.215)

What kind of (toothbrush/toothpaste) should I use?
¿Qué clase de (cepillo de dientes/(pasta de dientes/pasta dental/
crema dental)) debo usar? (Audio 5.216)

How much toothpaste should (I/they) use?
¿Cuánta pasta dental (debo/deben) usar? (Audio 5.217)

PATIENT RESPONSES
RESPUESTAS DE PACIENTES (AUDIO 5.218)

My (tooth/gum/mouth) is okay.
Mi (diente/encía/boca) está bien. (Audio 5.219)

My (tooth/gum/mouth) hurts here.
Mi (diente/encía/boca) me duele aquí. (Audio 5.220)

When I (bite/chew/eat), this tooth hurts.
Cuando (muerdo/mastico/como), este diente me duele.
(Audio 5.221)

My tooth hurts with (cold/heat/sweets).
Mi diente me duele con (frío/caliente/lo dulce). (Audio 5.222)

I have an (abscess/gum boil) in this tooth. Right here.
Tengo un (absceso/flemón) en este diente. Aquí. (Audio 5.223)

I have (bleeding/an infection) here.
Tengo (sangrado/una infección) aquí. (Audio 5.224)

I had a radiograph taken of the tooth.
Me tomaron una radiografía del diente. (Audio 5.225)

Be careful with my (tooth/gum/mouth).
Tenga cuidado con mi (diente/encía/boca). (Audio 5.226)

I've been without teeth for (_____ months/_____ years).
He estado sin dientes por (_____ meses/_____ años). (Audio 5.227)

I don't want a new denture.
No quiero una nueva (dentadura/placa). (Audio 5.228)

I want a new denture.
Quiero una nueva dentadura. (Audio 5.229)

I like the way my old denture (felt/looked).
Me gusta como mi dentadura vieja se (sentía/veía). (Audio 5.230)

My denture is (broken/loose/lost).
Mi dentadura está (quebrada/rota/suelta/perdida). (Audio 5.231)

My denture hurts my gum when I (eat/smile/speak).
Mi dentadura me lastima las encías cuando (como/sonrío/hablo).
(Audio 5.232)

I (brush/floss) _____ times a day.
Yo me (cepillo/limpio con hilo dental) _____ veces al día.
(Audio 5.233)

I use a (hard/soft) toothbrush.
Yo uso un cepillo de dientes (duro/suave). (Audio 5.234)

Flossing is too hard.
Limpiarse con hilo dental es demasiado difícil. (Audio 5.235)

I have no time for flossing.
Yo no tengo tiempo para limpiarme los dientes con hilo dental.
(Audio 5.236)

I am concerned about (my/my child's) _____. **(See Box 5.10)**
Me preocupa(n) _____ en (mí/mi niño(a)). (Vea el Cuadro 5.10)
(Audio 5.237)

I have never had my teeth cleaned.
Nunca me han hecho limpieza dental. (Audio 5.238)

It's been a long time since my last cleaning.
Ha pasado mucho tiempo desde mi última limpieza. (Audio 5.239)

My teeth are sensitive.
Mis dientes son sensibles. (Audio 5.240)

Don't touch this area when you are cleaning.
No toque esta área cuando esté limpiando. (Audio 5.241)

Box 5.10 **Conditions that** **patients may be** **concerned about** **(Audio 5.334)**	**Cuadro 5.10** **Condiciones que pueden** **preocupar** **a los pacientes** **(Audio 5.334)**
• Bad breath (Audio 5.335)	• El mal aliento (Audio 5.335)
• Bleeding gums (Audio 5.336)	• Las encías sangrando (Audio 5.336)
• Cavities (Audio 5.337)	• Las caries (Audio 5.337)
• Dry mouth (Audio 5.338)	• La boca reseca (Audio 5.338)
• Exposed root (Audio 5.339)	• La raíz expuesta (Audio 5.339)
• Fillings (Audio 5.340)	• (Los rellenos/empastes/ las calzas) (Audio 5.340)
• Stain (Audio 5.341)	• La mancha (Audio 5.341)
• Tartar/calculus (Audio 5.342)	• El sarro/el cálculo (Audio 5.342)

Box 5.11
Possible patient
needs during
treatment
(Audio 5.343)

Cuadro 5.11
Posibles necesidades del
paciente durante
el tratamiento
(Audio 5.343)

- More anesthesia
  (Audio 5.344)
- More rinsing (Audio 5.345)
- More suction (Audio 5.346)
- Nitrous oxide (Audio 5.347)
- To sit upright (Audio 5.348)
- To spit (Audio 5.349)
- Warm water rinse
  (Audio 5.350)

- Más anestesia (Audio 5.344)
- Más enjuague (Audio 5.345)
- Más succión (Audio 5.346)
- Óxido nitroso (Audio 5.347)
- Sentarme derecho(a)
  (Audio 5.348)
- Escupir (Audio 5.349)
- Enjuague de agua tibia
  (Audio 5.350)

My gums are bleeding.
Mis encías están sangrando. (Audio 5.242)

Does a cleaning remove the tooth?
¿Una limpieza remueve el diente? (Audio 5.243)

I need _____. (See Box 5.11)
Necesito _____. (Vea el Cuadro 5.11) (Audio 5.244)

Chapter 6
Dental Hygiene and Preventive Dentistry

Capítulo 6
Higiene Dental y Odontología Preventiva (Audio 6.1)

PREVENTIVE DENTISTRY
ODONTOLOGÍA PREVENTIVA (AUDIO 6.2)

I am a dental hygienist.
Yo soy higienista dental. (Audio 6.3)

We want to help (you/your family) keep (your/their) teeth and gums healthy.
Queremos ayudarle a (usted/su familia) a mantener sus dientes y encías saludables. (Audio 6.4)

We want to help (you/your family) keep (your/their) smile(s).
Queremos ayudarle a (usted/su familia) a mantener su sonrisa. (Audio 6.5)

Regular dental (checkups/examinations) and cleanings prevent dental disease.
(Las revisiones/Los exámenes) dentales y limpiezas regulares previenen la enfermedad dental. (Audio 6.6)

(Your dentist/We) can help prevent problems and catch any problems while they are easy to treat.
(Su dentista puede/Nosotros podemos) ayudarle a prevenir y a detectar cualquier problema mientras son fáciles de tratar. (Audio 6.7)

Do you have any questions about your dental health?
¿Tiene alguna pregunta sobre su salud dental? (Audio 6.8)

Do you have any questions about how to take care of your teeth?
¿Tiene alguna pregunta sobre cómo cuidar sus dientes? (Audio 6.9)

Let's talk about preventing dental disease.
Hablemos sobre la prevención de enfermedades dentales. (Audio 6.10)

There are two sets of teeth: (baby/primary) and (adult/permanent).
Hay dos grupos de dientes: los (de leche/primarios) y los (de adulto/permanentes). (Audio 6.11)

The permanent teeth begin to erupt around the age of 6.
Los dientes permanentes comienzan a salir alrededor de los 6 años. (Audio 6.12)

The first permanent teeth to erupt are the first molars.
Los primeros dientes permanentes en salir son los primeros molares. (Audio 6.13)

The first permanent molars come in behind the baby teeth. No baby teeth are lost.
Los primeros molares permanentes salen detrás de los dientes de leche. No se pierde ningún diente de leche. (Audio 6.14)

Except for the third molars, all the permanent teeth have erupted by about age 13.
Conexcepción de los terceros molares, todos los dientes permanentes ya han salido para aproximadamente la edad de 13 años. (Audio 6.15)

The third molars are also called "wisdom teeth."
A los terceros molares también se les llama "muelas cordales/muleas del juicio." (Audio 6.16)

Third molars erupt between the ages 17 and 21.
Los terceros molares salen entre los 17 y 21 años. (Audio 6.17)

Sometimes third molars are not positioned in the jaw correctly.
A veces los terceros molares no están posicionados correctamente en la mandíbula. (Audio 6.18)

Sometimes wisdom teeth have to be removed.
A veces las (muelas cordales/muleas del juicio) tienen que ser extraídas. (Audio 6.19)

Teeth are made of _____. (See Box 6.1)
Los dientes son hechos de _____. (Vea el Cuadro 6.1) (Audio 6.20)

The crown is the top part of the tooth, which you see.
La corona es la parte superior del diente, la que usted ve. (Audio 6.21)

Box 6.1
Tooth anatomy (Audio 6.419)

- Anterior (Audio 6.420)
- Cementum (Audio 6.421)
- Canine (eye tooth) (cuspid) (Audio 6.422)
- Cusps (cusp tips) (Audio 6.423)
- Dentin (Audio 6.424)
- Enamel (Audio 6.425)
- Incisor (Audio 6.426)
- Molar (wisdom tooth) (Audio 6.427)
- Nerve (Audio 6.428)
- Posterior (Audio 6.429)
- Premolar (bicuspid) (Audio 6.430)
- Pulp (Audio 6.431)

Cuadro 6.1
Anatomía del diente (Audio 6.419)

- Anterior (Audio 6.420)
- Cemento (Audio 6.421)
- Canino (cúspide canina) (Audio 6.422)
- Cúspide (Audio 6.423)

- Dentina (Audio 6.424)
- Esmalte (Audio 6.425)
- Incisivo (Audio 6.426)
- Molar (muela cordal/muela del juicio) (Audio 6.427)
- Nervio (Audio 6.428)
- Posterior (Audio 6.429)
- Premolar (bicúspide) (Audio 6.430)
- Pulpa (Audio 6.431)

The gumline is the border between the tooth and gums.
El borde de la encía es el borde entre el diente y las encías.
(Audio 6.22)

Healthy gums are not red and do not bleed.
Las encias saludables nos son rojas y no sangran. (Audio 6.23)

Healthy gums are pinkish and do not bleed.
Las encías saludables son rosadas y no sangran. (Audio 6.24)

(The space around the tooth/The space between the tooth and gum) is shallow (0 to 3 millimeter(s)).
(El espacio alrededor del diente/La depresión entre el diente y la encía) es poco profundo(a) (0 a 3 milímetro(s)). (Audio 6.25)

The root is the part of the tooth located in the jawbone.
La raíz es la parte del diente ubicada en el hueso de la mandíbula.
(Audio 6.26)

You can't see roots in a healthy mouth.
En una boca saludable no se ven las raíces. (Audio 6.27)

Enamel is the outermost layer of the tooth crown.
El esmalte es la capa más externa de la corona del diente.
(Audio 6.28)

Enamel is the hardest tissue in the body.
El esmalte es el tejido más duro en el cuerpo. (Audio 6.29)

Enamel can be damaged by acid from bacteria.
El esmalte puede ser dañado por el ácido de las bacterias.
(Audio 6.30)

Dentin is the layer under the enamel and on the root.
La dentina es la capa debajo del esmalte y sobre la raíz. (Audio 6.31)

Dentin can be damaged if caries goes through the enamel.
La dentina puede ser dañada si caries atraviesa el esmalte.
(Audio 6.32)

Dentin damage can lead to pulp damage.
El daño a la dentina puede causar daño a la pulpa. (Audio 6.33)

Cementum covers the tooth root.
El cemento cubre la raíz del diente. (Audio 6.34)

**Pulp is in the center of the tooth where the blood vessels
and nerves are located**.
La pulpa está en el centro del diente donde se encuentran los vasos
sanguíneos y los nervios. (Audio 6.35)

If decay reaches the pulp, you will feel pain.
Si la descomposición alcanza la pulpa, usted sentirá dolor.
(Audio 6.36)

PLAQUE
PLACA BACTERIANA (AUDIO 6.37)

**Plaque is a sticky film of bacteria that forms daily on the
teeth and gums**.
La placa es una película pegajosa de bacteria que se forma
diariamente en los dientes y las encías. (Audio 6.38)

Plaque can be stained so that you can see it on the teeth.
Es posible teñir la placa para que usted pueda verla en los dientes.
(Audio 6.39)

Plaque needs to be removed from the teeth and gums daily.
La placa bacteriana debe eliminarse diariamente de los dientes y encias. (Audio 6.40)

Plaque is removed by brushing and flossing.
La placa se remueve al cepillar y limpiar con hilo dental. (Audio 6.41)

Plaque produces an acid that can cause (decay/cavity/ caries). Certain types of plaque produce a toxin that can cause (gum disease/periodontal disease).
La placa produce un ácido que puede causar (descomposición/ cavidad/caries). Ciertos tipos de placa producen una toxina que puede causar enfermedad (de las encías/periodontal). (Audio 6.42)

You have (slight/moderate) plaque on your teeth.
Usted tiene placa (leve/moderada) en sus dientes. (Audio 6.43)

You have a heavy amount of plaque on your teeth.
Usted tiene mucha placa bacteriana en sus dientes. (Audio 6.44)

Your plaque is mostly located _____. (See Box 6.2)
Su placa está mayormente localizada _____. (Vea el Cuadro 6.2)
(Audio 6.45)

CARIES
CARIES (AUDIO 6.46)

The acids generated by plaque from food lead to tooth decay, resulting in the formation of a cavity.
Los ácidos generados por la placa de los alimentos provocan descomposicíon de los dientes, lo que resulta en la formación de una caries. (Audio 6.47)

You will not feel early (caries/cavities/tooth decay).
Al principio, no sentirá (las caries/las cavidades/la descomposición dental). (Audio 6.48)

**Box 6.2
Locations of plaque
(Audio 6.432)**

- On the tongue side of the teeth (Audio 6.433)
- On the back teeth (Audio 6.434)
- On the inside of the lower front teeth (Audio 6.435)

- On the biting surfaces (Audio 6.436)
- At the gumline (Audio 6.437)
- Between teeth (Audio 6.438)
- Above the gumline (supragingival) (Audio 6.439)
- Below the gumline (subgingival) (Audio 6.440)

**Cuadro 6.2
Localizaciones de placa
(Audio 6.432)**

- En la parte interior de los dientes (Audio 6.433)
- En los dientes de atrás (Audio 6.434)
- En el interior de los dientes de abajo delanteros (Audio 6.435)
- En las superficies de mordida (Audio 6.436)
- En el borde de las encías (Audio 6.437)
- Entre los dientes (Audio 6.438)
- Sobre el borde de la encía (supragingival) (Audio 6.439)
- Bajo el borde de la encía (subgingival) (Audio 6.440)

Tooth caries can lead to tooth loss when the pulp becomes infected.
La caries dental puede causar la pérdida de dientes cuando la pulpa se infecta. (Audio 6.49)

Most tooth decay occurs between teeth.
La mayoría de la descomposición dental ocurre entre los dientes. (Audio 6.50)

Pits and grooves make the chewing surfaces prone to decay.
Los hoyos y las ranuras hacen que las superficies de masticación sean propensas a pudrirse. (Audio 6.51)

Tooth decay can start around the margins of (poor/older) fillings.
Las caries dental pueden comenzar alrededor de los bordes de (empastes/rellenos) (malos/viejos). (Audio 6.52)

Tooth decay can occur where plaque is left at the gumline.
La descomposición dental puede ocurrir en el borde de la encía,
donde queda placa. (Audio 6.53)

Being softer, the roots are prone to decay.
Las raíces son propensas a la descomposición ya que son menos
duras. (Audio 6.54)

**Radiographs help show early (decay/cavities) between the
teeth**.
Las radiografías ayudan a mostrar (la descomposición/las caries)
temprana entre los dientes. (Audio 6.55)

**Caries on the chewing surfaces does not show up on
radiographs until it has become large**.
Las caries en las superficies de masticación no se ve en las
radiografías hasta que llega a ser grande. (Audio 6.56)

You are at (low/moderate/high) risk for (caries/cavities).
Su riesgo de tener (caries/cavidades) es (bajo/moderado/alto).
(Audio 6.57)

**Our estimate of your risk for (caries/cavity) is based on
your (dental work/diet/health/history/plaque)**.
Nuestro estimado de su riesgo de tener (caries/cavidades) se basa
en su (trabajo dental/dieta/salud/historial/placa). (Audio 6.58)

**The (dentist/office/clinic) has new technology to discover
early tooth decay**.
((El/La) dentista/La oficina/La clínica) tiene nueva tecnología para
descubrir la descomposición dental temprana. (Audio 6.59)

In order to save the tooth, this cavity needs to be repaired.
Para salvar el diente, esta caries debe ser reparada. (Audio 6.60)

PERIODONTAL DISEASE
ENFERMEDAD PERIODONTAL (AUDIO 6.61)

**Plaque produces a (poison/toxin) that causes severe
inflammation of the (gums/gingiva)**.
La placa produce (un veneno/una toxina) que causa la inflamación
severa de las encías. (Audio 6.62)

(Tartar/Calculus) is a hard deposit of calcium and phosphate. It creates areas above and beneath the (gums/gingiva) in which plaque can live.

El (sarro/cálculo) es un depósito duro de calcio y fosfato. Ésto crea áreas sobre y debajo de (las encías/la gingiva) en donde puede vivir la placa. (Audio 6.63)

Does (tartar/calculus) build up on your teeth?

¿Acumula (sarro/cálculo) en sus dientes? (Audio 6.64)

You have (slight/moderate) (tartar/calculus).

Usted tiene (sarro/cálculo) (liviano/moderado/). (Audio 6.65)

You have a heavy amount of calculus.

Usted tiene una gran cantidad de (cálculo/sarro). (Audio 6.66)

Diseased (gums/gingivae) are red, sore, or bleed easily.

Las encías enfermas están rojas, adoloridas, o sangran fácilmente. (Audio 6.67)

Early (gum disease/periodontal disease) is called gingivitis.

La enfermedad (de las encías/periodontal) temprana se llama gingivitis. (Audio 6.68)

(Gum disease/Periodontal disease) involving only the (gums/gingiva) is called gingivitis.

La enfermedad (de las encías/periodontal) que sólo involucra a las encías se llama gingivitis. (Audio 6.69)

Gingivitis can be reversed.

La gingivitis puede ser curada. (Audio 6.70)

You will not feel early (gum disease/periodontal disease).

Al principio, no sentirá la enfermedad (de las encías/periodontal). (Audio 6.71)

After a while diseased (gums/gingiva) may pull away from the teeth, forming pockets that fill with more plaque.

Después de un tiempo, las encías enfermas pueden apartarse de los dientes, formando bolsillos que se llenan con más placa. (Audio 6.72)

If the diseased (gums are/gingiva is) not treated, the bone around the teeth can be destroyed.

Si las encías enfermas no se tratan, el hueso alrededor de los dientes puede deteriorarse. (Audio 6.73)

When bone is destroyed by (gum disease/periodontal disease), the teeth may become loose and then be lost.
Cuando el hueso se destruye por la enfermedad (de las encías/ periodontal), los dientes pueden aflojarse y después perderse. (Audio 6.74)

Bone can be lost between the teeth and roots due to (gum disease/periodontal disease).
Se puede perder el hueso entre los dientes y las raíces debido a la enfermedad (de las encías/periodontal). (Audio 6.75)

Extensive (gum disease/periodontal disease) destroying bone around the teeth is called periodontitis.
La enfermedad extensiva (de las encías/periodontal) que destruye el hueso alrededor de los dientes se llama periodontitis. (Audio 6.76)

Treatment for (gum disease/periodontal disease) depends on the amount of bone lost.
El tratamiento para la enfermedad (de las encías/periodontal) depende de la cantidad de hueso que se haya perdido. (Audio 6.77)

Periodontitis can be stopped, but any damage that has occurred before the disease is stopped can't be reversed.
La periodontitis puede ser interrumpida, pero cualquier daño que haya ocurrido antes de parar la enfermedad no puede ser revertido. (Audio 6.78)

You are at (low/moderate/high) risk for (gum disease/ periodontal disease).
Usted tiene un riesgo (bajo/moderado/alto) de enfermedad (de las encías/periodontal). (Audio 6.79)

Our estimate of your risk for (gum disease/periodontal disease) is based on your _____. (See Box 6.3)
Nuestro estimado de su riesgo de enfermedad (de las encías/ periodontal) se basa en su _____. (Vea el Cuadro 6.3) (Audio 6.80)

Here's a (mirror/camera); let's look for signs of gum disease.
Aquí tiene (un espejo/una cámara); vamos a buscar señales de enfermedad de las encías. (Audio 6.81)

Let's check your radiographs for bone loss.
Vamos a examinar sus radiografías para la pérdida de hueso. (Audio 6.82)

Box 6.3
Periodontal disease risk factors (Audio 6.441)

- Dental health (Audio 6.442)
- Diabetes (Audio 6.443)
- Genetics (Audio 6.444)
- Health (Audio 6.445)
- Mouth (Audio 6.446)
- History (Audio 6.447)
- Plaque (Audio 6.448)
- Smoking (Audio 6.449)
- Tartar/calculus (Audio 6.450)
- Tobacco use (Audio 6.451)

Cuadro 6.3
Factores de riesgo de enfermedad periodontal (Audio 6.441)

- Salud dental (Audio 6.442)
- Diabetes (Audio 6.443)
- Genética (Audio 6.444)
- Salud (Audio 6.445)
- Boca (Audio 6.446)
- Historial (Audio 6.447)
- Placa bacteriana (Audio 6.448)
- Fumar (Audio 6.449)
- Sarro/cálculo (Audio 6.450)
- Uso de tabaco (Audio 6.451)

The (dentist/office/clinic) has new technology to detect early (gum disease/periodontal disease).
((El/La) dentista/La oficina/La clínica) tiene una tecnología nueva para dectectar la enfermedad (de las encías/periodontal) temprana. (Audio 6.83)

ATTRITION
DESGASTE (AUDIO 6.84)

The biting surfaces can wear down.
Las superficies para morder se pueden desgastar. (Audio 6.85)

The wearing of tooth surfaces due to normal use is called attrition.
El desgaste de las superficies de los dientes debido al uso normal se llama desgaste. (Audio 6.86)

The worn biting surfaces can stain permanently.
Las superficies para morder desgastadas pueden mancharse permanentemente. (Audio 6.87)

ABRASION
ABRASIÓN (AUDIO 6.88)

The wearing of tooth surfaces caused by biting/chewing abrasive substances or by other habits is called abrasion.
El desgaste de las superficies del diente causado por morder/masticar sustancias abrasivas o por otros hábitos, se llama abrasión. (Audio 6.89)

Using a toothpick is an example of a habit that can cause abrasion.
El uso de un palillo de dientes es un ejemplo de un hábito que causa abrasión. (Audio 6.90)

RECESSION
RECESIÓN (AUDIO 6.91)

When the gumline moves toward the root of a tooth, this process is called recession.
Cuando el borde de la encía se mueve hacia la raíz del diente, este proceso se llama recesión. (Audio 6.92)

Roots are exposed in recession.
Si hay recesión, las raíces están expuestas. (Audio 6.93)

Roots can recede due to_____. (See Box 6.4)
Las raíces pueden retroceder debido a _____. (Vea el Cuadro 6.4) (Audio 6.94)

Teeth can become sensitive due to recession.
Los dientes pueden volverse sensibles debido a la recesión. (Audio 6.95)

The roots can become permanently stained.
Las raíces pueden quedar manchadas permanentemente. (Audio 6.96)

Roots are covered with cementum.
Las raíces estan cubiertas con cemento. (Audio 6.97)

The thin cementum layer protects the tooth root.
La capa fina de cemento proteje la raíz del diente. (Audio 6.98)

Box 6.4
Reasons for gum recession (Audio 6.452)

- Age (Audio 6.453)
- Bite problems (Audio 6.454)

- Hard toothbrushing (Audio 6.455)
- Healing of gum tissue following an infection (Audio 6.456)
- Tooth position (Audio 6.457)
- Surgery (Audio 6.458)

Cuadro 6.4
Razones para la receción de las encías (Audio 6.452)

- La edad (Audio 6.453)
- Problemas para morder (Audio 6.454)
- El cepillado fuerte (Audio 6.455)
- La curación del tejido de la encía luego de una infección (Audio 6.456)
- La posición de un diente (Audio 6.457)
- La cirugía (Audio 6.458)

When the cementum is lost, the tooth can become sensitive.
Cuando se pierde el cemento, el diente puede volverse sensible. (Audio 6.99)

When you eat or drink, you can experience discomfort due to the exposed roots.
Cuando usted come o bebe, puedes sentir molestia debido a que las raíces están expuestas. (Audio 6.100)

When they become exposed, roots may also become sensitive to heat and cold.
Cuando están expuestas, las raíces también pueden volverse sensibles a lo calientey al frío. (Audio 6.101)

ORAL CANCER
CÁNCER ORAL (AUDIO 6.102)

Regular dental exams allow early detection of mouth cancer.
Los exámenes dentales regulares permiten la detección temprana del cáncer oral. (Audio 6.103)

Tobacco use and excessive consumption of alcohol are risk factors for mouth cancer.

El uso de tabaco y el consumo excesivo de alcohol son factores de riesgo para el cáncer oral. (Audio 6.104)

Excessive exposure to the sun can result in lip cancer.

La exposición excesiva al sol puede resultar en cáncer de los labios. (Audio 6.105)

You are at high risk for mouth cancer due to_____. (See Box 6.5)

Usted tiene alto riesgo de cáncer de la boca debido a _____. (Vea el Cuadro 6.5) (Audio 6.106)

Frequent self-examination and regular visits to your dentist will reduce your risk of mouth cancer. (See Box 6.6)

El autoexamen frecuente y visitas regulares a su dentista reducirán su riesgo de cáncer de boca. (Vea el Cuadro 6.6) (Audio 6.107)

Contact the dentist if you have _____. (See Box 6.7)

Llame (al/a la) dentista si tiene _____. (Vea el Cuadro 6.7) (Audio 6.108)

The (dentist/office/clinic) has new technology to discover mouth cancer in its early stages.

((El/La) dentista/La oficina/La clínica) tiene nueva tecnología para detectar el cáncer de la boca en su etapa temprana. (Audio 6.109)

Box 6.5 **Oral cancer risk factors (Audio 6.459)**	**Cuadro 6.5** **Factores de riesgo para el cáncer oral (Audio 6.459)**
• Alcohol (Audio 6.460)	• El alcohol (Audio 6.460)
• Habits (Audio 6.461)	• Los hábitos (Audio 6.461)
• History (Audio 6.462)	• El historial (Audio 6.462)
• Sun exposure (tanning bed) (Audio 6.463)	• La exposición al sol (cama de bronceado) (Audio 6.463)
• Tobacco (Audio 6.464)	• El tabaco (Audio 6.464)

Box 6.6
Self-examination steps (Audio 6.465)

- Prepare: Wash your hands, take out any removable dental appliances, and stand in front of a mirror in a well-lit room, wearing your eyeglasses if needed. (Audio 6.466)
- As you look, run your index finger along your outer lower lip while you smile; then do the same for your outer upper lip. (Audio 6.467)
- Using both index fingers and thumbs, pull down the sides of your lower lip on both sides of your face and look at the inner lower lip; then do the same for the inner upper lip. (Audio 6.468)

- Pull back your outer right cheek with two fingers and look at the right inner cheek; then do the same for the left inner cheek. (Audio 6.469)
- With your index finger, feel along the length of your bottom gums and mouth and underneath your tongue while you look. Be sure to examine areas without teeth, as well as those around your teeth; then do the

Cuadro 6.6
Pasos para la autoexaminación (Audio 6.465)

- Prepárese: Lávese las manos, remueva cualquier aparato dental removible, y párese frente a un espejo en un cuarto bien iluminado, usando sus lentes si es necesario. (Audio 6.466)
- Mientras mira, pase su dedo índice a lo largo del exterior de su labio inferior mientras sonríe; luego haga lo mismo con su labio superior. (Audio 6.467)
- Usando ambos dedos índices y pulgares, hale hacia abajo los lados de su labio inferior a ambos lados de su cara y observe el interior del labio inferior; luego haga lo mismo con el interior del labio superior. (Audio 6.468)
- Hale la mejilla derecha con dos dedos y observe su interior; luego haga lo mismo con la mejilla izquierda. (Audio 6.469)
- Con su dedo índice, sienta a lo largo de sus encías inferiores y su boca y debajo de su lengua mientras observa. Asegúrese de examinar las áreas sin dientes, al igual que las de alrededor de sus dientes; luego haga

Box 6.6
Self-examination steps—cont'd

same for the top gums and the roof of your mouth. (Audio 6.470)
- To see the roof of your mouth, you may need to tip your head back slightly. (Audio 6.471)
- Stick out your tongue and look at the top of it. (Audio 6.472)
- Putting your index finger on the surface of your tongue, in the middle, gently press, say "ah," and look at your throat. (Audio 6.473)
- Taking your two fingers, pull the tip of your tongue to the right and look at the left side; then pull your tongue to the left, looking at the right side. (Audio 6.474)

- Touch your tongue to the roof of your mouth, and look at the underside of your tongue. (Audio 6.475)

Cuadro 6.6
Pasos para la autoexaminación— continuación

lo mismo con las encías superiores y el cielo de la boca/paladar. (Audio 6.470)
- Para ver su paladar, puede que necesite inclinar la cabeza hacia atrás un poco. (Audio 6.471)
- Saque la lengua y observe la superficie de la lengua. (Audio 6.472)
- Colocando su dedo índice en la superficie de su lengua, en el medio, presione levemente, diga "a," y observe su garganta. (Audio 6.473)
- Tomando sus dos dedos, hale la punta de su lengua hacia la derecha y observe el lado izquierdo; luego hale la lengua hacia la izquierda, observando el lado derecho. (Audio 6.474)
- Toque con su lengua el cielo de la boca y observe la parte debajo de la lengua. (Audio 6.475)

BRUSHING
CEPILLADO (AUDIO 6.110)

How often do you brush?
¿Con cuánta frecuencia se cepilla? (Audio 6.111)

Box 6.7
Reasons to call the dentist (Audio 6.476)

- A sore or irritation that does not heal (Audio 6.477)
- Color change, such as the development of red and white areas (Audio 6.478)

- Constant pain, soreness, or numbness (Audio 6.479)

- A lump, thickening, rough spot, crust, or small ulcer that does not heal (Audio 6.480)
- Difficulty that does not get better in chewing, swallowing, speaking, or moving the jaw or tongue (Audio 6.481)
- A change in bite that does not correct itself (Audio 6.482)
- A sudden change in denture fit (Audio 6.483)

Cuadro 6.7
Razones para llamar (al/a la) dentista (Audio 6.476)

- Una (úlcera/llaga) o irritación que no sana (Audio 6.477)
- Un cambio de color, tal como el desarrollo de áreas de color rojo y blanco (Audio 6.478)
- Dolor constante, molestias o entumecimiento (Audio 6.479)
- Un bulto, engrosamiento, zona áspera, o úlcera pequeña que no sana (Audio 6.480)
- Dificultad que no se mejora al masticar, tragar, hablar, o mover la mandíbula o la lengua (Audio 6.481)
- Un cambio en la mordida que no se corrige por sí mismo (Audio 6.482)
- Un cambio repentino en el ajuste de su dentadura (Audio 6.483)

Do you use a hard or soft toothbrush?
¿Usa un cepillo duro o suave? (Audio 6.112)

Brush your teeth twice a day with a soft brush.
Cepíllese los dientes dos veces al día con un cepillo suave.
(Audio 6.113)

Brushing with a soft brush helps remove plaque from the tooth and (gums/gingiva).
El cepillarse con un cepillo suave ayuda a remover la placa del diente y de las encías. (Audio 6.114)

Plaque can be stained so that we can see which areas you are missing with the toothbrush.

La placa se puede teñir para que podamos ver qué áreas no está alcanzando con el cepillo. (Audio 6.115)

Can you show me how you brush?

¿Puede mostrarme cómo se cepilla? (Audio 6.116)

Can I show you how to brush? (See Box 6.8 and Fig. 6.1)

¿Puedo mostrarle cómo cepillarse? (Vea el Cuadro 6.8 y la Figura 6.1) (Audio 6.117)

You brush your teeth very well.

Usted se cepilla muy bien. (Audio 6.118)

Can I share some brushing tips?

¿Puedo compartir algunos consejos de cepillado con usted? (Audio 6.119)

You are missing here with your toothbrush.

Está faltando cepillarse aquí. (Audio 6.120)

Use a pea-sized amount of toothpaste on the brush.

Use la cantidad de pasta de dientes del tamaño de un guisante en su cepillo. (Audio 6.121)

Use toothpaste with fluoride.

Use una pasta de dientes con floruro. (Audio 6.122)

Tartar-control toothpaste helps prevent (tartar/calculus) by keeping plaque from hardening.

La pasta de dientes con control de sarro ayuda a prevenir el (sarro/cálculo) evitando el endurecimiento de la placa. (Audio 6.123)

It's not the toothpaste that cleans, but the effort that you put behind the brushing.

No es la pasta la que limpia, sino el esfuerzo detrás del cepillado. (Audio 6.124)

Can I show you how to clean your tongue?

¿Puedo mostrarle cómo limpiarse la lengua? (Audio 6.125)

Would you like to try and clean your tongue?

¿Le gustaría tratar de limpiarse la lengua? (Audio 6.126)

Box 6.8
Toothbrushing steps
(Audio 6.484)

- Hold your brush at an angle against the gums and move the brush back and forth in short strokes. Positioning your brush correctly helps remove the plaque without damaging your teeth and gums. (Audio 6.485)
- Brush the outer tooth surfaces, the inner tooth surfaces, and the chewing surfaces. (Audio 6.486)
- Place the brush against the chewing surface and use a gentle back-and-forth scrubbing motion. Be thorough when brushing, making sure to remove plaque from all areas. (Audio 6.487)

- Use the "toe" of the brush to clean the inside of the front teeth with an up-and-down stroke. Cleaning the inside of the lower front teeth will keep them from becoming covered with tartar and stains. (Audio 6.488)
- Clean the top of your tongue. Cleaning your tongue will remove plaque and freshen your breath. (Audio 6.489)

Cuadro 6.8
Pasos para el cepillado
dental (Audio 6.484)

- Ponga el cepillo a un ángulo contra las encías y muévalo hacia delante y atrás con movimientos cortos. El posicionar su cepillo correctamente remueve la placa sin dañar sus dientes y encías. (Audio 6.485)
- Cepille las superficies externas de los dientes, las superficies internas, y las superficies de masticación. (Audio 6.486)
- Coloque el cepillo contra las superficies de masticación y use un movimiento suave hacia delante y atrás. Sea minucioso cuando se cepille, asegurándose de eliminar la placa de todas las zonas. (Audio 6.487)

- Use la "punta" del cepillo para limpiar el interior de los dientes del frente con un movimiento de arriba a abajo. El limpiar el interior de los dientes inferiores del frente los mantendrá libres de sarro y manchas. (Audio 6.488)
- Limpie la superficie de su lengua. El limpiar su lengua removerá la placa y refrescará su aliento. (Audio 6.489)

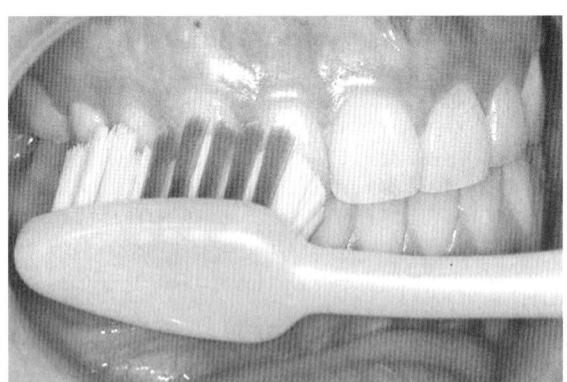

Fig. 6.1 Modified bass technique. Técnica de bass modificada.

Crowded teeth are harder to brush.
Los dientes más juntos son los más difíciles de cepillar. (Audio 6.127)

How often do you change your toothbrush?
¿Con qué frecuencia cambia su cepillo de dientes? (Audio 6.128)

Your removable (appliance/denture) should be taken out before brushing.
Antes de cepillarse, debe quitarse (los aparatos/las dentaduras) removibles. (Audio 6.129)

Toothbrush Recommendations
Recomendaciones para el Cepillo de Dientes (Audio 6.130)

Change your toothbrush every _____ months.
Cambie su cepillo de dientes cada _____ meses. (Audio 6.131)

Bacteria and viruses can grow on your toothbrush.
Las bacterias y los virus pueden crecer en su cepillo de dientes. (Audio 6.132)

Change your toothbrush more often if you have _____. (See Box 6.9)
Cambie su cepillo de dientes con más frecuencia si tiene _____. (Vea el Cuadro 6.9) (Audio 6.133)

Box 6.9
**Reasons to change
your toothbrush
more frequently
(Audio 6.490)**

- Braces (Audio 6.491)

- Canker sore (aphthous
  ulcer) (Audio 6.492)
- Cold or flu (Audio 6.493)

- Cold sore (fever
  blister) (herpes labialis)
  (Audio 6.494)
- Gum disease/periodontal
  disease (Audio 6.495)

- Infections (Audio 6.496)
- Sinus infection (Audio 6.497)

Cuadro 6.9
**Razones para cambiar
su cepillo de dientes
más frecuentemente
(Audio 6.490)**

- Frenillos (frenos/brackets)
  (Audio 6.491)
- Afta (úlcera/aftosa/fuego)
  (Audio 6.492)
- Resfriado o influenza
  (Audio 6.493)
- Úlcera en los labios (vesícula
  febril) (herpes labial)
  (Audio 6.494)
- Enfermedad de las encías/
  enfermedad periodontal
  (Audio 6.495)
- Infecciones (Audio 6.496)
- Infección de sinusitis
  (Audio 6.497)

Don't share your toothbrushes.
No comparta su cepillo de dientes. (Audio 6.134)

**Have a separate toothbrush for each time of the day that
you brush**.
Tenga un cepillo de dientes distinto para cada momento del día en
que se cepilla. (Audio 6.135)

All family members should have their own toothbrushes.
Todos los miembros de la familia deben tener su propio cepillo de
dientes. (Audio 6.136)

There are many different kinds of toothbrushes.
Hay muchas clases diferentes de cepillos de dientes. (Audio 6.137)

Our (office/clinic) recommends this toothbrush.
Nuestra (oficina/clínica) recomienda este cepillo. (Audio 6.138)

Here is a toothbrush for (you/your child).
Aquí tiene un cepillo para (usted/su niño(a)). (Audio 6.139)

Many patients enjoy using a powered brush.
A muchos pacientes les gusta usar un cepillo eléctrico. (Audio 6.140)

As a caregiver, it is recommended you use a powered toothbrush.
Como cuidador, se recomienda que usted utilice un cepillo de dientes eléctrico. (Audio 6.141)

FLOSSING
LIMPIARSE CON HILO DENTAL (AUDIO 6.142)

Do you floss?
¿Usted se limpia los dientes con hilo dental? (Audio 6.143)

How often do you floss?
¿Con cuánta frecuencia se limpia con hilo dental? (Audio 6.144)

Can you show me how you floss?
¿Me puede mostrar cómo se limpia con hilo dental? (Audio 6.145)

You floss very well.
Usted se limpia muy bien con hilo dental. (Audio 6.146)

Can I share some flossing tips?
¿Puedo compartir algunos consejos sobre la limpieza con hilo dental? (Audio 6.147)

Can I show you how to floss? (See Boxes 6.10 and 6.11)
¿Puedo mostrarle cómo usar hilo dental? (Vea los Cuadros 6.10 y 6.11) (Audio 6.148)

Floss your teeth once a day.
Limpie sus dientes con hilo dental una vez al día. (Audio 6.149)

Flossing helps remove plaque from between the teeth.
El limpiarse con hilo dental ayuda a remover la placa entre los dientes. (Audio 6.150)

Floss can reach the spaces between your teeth that a brush can't.
El hilo dental puede alcanzar los espacios entre los dientes a los que el cepillo no llega. (Audio 6.151)

Box 6.10
Flossing steps
(Audio 6.498)

- Break off about a foot and a half of floss, and wind most of it around one of your middle fingers. (Audio 6.499)

- Wind the remaining floss around the same finger of the opposite hand so that it will take up the floss as it becomes dirty. (Audio 6.500)

- After winding the floss, hold the floss tightly between your thumbs and forefingers. (Audio 6.501)

- Using a gentle motion, guide the floss below the contacts of your teeth. (Audio 6.502)

- Curve the floss into a "C" shape against one tooth and gently slide the floss into the space between the gum and the tooth. (Audio 6.503)

- Hold the floss tightly against the tooth and gently rub the side of the tooth with an up-and-down motion. (Audio 6.504)

- Floss each tooth thoroughly with a clean section of floss. (Audio 6.505)

Cuadro 6.10
Pasos para limpiarse con hilo dental (Audio 6.506)

- Corte un pedazo de hilo dental de aproximadamente un pie y medio de largo, y enrolle la mayor parte de él alrededor de uno de sus dedos medios. (Audio 6.499)

- Enrolle la parte restante del hilo dental alrededor del mismo dedo en la mano opuesta de manera que acumule el hilo dental a medida que se ensucia. (Audio 6.500)

- Después de enrollar el hilo dental, sosténga el hilo firmemente entre sus dedos pulgares e índices. (Audio 6.501)

- Usando un movimento suave, guíe el hilo dental debajo de los contactos de sus dientes. (Audio 6.502)

- Curve el hilo dental en forma de "C" contra un diente y suavemente deslize el hilo dental en el espacio entre la encía y el diente. (Audio 6.503)

- Sostenga el hilo dental firmemente contra el diente y suavemente frote el lado de su diente con un movimiento de arriba hacia abajo. (Audio 6.504)

- Limpie cada diente por completo con una sección limpia del hilo dental. (Audio 6.505)

Box 6.11
Alternate flossing steps
(Audio 6.506)

- Break off a 12-inch piece of floss. (Audio 6.507)

- Tie it in a loop just wide enough to comfortably hold in both hands with your hands close together. (Audio 6.508)

- Hold the floss in both hands with the fingers on the inside of the circle. (Audio 6.509)

- Using the thumb and first finger of each hand, guide the floss with a gentle motion below the contacts of your teeth. (Audio 6.510)

- Curve the floss into a "C" shape against one tooth and gently slide the floss into the space between the gum and the tooth. (Audio 6.511)

- Hold the floss tightly against the tooth and gently rub the side of the tooth with an up-and-down motion. (Audio 6.512)

- Floss each tooth thoroughly with a clean section of floss. (Audio 6.513)

Cuadro 6.11
Pasos alternativos
para limpiarse con hilo
dental (Audio 6.506)

- Corte un pedazo de hilo dental de 12 pulgadas de largo. (Audio 6.507)

- Amárrelo en un lazo, lo suficientemente ancho como para aguantarlo con ambas manos cómodamente con las manos cerca una de la otra. (Audio 6.508)

- Aguante el hilo dental en ambas manos con los dedos en el interior del círculo. (Audio 6.509)

- Usando el dedo pulgar y el primer dedo de cada mano, guíe el hilo dental con un movimiento suave por debajo de los contactos entre sus dientes. (Audio 6.510)

- Doble el hilo dental en forma de "C" contra un diente y suavemente deslize el hilo dental en el espacio entre la encía y el diente. (Audio 6.511)

- Sostenga el hilo dental firmemente contra el diente y suavemente frote el lado de su diente con un movimiento de arriba hacia abajo. (Audio 6.512)

- Limpie cada diente por completo con una sección limpia del hilo dental. (Audio 6.513)

Plaque that remains on the teeth can become stained.
La placa que se queda en el diente puede mancharse. (Audio 6.152)

Flossing is not hard to do.
Limpiarse con hilo dental no es difícil. (Audio 6.153)

Flossing does not take a long time.
Limpiarse con hilo dental no toma mucho tiempo. (Audio 6.154)

Never snap the floss into the (gums/gingiva).
Nunca fuerce el hilo dental hacia las encías. (Audio 6.155)

Don't use your floss with a back-and-forth sawing motion.
No use el hilo dental con un movimiento de adelante hacia atrás.
(Audio 6.156)

Do not try to cut your (gums/gingiva) with your floss.
No intente cortar las encías con el hilo dental. (Audio 6.157)

You need to shape the floss better around this tooth here.
Necesita pasarse el hilo dental con mejor forma alrededor de este
diente. (Audio 6.158)

Don't forget to floss the back side of your last tooth.
No se olvide de limpiar la parte de atrás de su ultimo diente.
(Audio 6.159)

Floss is not reusable.
El hilo dental no es reusable. (Audio 6.160)

Floss Recommendations
Recomendaciones para el Hilo Dental (Audio 6.161)

There are many different kinds of floss.
Hay muchos tipos diferentes de hilo dental. (Audio 6.162)

You need to use dental tape since it is wider than floss.
Usted necesita usar cinta dental ya que es más ancha que el hilo
dental. (Audio 6.163)

**You need to use a coated floss since your teeth are very
close together**.
Debe utilizar un hilo dental recubierto ya que sus dientes están muy
juntos. (Audio 6.164)

Our (office/clinic) recommends this kind of floss.
Nuestra (oficina/clínica) recomienda este tipo de hilo dental.
(Audio 6.165)

Here's a sample of floss for (you/your child).
Aquí tiene una muestra de hilo dental para (usted/su niño(a)).
(Audio 6.166)

Floss Alternatives
Alternativas para Limpiarse con Hilo Dental (Audio 6.167)

There are ways to clean your (bridge/implant).
Hay maneras de limpiar su (puente/implante). (Audio 6.168)

Let me show you how to clean your (bridge/implant).
Permítame mostrarle cómo se limpia su (puente/implante).
(Audio 6.169)

Would you like to try to clean your (bridge/implant)?
¿Le gustaría tratar de limpiar su (puente/implante)? (Audio 6.170)

Use a (bridge/floss) threader to clean here.
Use un enhebrador de (puente/hilo dental) para limpiar aquí.
(Audio 6.171)

Here's a sample of (bridge/floss) threaders for you.
Aquí tiene una muestra de enhebradores de (puente/hilo dental)
para usted. (Audio 6.172)

Floss holders help if you have difficulty.
Los porta hilo dental ayudan si usted tiene dificultad. (Audio 6.173)

People who have difficulty flossing may use other aids.
Las personas que tienen dificultad para usar el hilo dental pueden
usar otros dispositivos. (Audio 6.174)

Other aids include small brushes, picks, or sticks.
Otros dispositivos incluyen cepillos pequeños, limpiadientes o
palillos. (Audio 6.175)

Interdental aids also help clean out plaque between the roots.
Los dispositivos interdentales también ayudan a limpiar la placa
entre las raíces. (Audio 6.176)

Can I show you how to use this interdental aid?
¿Le puedo mostrar cómo se usa este dispositivo interdental?
(Audio 6.177)

Here's a sample of interdental aids that we recommend.
Aquí tiene una muestra de los dispositivos interdentales que
recomendamos. (Audio 6.178)

Flossing and Children
El Limpiarse con Hilo Dental y los Niños (Audio 6.179)

Start flossing when your child's teeth begin to touch.
Comience a usar el hilo dental cuando los dientes de su niño(a)
comiencen a tocarse. (Audio 6.180)

Floss your child's teeth once daily until (he/she) can do it.
Limpie los dientes de su niño(a) con hilo dental una vez al día hasta
que (él/ella) lo pueda hacer por su cuenta. (Audio 6.181)

**If you show your child that you floss, it is more likely that
(he/she) will floss too.**
Si usted le muestra a su niño(a) que usted se limpia con hilo dental,
es más probable que (él/ella) también lo haga. (Audio 6.182)

You will need to show your child how to floss.
Usted necesitará mostrarle a su niño(a) cómo se usa el hilo dental.
(Audio 6.183)

**Watch your child's flossing until you're certain that (he/she)
is doing it correctly.**
Supervise a su niño(a) mientras se limpia con hilo dental hasta que
esté seguro(a) de que (él/ella) lo hace correctamente. (Audio 6.184)

I will be showing your child how to floss.
Voy a mostrarle a su niño(a) cómo se usa el hilo dental. (Audio 6.185)

**We need to use floss to remove the sugar bugs from
between our teeth.**
Necesitamos usar el hilo dental para sacar los gusanos de azucar
que aparecen entre nuestros dientes. (Audio 6.186)

**With braces it is harder to floss around the teeth, but you
will need to do it.**
Con (frenillos/frenos/brackets) es más difícil usar el hilo dental
alrededor de los dientes, pero necesitas hacerlo. (Audio 6.187)

Not flossing braces can lead to tooth decay or (gum/ periodontal) disease.
No limpiarse los (frenillos/frenos/brackets) con hilo dental puede resultar en la descomposición de los dientes o en enfermedad (de las encías/periodontal). (Audio 6.188)

Back teeth (molars) are the most difficult for children to floss correctly.
Los dientes de atrás (molares) son los más difíciles para que los niños usen el hildo dental correctamente. (Audio 6.189)

BAD BREATH (HALITOSIS)
MAL ALIENTO (HALITOSIS) (AUDIO 6.190)

_____ can cause bad breath. (See Box 6.12)
_____ puede(n) causar mal aliento. (Vea el Cuadro 6.12) (Audio 6.191)

Keeping your teeth clean can help keep your breath fresh.
Mantener sus dientes limpios puede ayudar a mantener fresco su aliento. (Audio 6.192)

Not cleaning your teeth regularly can contribute to bad breath.
No mantener sus dientes limpios puede contribuir al mal aliento. (Audio 6.193)

Not cleaning around braces can lead to bad breath.
El no limpiar alrededor de los (frenillos/frenos/brackets) puede causar mal aliento. (Audio 6.194)

Bad breath can be a sign of a medical problem.
El mal aliento puede ser una señal de un problema médico. (Audio 6.195)

Mouthwashes don't have a long-lasting effect on bad breath.
Los enjuagues bucales no tienen un efecto duradero en el mal aliento. (Audio 6.196)

Cleaning your tongue can freshen your breath.
El limpiar su lengua puede refrescar su aliento. (Audio 6.197)

There are many products for fighting bad breath.
Hay muchos productos para combatir el mal aliento. (Audio 6.198)

Box 6.12
Possible reasons for bad breath (Audio 6.514)

- A dirty denture (Audio 6.515)
- Dry mouth (Audio 6.516)
- Garlic and onions (Audio 6.517)
- Gums bleeding (Audio 6.518)
- Gum disease (Audio 6.519)

- Gum infection (Audio 6.520)

- Plaque (Audio 6.521)

- Tartar/calculus (Audio 6.522)

- Tobacco (Audio 6.523)
- Medication (Audio 6.524)

- Sulfur-producing bacteria (Audio 6.525)
- Not flossing (Audio 6.526)

- Poor brushing habits (Audio 6.527)
- Not brushing (Audio 6.528)
- Sinus drainage (postnasal drip) (Audio 6.529)
- Tonsil infections (Audio 6.530)

Cuadro 6.12
Posibles razones para el mal aliento (Audio 6.514)

- La dentadura sucia (Audio 6.515)
- La boca seca (Audio 6.516)
- El ajo y las cebollas (Audio 6.517)
- El sangrado de las encías (Audio 6.518)
- La enfermedad de las encías (Audio 6. 519)
- La infección de las encías (Audio 6.520)
- La placa bacteriana (Audio 6.521)
- El sarro/El cálculo (Audio 6.522)
- El tabaco (Audio 6.523)
- El medicamento (Audio 6.524)
- Las bacterias que producen el azufre (Audio 6.525)
- El no usar el hilo dental (Audio 6.526)
- Los malos hábitos de cepillar (Audio 6.527)
- El no cepillar (Audio 6.528)
- El drenaje del seno (drenaje post-nasal) (Audio 6.529)
- Las infecciones de las amígdalas (Audio 6.530)

Our (office/clinic) recommends these products for bad breath.
Nuestra (oficina/clínica) recomienda estos productos para el mal aliento. (Audio 6.199)

Dry mouth can make our breath less than pleasant.
Una boca seca puede causar que nuestro aliento no sea agradable. (Audio 6.200)

Sodium lauryl sulfate (in many dental products) can cause our mouth to become dry.
El sulfato de laurilo de sodio (en muchos productos dentales) puede causar que nuestra boca se reseque. (Audio 6.201)

"Morning breath" results from the decreased production of saliva during sleep.
"El mal aliento de la mañana" es resultado de la disminución de la producción de saliva mientras dormimos. (Audio 6.202)

Round dots can appear on the tonsils and can cause a bitter or bad taste and odor.
Pueden aparecer unos puntitos redondos en las amígdalas y pueden causar un sabor y un olor amargo o malo. (Audio 6.203)

The back of the tongue seems to be an odor-producing area.
La parte posterior de la lengua parece ser un zona productora del mal aliento. (Audio 6.204)

The central groove of the tongue can trap bacteria.
La ranura central de la lengua puede atrapar bacterias. (Audio 6.205)

(Some foods/ingredients) can increase sulfur production, which results in bad breath. (See Box 6.13)
(Algunas comidas/Algunos ingredientes) pueden aumentar la producción de azufre, lo que causa mal aliento. (Vea el Cuadro 6.13) (Audio 6.206)

What You Can Do About Bad Breath
Qué Puede Hacer sobre el Mal Aliento (Audio 6.207)

Keep your tongue clean.
Mantenga la lengua limpia. (Audio 6.208)

Box 6.13
Foods/ingredients that can increase sulfur production (Audio 6.531)

- Drying agents – especially alcohol (mouthwashes) (Audio 6.532)

- Dense protein foods (dairy foods; large quantities of chicken, beef, or fish) (Audio 6.533)

- Sugary and acidic foods and drinks (coffee and all fruit and vegetable drinks) (Audio 6.534)

Cuadro 6.13
Comidas/ingredientes que pueden aumentar la producción de azufre (Audio 6.531)

- Agentes resecantes-especialmente el alcohol (enjuagues bucales) (Audio 6.532)

- Comidas densas en proteína (productos lácteos; cantidades grandes de pollo, carne de res, o pescado) (Audio 6.533)

- Comidas azucaradas y ácidas y bebidas (el café y todas las bebidas de frutas y vegetales) (Audio 6.534)

Drink more water (not coffee, juice, or carbonated beverages).
Beba más agua (que no sea café, jugo, o bebidas carbonatadas). (Audio 6.209)

Watch out for the obvious: onions, garlic, and tobacco.
Tenga cuidado con lo obvio: cebollas, ajo, y tabaco. (Audio 6.210)

Don't overdo your consumption of protein, alcoholic beverages, or coffee.
No consuma demasiada proteína, bebidas alcohólicas, o café. (Audio 6.211)

Avoid sugar in breath mints, gum, candy, alcohol, and juice.
Evite el azúcar en las mentas para el aliento, el chicle, los dulces, el alcohol, y el jugo. (Audio 6.212)

Avoid smoking.
Evite fumar. (Audio 6.213)

TONGUE SCRAPING
RASPADO DE LA LENGUA (AUDIO 6.214)

Bacteria are present in the fibers of the tongue naturally.
Las bacterias están presentes naturalmente en las fibras de la lengua.
(Audio 6.215)

Tongue scraping can give you better breath and improve the taste in your mouth.
El raspado de la lengua puede darle mejor aliento y mejorar el sabor en la boca. (Audio 6.216)

You can use a very soft brush to clean your tongue.
Puede usar un cepillo muy suave para limpiarse la lengua.
(Audio 6.217)

Special tongue scrapers can be purchased in stores.
Se pueden comprar raspadores de lengua especiales en las tiendas.
(Audio 6.218)

You can use a round-ended spoon turned upside down to scrape the flat surface of your tongue.
Puede usar una cuchara de punta redonda volteada boca abajo para raspar la superficie plana de su lengua. (Audio 6.219)

Do not scrape or brush too hard; be gentle.
No raspe o cepille duro; hágalo suavemente. (Audio 6.220)

You can injure your tongue or make it hurt or burn.
Usted puede lastimarse la lengua o hacerla doler o arder.
(Audio 6.221)

Scraping too hard can make your tongue feel dry.
El raspar muy duro puede causar que su lengua se sienta reseca.
(Audio 6.222)

Be careful not to reach too far back on your tongue; tongue scraping can make you gag.
Tenga cuidado de no raspar muy atrás en su lengua; el raspar la lengua puede causar náuseas. (Audio 6.223)

Too much bacteria or altered bacteria can cause odors.
Demasiada bacteria o bacteria alterada puede causar malos olores.
(Audio 6.224)

Mouthwash does not get your tongue clean.
El enjuague bucal no limpia la lengua. (Audio 6.225)

Mouthwash (with alcohol) can actually dry out your tongue and oral tissue.
El enjuague bucal (con alcohol) puede resecar la lengua y el tejido oral. (Audio 6.226)

FLUORIDE
FLUORURO/FLÚOR (AUDIO 6.227)

Fluoride makes your teeth decay resistant.
El fluoruro hace que los dientes sean más resistentes a la descomposición. (Audio 6.228)

Fluoride in (toothpaste/rinses/water) helps protect your teeth from cavities.
El fluoruro en (la pasta de dientes/los enjuagues/el agua) ayuda a proteger los dientes contra las caries. (Audio 6.229)

Fluoride helps protect your teeth from cavities.
El fluoruro ayuda a proteger sus dientes contra las caries. (Audio 6.230)

Follow the dentist's instructions so that your child gets the right amount of fluoride.
Siga las instrucciones (del dentista/de la dentista) para que su niño(a) obtenga la cantidad de fluoruro correcta. (Audio 6.231)

Prescription fluoride _____ (are/is) needed to help protect your child's teeth from decay. (See Box 6.14)
Necesita fluoruro recetado en _____ para ayudar en proteger los dientes de su niño(a) de la descomposición. (Vea el Cuadro 6.14) (Audio 6.232)

Regular mouthwash does not contain fluoride.
El enjuague bucal regular no contiene fluoruro. (Audio 6.233)

Check your well water for fluoride content. When we receive the report, we will give you the right prescription.
Averigüe cuál es el contenido de fluoruro en su agua de pozo. Cuando recibamos el informe, le daremos la receta correcta. (Audio 6.234)

**Box 6.14
Types of fluoride
prescriptions
(Audio 6.535)**

- Chewable tablets
  (Audio 6.536)
- Drops (Audio 6.537)
- Gels (Audio 6.538)
- Lozenges (Audio 6.539)
- Rinses (Audio 6.540)
- Toothpaste (Audio 6.541)

- Varnish (Audio 6.542)

**Cuadro 6.14
Tipos de recetas de
fluoruro (Audio 6.535)**

- Pastillas masticables
  (Audio 6.536)
- Gotas (Audio 6.537)
- Geles (Audio 6.538)
- Tabletas (Audio 6.539)
- Enjuagues (Audio 6.540)
- Pasta de dientes
  (Audio 6.541)
- Barniz (Audio 6.542)

Fluoride can help with your teeth sensitivity.
El fluoruro le puede ayudar con la sensibilidad de dientes.
(Audio 6.235)

**Because of your dry mouth, you need fluoride supplements
to help protect your teeth from decay.**
Como tiene la boca seca, necesita suplementos de fluoruro para
ayudar a proteger sus dientes de la descomposición. (Audio 6.236)

ORAL HABITS
HÁBITOS ORALES (AUDIO 6.237)

Piercing the tongue or lips can cause dental damage.
El perforar la lengua o los labios y ponerse piercing puede dañar los
dientes. (Audio 6.238)

**Chewing on hard objects like _____ can crack a tooth or
filling. (See Box 6.15)**
El masticar objetos duros como _____ puede fracturar un diente o
un empaste/relleno/calza. (Vea el Cuadro 6.15) (Audio 6.239)

(Grinding/Clenching) the teeth can cause tooth damage.
El (rechinar/crujir/apretar) los dientes puede causar daños a los
dientes. (Audio 6.240)

Box 6.15
Objects that can cause cracks in teeth or dental work (Audio 6.543)

- Ice (Audio 6.544)
- Metal (Audio 6.545)
- Pencils (Audio 6.546)
- Toothpicks (Audio 6.547)

Cuadro 6.15
Objectos que pueden causar fracturas en los dientes o en el trabajo dental (Audio 6.548)

- Hielo (Audio 6.544)
- Metal (Audio 6.545)
- Lápices (Audio 6.546)
- Palillos (Audio 6.547)

Excessive vomiting can cause tooth damage.
El vómito excesivo puede causar daños a los dientes. (Audio 6.241)

Playing sports can damage the teeth. This includes sports like basketball, baseball, gymnastics, and volleyball.
El jugar deportes puede dañar los dientes. Esto incluye deportes como el baloncesto, el béisbol, la gimnasia, y el voleibol. (Audio 6.242)

Custom-made mouthguards can protect teeth during sports.
Los protectores bucales hechos a la medida pueden proteger los dientes durante los deportes. (Audio 6.243)

Frequent swimming in pools can damage your teeth and (gums/gingiva) and can cause unusual stains.
El nadar frecuentemente en piscinas puede dañar los dientes y las encías, y puede causar manchas inusuales. (Audio 6.244)

Aspirin placed near a toothache can severely burn the gums. You need to swallow the aspirin.
La aspirina puesta en el área de un dolor de muelas puede quemar las encías gravemente. Usted debe tragarse la aspirina. (Audio 6.245)

Drinking coffee and tea stains the teeth.
El tomar café y té mancha los dientes. (Audio 6.246)

Chewing on only one side of your mouth can create a muscle imbalance.
El masticar por sólo un lado de la boca puede crear un desequilibrio muscular. (Audio 6.247)

ASSESSMENT OF ORAL HYGIENE HABITS
EVALUACIÓN DE LOS HÁBITOS DE HIGIENE ORAL (AUDIO 6.248)

Do you brush your teeth every day?
¿Se cepilla los dientes todos los días? (Audio 6.249)

How many times a day do you brush your teeth?
¿Cuántas veces al día se cepilla los dientes? (Audio 6.250)

Show me how you brush your teeth.
Muéstreme cómo se cepilla los dientes. (Audio 6.251)

Are you able to floss your teeth?
¿Puede limpiarse los dientes con hilo dental? (Audio 6.252)

Do you floss your teeth every day?
¿Se limpia los dientes con hilo dental todos los días? (Audio 6.253)

How often do you floss?
¿Con cuánta frecuencia se limpia los dientes con hilo dental?
(Audio 6.254)

Do your gums bleed when you (brush/floss) your teeth?
¿Le sangran las encías cuando se (cepilla/limpia con hilo dental) los
dientes? (Audio 6.255)

Show me how you floss your teeth.
Muéstreme cómo se limpia los dientes con hilo dental.
(Audio 6.256)

Would you like me to show you how to floss your teeth?
¿Le gustaría que le enseñe cómo limpiarse los dientes con hilo
dental? (Audio 6.257)

Do you use any special brush or tool to clean your teeth?
¿Usa algún cepillo o herramienta especial para limpiarse los dientes?
(Audio 6.258)

What special brush or tool do you use to clean your teeth?
¿Qué cepillo o herramienta especial usa para limpiarse los dientes?
(Audio 6.259)

Do you use an interproximal brush?
¿Usa un cepillo interproximal? (Audio 6.260)

Do you use a (cylindrical/tapered) interproximal brush?
¿Usa un cepillo interproximal (cilíndrico/cónico)? (Audio 6.261)

How do you clean under your bridge?
¿Cómo se limpia debajo del puente? (Audio 6.262)

Would you like me to show you how to clean under your bridge?
¿Le gustaría que le mostrara cómo limpiarse debajo del puente? (Audio 6.263)

Do you use a manual or powered toothbrush?
¿Usa un cepillo de dientes manual o eléctrico? (Audio 6.264)

How often do you change your toothbrush?
¿Con cuánta frecuencia cambia su cepillo de dientes? (Audio 6.265)

You brush your teeth too hard.
Usted se cepilla los dientes demasiado fuerte. (Audio 6.266)

You have worn away the tooth and (gums/gingiva) by brushing too hard.
Usted ha desgastado el diente y las encías por cepillarse muy fuerte. (Audio 6.267)

Do you know what causes (dental decay/a cavity/caries)?
¿Usted sabe lo que causa (la descomposición dental/una cavidad/las caries)? (Audio 6.268)

Do you know what causes (gum disease/periodontal disease)?
¿Usted sabe lo que causa la enfermedad (de las encías/periodontal)? (Audio 6.269)

You have many areas of plaque accumulation.
Usted tiene muchas áreas de acumulación de placa. (Audio 6.270)

It is important that you remove plaque daily.
Es importante que usted remueva la placa a diario. (Audio 6.271)

You need to do a better job with your plaque control.
Usted necesita controlar la placa de una mejor manera. (Audio 6.272)

I will paint your teeth with this red liquid so that you can easily see the plaque.
Yo le pintaré los dientes con este líquido rojo para que pueda ver fácilmente la placa. (Audio 6.273)

Rinse with this water.
Enjuáguese con esta agua. (Audio 6.274)

Look into the mirror.
Mírese en el espejo. (Audio 6.275)

All the red areas are areas of plaque.
Todas las áreas rojas son áreas de placa. (Audio 6.276)

Can you see the red areas on your teeth?
¿Puede ver las áreas rojas en sus dientes? (Audio 6.277)

Can you see the plaque on your teeth?
¿Puede ver la placa en sus dientes? (Audio 6.278)

Have there been any changes in your oral hygiene habits?
¿Ha habido algún cambio en sus hábitos de higiene oral? (Audio 6.279)

Have there been any changes in your (health/diet/ medications)?
¿Ha habido cambios en su(s) (salud/dieta/medicamentos)? (Audio 6.280)

TOBACCO USE AND CESSATION
USO Y CESACIÓN DEL TABACO (AUDIO 6.281)

Tobacco products, such as _____, stain the teeth and tongue. (See Box 6.16)
Los productos de tabaco, tales como _____, manchan los dientes y la lengua. (Vea el Cuadro 6.16) (Audio 6.282)

Chewing tobacco contains sand and grit, which can wear down your teeth.
El (tabaco de mascar/tabaco sin humo) contiene arena y gravilla, que puede desgastar sus dientes. (Audio 6.283)

Box 6.16
Tobacco products
(Audio 6.548)

- Bidis (a type of cigar/ cigarette flavored with chocolate) (Audio 6.549)
- Chew (Audio 6.550)
- Chewing tobacco (Audio 6.551)

- Cigar (Audio 6.552)

- Cigarettes (Audio 6.553)
- Pipe (Audio 6.554)
- Smokeless tobacco (Audio 6.555)
- Tobacco leaves (Audio 6.556)

Cuadro 6.16
Productos de tabaco
(Audio 6.548)

- Los bidis (un tipo de cigarro/ cigarrillo con sabor de chocolate) (Audio 6.549)
- Masticar (Audio 6.550)
- El tabaco para masticar/ taboco para mascar (Audio 6.551)
- Los puros/habanos/cigarros (Audio 6.552)
- Los cigarrillos (Audio 6.553)
- La pipa (Audio 6.54)
- El tabaco sin humo (Audio 6.555)
- Las hojas de tabaco (Audio 6.556)

Chewing tobacco contains sugar, which will cause tooth decay when held against your teeth.
El (tabaco de mascar/tabaco sin humo) contiene azúcar, la que causará la descomposición de los dientes cuando se sostiene al lado de los dientes. (Audio 6.284)

Tobacco can contribute to (tartar/calculus) buildup.
El tabaco puede contribuir a la acumulación de (sarro/cálculo). (Audio 6.285)

Tobacco delays healing after a(n) (cleaning/extraction/ surgery).
El tabaco atrasa la curación después de una (limpieza/extracción/ cirugía). (Audio 6.286)

Tobacco increases your risk of gum disease and mouth cancer.
El tabaco aumenta el riesgo de enfermedad de las encías y cáncer de la boca. (Audio 6.287)

_____ (is/are) not a safe alternative to cigarettes. (See Box 6.16)
_____ no (es/son) alternativa(s) segura(s) al cigarrillo/cigarro. (Vea el Cuadro 6.16) (Audio 6.288)

Many products are available to help you quit tobacco use.
Hay muchos productos disponibles para ayudarle a dejar el tabaco. (Audio 6.289)

Can we assist you in quitting your tobacco use?
¿Le podemos ayudar a dejar el tabaco? (Audio 6.290)

We will work with your medical doctor to help you quit.
Trabajaremos con su doctor(a) para ayudarle a dejar el tabaco. (Audio 6.291)

Our (office/clinic) recommends these products for quitting tobacco use.
Nuestra (oficina/clínica) recomienda estos productos para dejar el tabaco. (Audio 6.292)

The dentist recommends _____to help you quit tobacco use. (See Box 6.17)
El/La dentista recomienda _____ para ayudarle a dejar el tabaco. (Vea el Cuadro 6.17) (Audio 6.293)

Successfully quitting tobacco use can take many attempts.
El dejar el tabaco con éxito puede tomar muchos intentos. (Audio 6.294)

The more times you try to quit, the more likely it is that the next attempt will work.
Mientras más veces lo trate de dejar, más probable será que el próximo intento funcionará. (Audio 6.295)

Keep on quitting!
!Siga dejándolo! (Audio 6.296)

Box 6.17
Ways to quit using tobacco (Audio 6.557)

- Contacting your doctor (medical consult) (Audio 6.558)
- Medicine (antidepressant) (Audio 6.559)
- Nicotine gum (Audio 6.560)
- Nicotine inhaler (Audio 6.561)
- Nicotine lozenge (Audio 6.562)
- Nicotine patch (Audio 6.563)
- Therapy (Audio 6.564)

Cuadro 6.17
Maneras de dejar de usar tabaco (Audio 6.557)

- Contactarse con su médico(a) (un especialista médico) (Audio 6.558)
- La medicina (un antidepresivo) (Audio 6.559)
- La goma/chicle de mascar de nicotina (Audio 6.560)
- El inhalador de nicotina (Audio 6.561)
- Las tabletas de nicotina (Audio 6.562)
- El parche de nicotina (Audio 6.563)
- La terapia (Audio 6.564)

DENTAL HYGIENE
HIGIENE DENTAL (AUDIO 6.297)

Adult Prophylaxis and Scaling
Profilaxis y Raspado para Adultos (Audio 6.298)

I will be doing (a cleaning/adult prophylaxis/a scaling).
Estaré haciendo (una limpieza/una profilaxis para adultos/un raspado). (Audio 6.299)

Have you ever had your teeth cleaned? When?
¿Le han hecho alguna vez una limpieza dental? ¿Cuándo? (Audio 6.300)

I will be (cleaning/scaling) your teeth with dental instruments.
Estaré (limpiando/raspando) sus dientes con instrumentos dentales. (Audio 6.301)

I will be using special instruments to (clean/scale) your implant.
Utilizaré instrumentos especiales para (limpiar/raspar) su implante.
(Audio 6.302)

(Cleaning/Scaling) your teeth removes bacteria and hard deposits and will make your teeth and (gums/gingiva) healthy.
El (limpiar/raspar) sus dientes remueve la bacteria y depósitos duros y hará que sus dientes y encías estén saludables. (Audio 6.303)

You will need to have a deep cleaning because of your (gum disease/periodontal disease).
Usted necesitará una limpieza profunda por su (enfermedad de las encías/enfermedad periodontal). (Audio 6.304)

This deep cleaning of your teeth is more extensive than a usual teeth cleaning.
Esta limpieza profunda de los dientes es más extensa que una limpieza dental normal. (Audio 6.305)

I will be scaling deep in the pockets around your teeth.
Estaré raspando en los bolsillos alrededor de sus dientes.
(Audio 6.306)

Removal of deposits deep in the pockets of the teeth will make your teeth and gums healthy.
La eliminación de depósitos en la profundidad de los bolsillos de los dientes hará sus dientes y encías más sanas. (Audio 6.307)

(Cleaning/Scaling) does not remove any of the tooth.
El (limpiar/raspar) no elimina nada del diente. (Audio 6.308)

I can't scale your teeth today since you have (an abscess/a gum boil/a canker sore/an infection).
No puedo raspar sus dientes hoy ya que tiene (un absceso/un flemón/un fuego/una infección). (Audio 6.309)

If your (gums/gingiva) bleed(s), it is not due to a rough cleaning but to poor health.
Si le sangran las encías, no es debido a una limpieza dura sino a la mala salud. (Audio 6.310)

Are your teeth sensitive to (cleaning/scaling)?
¿Son sus dientes sensibles (a la limpieza/al raspado)? (Audio 6.311)

Are you comfortable while I (clean/scale) your teeth?
¿Está cómodo(a) mientras le (limpio/raspo) los dientes?
(Audio 6.312)

**Let me know if you are uncomfortable while I (clean/scale)
your teeth.**
Hágame saber si está incómodo(a) mientras le (limpio/raspo) los
dientes. (Audio 6.313)

I will be gentle while I (clean/scale) your teeth.
Seré cuidadoso(a) mientras le (limpio/raspo) los dientes.
(Audio 6.314)

**Most people receive an anesthetic before a scaling so that
they are comfortable and I can clean completely.**
La mayoría de las personas reciben un anestésico antes de un
raspado, para que puedan estar más cómodas, y yo pueda limpiar
completamente. (Audio 6.315)

**I will be numbing your teeth and (gums/gingiva) before
scaling.**
Le adormeceré los dientes y las encías antes del raspado.
(Audio 6.316)

**Numbing your teeth and (gums/gingiva) will make them
comfortable during scaling.**
El adormecerle los dientes y las encías los hará sentir más cómodos
durante el raspado. (Audio 6.317)

I am certified to numb your teeth and (gums/gingiva).
Estoy certificado(a) para adormecerle los dientes y las encías.
(Audio 6.318)

Do you (need/use) nitrous oxide gas during scaling?
¿Usted (necesita/utiliza) gas de óxido nitroso durante el raspado?
(Audio 6.319)

I am certified to use nitrous oxide.
Estoy certificado(a) para utilizar el óxido nitroso. (Audio 6.320)

I am checking your teeth for (tartar/calculus).
Estoy examinando sus dientes para (sarro/cálculo). (Audio 6.321)

I will be drying your teeth now.
Ahora le secaré los dientes. (Audio 6.322)

Drying the teeth helps me check for (tartar/calculus).
El secar los dientes me ayuda a ver (sarro/cálculo). (Audio 6.323)

I will be sharpening my scaling instruments.
Afilaré mis instrumentos de raspado. (Audio 6.324)

Sharp scaling instruments help me remove (tartar/calculus).
Los instrumentos de raspado afilados me ayudan a eliminar (el sarro/el cálculo). (Audio 6.325)

I will be using an antiseptic rinse to heal your (gums/ gingiva).
Usaré un enjuague antiséptico para sanar sus encías. (Audio 6.326)

Irrigation of the (gums/gingiva) helps them heal after scaling.
La irrigación de las (encías/gingiva) ayuda a sanar las encias después del raspado. (Audio 6.327)

While I (clean/scale), I will rinse your mouth using water and suction.
Mientras (limpio/raspo), le enjuagaré la boca con agua y succión. (Audio 6.328)

Have I rinsed your mouth enough after the (cleaning/ scaling)?
¿He enjuagado su boca lo suficiente después (de la limpieza/del raspado)? (Audio 6.329)

Additions to Scaling
Adiciones al Raspado (Audio 6.330)

I will be root planing your teeth.
Estaré haciendo un alisado radicular en su diente. (Audio 6.331)

Root planing removes bacterial toxins and hard deposits and reduces inflammation.
El alisado radicular elimina las toxinas bacterianas y los depósitos duros y reduce la inflamación. (Audio 6.332)

I will be curetting your (gums/gingiva).
Estaré haciendo un curetaje en sus encías. (Audio 6.333)

Curetting the (gums/gingiva) removes diseased tissue, which will help to heal the (gums/gingiva).
El hacer un curetaje en sus encías elimina el tejido enfermo, lo que le ayudará a que las encías sanen. (Audio 6.334)

ULTRASONIC SCALING
CURETAJE ULTRASÓNICO (AUDIO 6.335)

This is an ultrasonic scaler.
Ésta es un(a) (cureta/escalador) ultrasónico(a). (Audio 6.336)

I will be using an ultrasonic scaler.
Usaré un(a) (cureta/escalador) ultrasónico(a). (Audio 6.337)

An ultrasonic scaler removes bacteria and (tartar/calculus) comfortably and efficiently.
Un raspador ultrasónico elimina bacterias y (sarro/cálculo) de manera cómoda y eficiente. (Audio 6.338)

The ultrasonic scaler uses sound waves and water to remove deposits.
El escalador ultrasónico utiliza ondas de sonido y agua para eliminar los depósitos. (Audio 6.339)

It uses water to keep the tooth cool and the area flushed out.
Utiliza agua para mantener el diente fresco y el área enjuagada. (Audio 6.340)

The ultrasonic scaler will cause your teeth to vibrate slightly.
La cureta (ultrasónica/raspador ultrasónico) hará que sus dientes vibren levemente. (Audio 6.341)

The ultrasonic scaler can be noisy when I use it here. It vibrates slightly and makes a whistling noise.
La cureta ultrasónica podría ser ruidosa cuando la utilizo aquí. Hace una leve vibración y un silbido. (Audio 6.342)

Are you comfortable as I use the ultrasonic scaler on your teeth?
¿Se siente cómodo mientras uso el raspador ultrasónico en sus dientes? (Audio 6.343)

Let me know if you are uncomfortable as I use the ultrasonic scaler.
Hágame saber si está incómodo(a) mientras utilizo la cureta ultrasónica. (Audio 6.344)

POSTSCALING INSTRUCTIONS
INTRUCCIONES PARA DESPUÉS DEL RASPADO (AUDIO 6.345)

After scaling, _____. (See Box 6.18)
Después del raspado _____. (Vea el Cuadro 6.18) (Audio 6.346)

Your (gums/gingiva) will heal faster after scaling if you keep your mouth clean.
Sus (encías/gingiva) se sanarán más rápidamente después del raspado si mantiene la boca limpia. (Audio 6.347)

(I/The dentist) recommend(s) warm saltwater rinses to heal the (gums/gingiva) after scaling.
(Yo/(El/La) dentista) recomiendo(a) enjuagues de agua tibia con sal para sanar las encías después del raspado. (Audio 6.348)

Box 6.18 **Descriptions of (gums/ gingiva) after scaling (Audio 6.565)**	**Cuadro 6.18** **Descripciones de las encías después del raspado (Audio 6.565)**
• Gums/gingiva may be sore (Audio 6.566)	• Las encías pueden quedar adoloridas (Audio 6.566)
• Gums/gingiva may bleed (Audio 6.567)	• Las encías pueden sangrar (Audio 6.567)
• Root decay may be found (Audio 6.568)	• Puede haber descomposición de la raíz (Audio 6.568)
• Teeth may be sensitive (Audio 6.569)	• Los dientes pueden quedar sensibles (Audio 6.569)
• You may need an over-the-counter pain reliever (Audio 6.570)	• Usted puede necesitar un analgésico sin receta para el dolor (Audio 6.570)

(I/The dentist) recommend(s) this (rinse/gel) to heal the (gums/gingiva) after the scaling.
(Yo/(El/La) dentista) recomiendo(a) este (enjuague/gel) para sanar las encías después del raspado. (Audio 6.349)

This (gel/rinse) to heal the (gums/gingiva) must be used ____ a day after brushing and flossing.
Este (gel/enjuague) para sanar las encías debe utilizarse ____ veces al día después de cepillar y limpiar con hilo dental. (Audio 6.350)

This (gel/rinse) to heal the (gums/gingiva) may temporarily stain your teeth.
Este (gel/enjuague) para sanar las encías puede manchar temporalmente sus dientes. (Audio 6.351)

The dentist recommends that you take an antibiotic (before/after) scaling.
El/La dentista recomienda que tome un antibiótico (antes/después) del raspado. (Audio 6.352)

Contact the (dentist/office/clinic) if you experience any swelling of the (gums/gingiva) after scaling.
Comuníquese con (el/la) (dentista/consultorio/clínica) si experiencia alguna inflamación de (las encías/gingiva) después del raspado. (Audio 6.353)

POLISHING THE TEETH
PULIR LOS DIENTES (AUDIO 6.354)

Are your teeth sensitive to polishing?
¿Son sus dientes sensibles al pulido? (Audio 6.355)

I will be using a rubber cup and pumice to polish. Here it is.
Usaré una taza de goma y una piedra pómez para pulir. Aquí está. (Audio 6.356)

I will be using (fine/medium/coarse) paste in your mouth.
Usaré una pasta (fina/mediana/dura) en su boca. (Audio 6.357)

I will be using a prophy jet to polish.
Usaré un aeropulidor para pulir. (Audio 6.358)

The prophy jet uses powder to polish.
El aeropulidor utiliza polvo para pulir. (Audio 6.359)

Polishing removes stains and helps whiten your teeth.
El pulir elimina las manchas y ayuda a blanquear sus dientes.
(Audio 6.360)

You have (slight/moderate) staining.
Usted tiene manchas (leve/moderada). (Audio 6.3561)

You have a lot of staining on your teeth.
Usted tiene muchas manchas en los dientes. (Audio 6.362)

Stains can be caused by _____ . (See Box 6.19)
Las manchas pueden ser causadas por _____. (Vea el Cuadro
6.19) (Audio 6.363)

**While polishing, I will be rinsing your mouth using water
and suction**.
Mientras pulo, le enjuagaré la boca con agua y succión. (Audio 6.364)

Box 6.19 **Staining etiology** **(Audio 6.571)**	**Cuadro 6.19** **Etiología de las** **manchas (Audio 6.571)**
• Bacteria (Audio 6.572)	• Bacteria (Audio 6.572)
• Betel nut (Audio 6.573)	• Nuez de areca (Audio 6.573)
• Coffee (Audio 6.574)	• Café (Audio 6.574)
• Cola/soda/pop (Audio 6.575)	• Cola/Soda/refresco (Audio 6.575)
• Fluoride (stannous) (Audio 6.576)	• Fluoruro (estañoso) (Audio 6.576)
• Food (Audio 6.577)	• Alimentos (Audio 6.577)
• Medications (Audio 6.578)	• Medicamentos (Audio 6.578)
• Plaque (Audio 6.579)	• Placa bacteriana (Audio 6.579)
• Rinse (chlorhexidine) (Audio 6.580)	• Enjuague (clorohexidina) (Audio 6.580)
• Tartar (Audio 6.581)	• Sarro/calculo (Audio 6.581)
• Tea (Audio 6.582)	• Té (Audio 6.582)
• Tobacco (Audio 6.583)	• Tabaco (Audio 6.583)

Rinsing your mouth during polishing removes the (pumice/ powder).
El enjuagar su boca durante el pulido elimina (la piedra pómez/el polvo). (Audio 6.365)

Are you comfortable while I polish?
¿Está cómodo(a) mientras pulo? (Audio 6.366)

Let me know if you are uncomfortable while I polish.
Hágame saber si está incómodo(a) mientras pulo. (Audio 6.367)

Is the rinse water comfortable for you?
¿Está el agua de enjuague cómoda para usted? (Audio 6.368)

Have I rinsed your mouth enough to remove the (pumice/ powder)?
¿He enjuagado su boca lo suficiente para eliminar (la piedra pómez/el polvo)? (Audio 6.369)

I will be flossing after polishing.
Después de pulir, le limpiaré con hilo dental. (Audio 6.370)

Flossing after polishing helps remove any (pumice/powder) between your teeth.
El limpiar con hilo dental después de pulir ayuda a eliminar (la piedra pómez/el polvo) de entre sus dientes. (Audio 6.371)

I can't remove the stain(s) _____. (See Box 6.20)
No puedo eliminar la(s) mancha(s) _____. (Vea el Cuadro 6.20) (Audio 6.372)

PERIODIC MAINTENANCE
MANTENIMIENTO PERIÓDICO (AUDIO 6.373)

It may have been a long time since your last cleaning, but you are here now to get your teeth and gums healthy.
Puede que haya pasado mucho tiempo desde su última limpieza, pero ahora está aquí para recuperar la salud de sus dientes y encías. (Audio 6.374)

I will be checking to see if your gums bleed.
Le examinaré para ver si le sangran las encías. (Audio 6.375)

Box 6.20
Types of stains that polishing cannot remove (Audio 6.584)

- On the top of your teeth (Audio 6.585)
- On the gum line (Audio 6.586)
- Between crowded teeth (Audio 6.587)
- From your tooth-colored fillings (Audio 6.588)

- From medication (Audio 6.589)
- From internal injury to the tooth (Audio 6.590)

Cuadro 6.20
Tipos de manchas que el pulido no puede eliminar (Audio 6.584)

- En la parte superior del diente (Audio 6.585)
- En el borde de las encías (Audio 6.586)
- Entre dientes apiñados (Audio 6.587)
- De sus (empastaduras/ empastes/rellenos/calzas) del color del diente (Audio 6.588)
- De medicamentos (Audio 6.589)
- De lesiones internas del diente (Audio 6.590)

Bleeding means that your gum disease is still active.
El sangrado indica que su enfermedad de las encías sigue activa.
(Audio 6.376)

I will be probing around your teeth to see if your pockets are deeper.
Sondearé alrededor de sus dientes para ver si sus bolsillos son más profundos. (Audio 6.377)

I will be measuring your gums to determine their health.
Estaré midiendo sus encías para determinar su salud. (Audio 6.378)

I will be recording the pocket measurements.
Registraré las medidas de los bolsillos. (Audio 6.379)

Deeper (pockets/probe readings) mean that more bone has been destroyed around your teeth.
Mientras más profundos(as) sean (los bolsillos/las medidas de la sonda) más hueso se ha destruido alrededor del diente.
(Audio 6.380)

I will probe your teeth every _____ months to check for bone loss.
Sondearé sus dientes cada _____ meses para evaluar su pérdida de hueso. (Audio 6.381)

I will be comparing your radiographs to see if more bone has been lost.
Compararé sus radiografías para ver si se ha perdido más hueso. (Audio 6.382)

We will need to space over _____ appointments the deep cleaning of your teeth.
Necesitaremos separar la limpieza profunda de sus dientes en _____ citas. (Audio 6.383)

You need to come in for your (cleanings/scalings) more often.
Usted necesita venir más seguido para sus (limpiezas/raspados). (Audio 6.384)

You will need to come in for a cleaning every _____ months.
Usted necesitará venir para una limpieza cada _____ meses. (Audio 6.385)

FLUORIDE TREATMENT
TRATAMIENTO DE FLUORURO (AUDIO 6.386)

I will be giving you a fluoride treatment.
Le daré un tratamiento de fluoruro. (Audio 6.387)

Fluoride will be applied to your teeth using a _____. (See Box 6.21)
El fluoruro será aplicado a sus dientes mediante un(a) _____. (Vea el Cuadro 6.21) (Audio 6.388)

What flavor of fluoride would you like? (See Box 6.22)
¿Qué sabor de fluoruro desea? (Vea el Cuadro 6.22) (Audio 6.389)

I have several flavors of fluoride that you may choose from. (See Box 6.22).
Tengo varios sabores de fluoruro entre los cuales puede elegir. (Vea el Cuadro 6.22). (Audio 6.390)

Box 6.21
Types of fluoride treatments
(Audio 6.591)

- Foam in a tray (Audio 6.592)

- Gel in a tray (Audio 6.593)

- Rinse (Audio 6.594)
- Varnish (Audio 6.595)

Cuadro 6.21
Tipos de tratamientos de fluoruro
(Audio 6.591)

- Espuma en una bandeja (Audio 6.592)
- Gel en una bandeja (Audio 6.593)
- Enjuague (Audio 6.594)
- Barniz (Audio 6.595)

Box 6.22
Fluoride flavors
(Audio 6.596)

- Bubble gum (Audio 6.597)
- Cherry (Audio 6.598)
- Chocolate (Audio 6.599)
- Grape (Audio 6.600)
- Mint (Audio 6.5601)
- Orange (Audio 6.602)
- Raspberry (Audio 6.603)
- Strawberry (Audio 6.604)
- Vanilla (Audio 6.605)

Cuadro 6.22
Sabores de fluoruro
(Audio 6.596)

- Chicle (Audio 6.597)
- Cereza (Audio 6.598)
- Chocolate (Audio 6.599)
- Uva (Audio 6.600)
- Menta (Audio 6.601)
- Naranja (Audio 6.602)
- Frambuesa (Audio 6.603)
- Fresa (Audio 6.604)
- Vainilla (Audio 6.605)

The fluoride treatment takes ____ minutes.
El tratamiento de fluoruro toma ____ minutos. (Audio 6.391)

During the treatment be careful to suction and not to swallow the fluoride.
Durante el tratamiento succione, pero no se trague el fluoruro.
(Audio 6.392)

Let's check the fit of this fluoride tray.
Veamos cómo le queda esta bandeja de fluoruro. (Audio 6.393)

Does the fluoride tray fit comfortably?
¿La bandeja de fluoruro le cabe cómodamente? (Audio 6.394)

Breathe through your nose during the fluoride treatment.
Respire por la nariz durante el tratamiento de fluoruro. (Audio 6.395)

Rinse with the fluoride in this cup but do not swallow it; just (spit/suction) it out.
Enjuáguese con el fluoruro en esta taza pero no se lo trague; sólo (escúpalo/succiónelo). (Audio 6.396)

Are you comfortable with the fluoride?
¿Está cómodo(a) con el fluoruro? (Audio 6.397)

Let me know if you are uncomfortable while I give you the fluoride.
Hágame saber si está incómodo(a) mientras le doy el fluoruro. (Audio 6.398)

Have you swallowed the fluoride?
¿Se tragó el fluoruro? (Audio 6.399)

Let me know if the fluoride makes you feel sick.
Hágame saber si el fluoruro le hace sentir enfermo(a). (Audio 6.400)

Do you feel (like vomiting/uncomfortable)?
¿Usted se siente (con ganas de vomitar/incómodo(a))? (Audio 6.401)

After the fluoride treatment you must wait ____ minutes before rinsing or eating.
Después del tratamiento de fluoruro, debe esperar ____ minutos antes de enjuagarse o comer. (Audio 6.402)

You can eat and drink after the application of fluoride varnish.
Usted puede comer y beber después de la aplicación del barniz de (flúor/fluoruro). (Audio 6.403)

Avoid eating anything hard, crunchy, or hot for the next _____ minutes/hours).
Evite comer cualquier cosa dura, crujiente, o caliente durante los próximos _____ (minutos/horas). (Audio 6.404)

The fluoride varnish leaves a temporary yellow coat on the teeth, which will remain until you brush it off later.
El barniz del fluoruro deja una capa amarilla temporal en los dientes, la que permanecerá en su lugar hasta que usted la cepille. (Audio 6.405)

Leave the fluoride varnish on until you brush.
Deje el barniz del fluoruro hasta que se cepille. (Audio 6.406)

DESENSITIZATION
DESENSIBILIZACIÓN (AUDIO 6.407)

I will be applying (gel/rinse/varnish) to reduce tooth sensitivity.
Le aplicaré un (gel/enjuague/barniz) para reducir la sensibilidad del diente. (Audio 6.408)

You may feel some slight sensitivity while I apply the desensitizer.
Usted puede sentir una cierta sensibilidad mientras le aplico el desensibilizador. (Audio 6.409)

The desensitizer will coat the exposed nerve ends on the root.
El desensibilizador cubrirá los extremos expuestos del nervio en la raíz. (Audio 6.410)

We recommend a (gel/rinse/toothpaste) to reduce tooth sensitivity.
Le recomendamos (un gel/un enjuague/una pasta dental) para reducir la sensibilidad del diente. (Audio 6.411)

This (gel/rinse/toothpaste) to reduce tooth sensitivity may temporarily stain the teeth.
(Este gel/Este enjuague/Esta pasta dental) para reducir la sensibilidad del diente puede manchar temporalmente los dientes. (Audio 6.412)

POSTAPPOINTMENT DISCUSSION
DISCUSIÓN DESPUÉS DE LA CITA (AUDIO 6.413)

I am finished with your (cleaning/scaling).
Ya terminé su (limpieza/raspado). (Audio 6.414)

The dentist will now examine your teeth.
El/La dentista/odontolgo(a) ahora le examinará los dientes. (Audio 6.415)

I will need to see you again in order to finish the scaling.
Necesitaré verle otra vez para terminar el raspado. (Audio 6.416)

Let's make your next (cleaning/scaling) appointment.
Vamos hacer su siguiente cita para (limpieza/raspado). (Audio 6.417)

Let's make your (recare/recall) appointment.
Vamos hacer su cita de mantenimiento. (Audio 6.418)

Chapter 7
Operative Dentistry

Capítulo 7
Odontología Operativa (Audio 7.1)

(Figure 7.1)

Tell me if you feel this. (Audio 7.2)
Dígame si siente esto. (Audio 7.2)

This is the handpiece I will use to remove the decay.
Este es (el aparato manual/la pieza de mano) que usaré para eliminar las caries. (Audio 7.3)

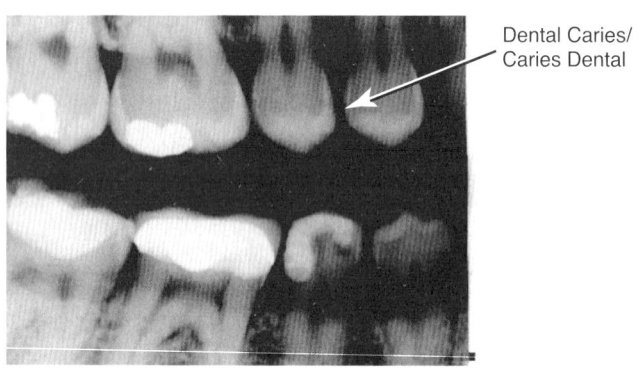

Dental Caries/
Caries Dental

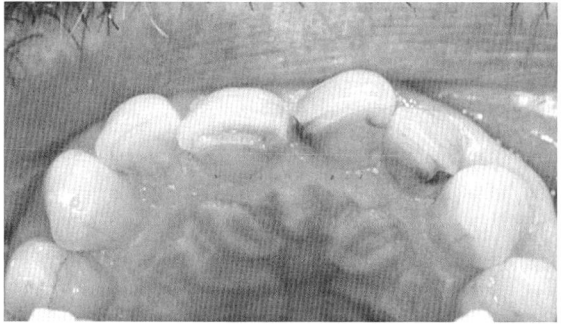

Fig. 7.1 Dental caries. Caries dental. *Courtesy Dr. Mohsen Taleghani.*

The handpiece makes a whistling sound.
El aparato manual hace un sonido que silba./ La pieza de mano
emite un silbido. (Audio 7.4)

The handpiece makes noise, but it will be comfortable.
El/la (aparato manual/pieza de mano) hace ruido, pero será cómodo.
(Audio 7.5)

The handpiece may vibrate your tooth.
El/la (aparato manual/ pieza de mano) puede hacer vibrar su diente.
(Audio 7.6)

**When I use the handpiece, it will spray water, which will
wash and cool the tooth**.
Cuando use el/la (aparato manual/pieza de mano), rociará agua, la
cual lavará y refrescará el diente. (Audio 7.7)

Please open wide.
Abra grande, por favor. (Audio 7.8)

Turn to your left.
Volte a su izquierda. (Audio 7.9)

Turn to your right.
Volte a su derecha. (Audio 7.10)

Let us know if this bothers you.
Háganos saber si esto le molesta. (Audio 7.11)

**If you need to (take a break/rest a moment), please raise
your (right/left) hand**.
Si necesita (tomar un descanso/descansar por un momento), por
favor levante la mano (derecha/izquierda). (Audio 7.12)

**We have removed all the decay, and we will now place the
filling**.
Hemos eliminado toda las caries y ahora colocaremos el (empaste/
relleno/calza). (Audio 7.13)

Grind your teeth on this (device/paper).
Rechine los dientes sobre este (aparato/papel). (Audio 7.14)

Bite (down/hard) on this device.
Muerda duro sobre este aparato. (Audio 7.15)

Slide your teeth (back and forward/left to right).
Deslice los dientes (hacia atrás y adelante/de izquierda a derecha).
(Audio 7.16)

Now slightly close your mouth.
Ahora, cierre ligeramente la boca. (Audio 7.17)

We are going to take an impression of your mouth.
Vamos a tomar una impresión de su boca. (Audio 7.18)

**We will place some (soft/pudding like) material in this tray,
and then we will place the tray in your mouth**.
Colocaremos algo de material (suave) en esta bandeja y entonces
colocaremos la bandeja en su boca. (Audio 7.19)

Open wide so I can place the tray in your mouth.
Abra grande para poder colocar la bandeja en su boca. (Audio 7.2)

Now bend your head forward.
Ahora inclina la cabeza hacia adelante. (Audio 7.21)

Open wide so I can remove the tray.
Abra grande para que yo pueda remover la bandeja. (Audio 7.22)

SPECIFIC RESTORATION: AMALGAM
RESTAURACIÓN ESPECÍFICA: AMALGAMA
(AUDIO 7.23)

The tooth will have an amalgam filling.
El diente tendrá una empaste/relleno de amalgama. (Audio 7.24)

Amalgam is a very safe filling material.
La amalgama es un material de empaste/relleno muy seguro.
(Audio 7.25)

**You must keep your mouth open while I put the amalgam
into your tooth**.
Usted debe mantener la boca abierta mientras le pongo la amalgama
en el diente. (Audio 7.26)

**We will scrape off a little bit of the filling to make it fit your
bite**.
Rasparemos un poco del relleno/empaste para que se ajuste a su
mordida. (Audio 7.27)

We will check your bite.
Examinaremos su mordida. (Audio 7.28)

Gently bite down on this marking paper.
Muerda suavemente sobre este papel para marcar. (Audio 7.29)

When you close your mouth, does it feel as though your teeth are coming together normally?
¿Cuándo cierra la boca, siente que sus dientes se juntan normalmente? (Audio 7.30)

When you gently bring your teeth together, does the filling feel high?
¿ Cuando junta los dientes suavemente, ¿se siente el/la (empaste/relleno/calza) alto/a? (Audio 7.31)

Do not chew on that side of your mouth for the next few hours.
No mastique por ese lado de la boca por las próximas horas. (Audio 7.32)

The filling material needs to set completely.
El material de (relleno/empaste) necesita fijarse totalmente. (Audio 7.33)

It takes a few hours for the filling to harden.
El relleno/empaste tarda unas horas en endurecerse. (Audio 7.34)

Do not bite down hard until the numbness in your mouth wears off.
No muerda fuerte hasta que desaparezca el entumecimiento en su boca. (Audio 7.35)

All ready to go!
¡Todo listo! (Audio 7.36)

SPECIFIC RESTORATION: COMPOSITE
RESTAURACIÓN ESPECÍFICA: COMPUESTO (AUDIO 7.37)

This tooth will have a (white/tooth-colored) filling, called a composite.
Este diente tendrá un empaste/relleno (blanco/del color del diente), llamado resina compuesta o composite. (Audio 7.38)

Keep your mouth open while I put the composite into your tooth.
Mantenga la boca abierta mientras coloco (la resina compuesta/el composite) en el diente. (Audio 7.39)

This light will (set/harden) the filling material.
Esta luz (fijará/endurecerá) el material de relleno/empaste. (Audio 7.40)

With the handpiece we will trim the composite to fit your bite.
Con (el aparato manual/la pieza de mano) rebajaremos (el composite/la resina) para ajustarlo a su mordida. (Audio 7.41)

Gently bite down on this marking paper.
Muerda suavemente en este papel para marcar. (Audio 7.42)

When you bring your teeth together, does the filling feel high?
Cuando junta los dientes, ¿se siente el (empaste/relleno) alto? (Audio 7.43)

We will now polish the filling.
Ahora puliremos el (empaste/relleno). (Audio 7.44)

The filling is completely set.
El (empaste/relleno) está listo. (Audio 7.45)

All ready to go!
¡Todo listo! (Audio 7.46)

Chapter 8
Cosmetic Dentistry

Capítulo 8
Odontología Cosmética (Audio 8.1)

We can place a _____ on that tooth to _____. (See Boxes 8.1 and 8.2)
Podemos colocar un(a) _____ en ese diente para _____. (Vea los Cuadros 8.1 y 8.2) (Audio 8.2)

Box 8.1
Types of cosmetic restorations (Audio 8.57)

- Filling (Audio 8.58)

- Veneer (Audio 8.59)

- Crown (Audio 8.60)
- Bridge (Audio 8.61)

Cuadro 8.1
Tipos de restauraciones cosméticas (Audio 8.57)

- Empaste/relleno/calza (Audio 8.58)
- Revestimiento/carilla (Audio 8.59)
- Corona (Audio 8.60)
- Puente (Audio 8.61)

Box 8.2
Results of cosmetic restoration (Audio 8.62)

- Make it look better (Audio 8.63)
- Make it look normal (Audio 8.64)
- Change the shape (Audio 8.65)
- Change the color (Audio 8.66)
- Close the gap (Audio 8.67)
- Fix the broken tooth (Audio 8.68)

Cuadro 8.2
Resultados de la restauración cosmética (Audio 8.62)

- Que (luzca/se vea) mejor/ (Audio 8.63)
- Que (luzca/se vea) normal(Audio 8.64)
- Cambiar la forma (Audio 8.65)
- Cambiar el color (Audio 8.66)
- Cerrar el espacio (Audio 8.67)
- Arreglar el diente roto/ quebrado (Audio 8.68)

A filling can be (shaped/tinted) to match your other teeth.
Un (empaste/relleno/calza) se puede (formar/teñir) para que sea igual a sus otros dientes. (Audio 8.3)

A veneer is a thin layer of (material/porcelain/resin) that will be (bonded/cemented) to your tooth.
(Una carilla/un revestimiento) es una capa fina de (material/porcelana/resina) que se (adherirá/cementará) a su diente. (Audio 8.4)

A crown is a (protective covering/cap) that will fit over your tooth.
Una corona es un revestimiento protector que encajará sobre su diente. (Audio 8.5)

In this next section, *crown* can be interchanged with *bridge*.
En la siguiente sección la palabra *corona* se puede intercambiar con *puente*. (Audio 8.6)

The crown can be completed today.
Le podemos hacer la corona hoy. (Audio 8.7)

We will need _____ appointments to make this crown.
Necesitaremos _____ citas para hacer esta corona. (Audio 8.8)

In order to place a crown we will need to remove a little of your tooth on all sides.
Para colocar una corona necesitaremos quitar un poco de su diente en todos los lados. (Audio 8.9)

Then we will need to take an impression of your tooth.
Luego, necesitaremos tomar una impresión de su diente.
(Audio 8.10)

We will now take the impression.
Ahora tomaremos la impresión. (Audio 8.11)

You will have a temporary crown on your tooth until the permanent crown is made. (See Figure 8.1)
Usted tendrá una corona temporal en el diente hasta que se le haga la corona permanente. (Vea la Imagen 8.1) (Audio 8.12)

Now we will remove the temporary crown in order to fit the permanent crown.
Ahora quitaremos la corona temporal para encajar la corona permanente. (Audio 8.13)

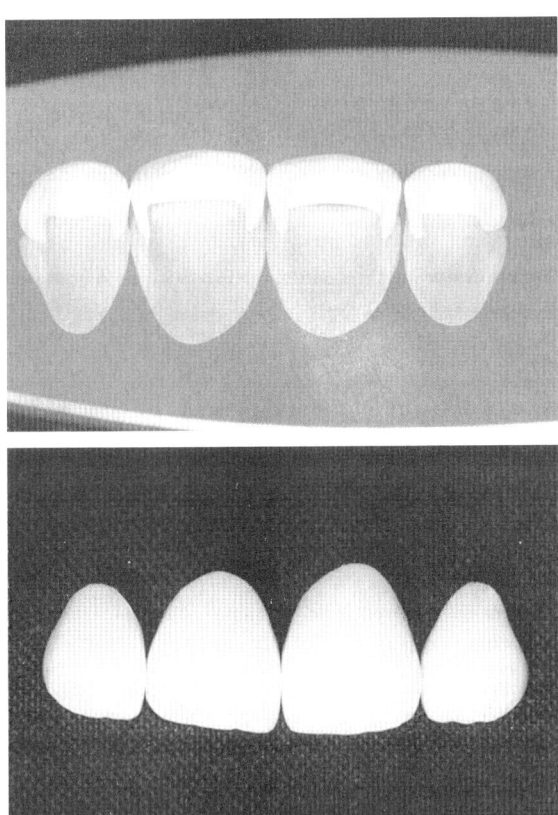

Fig. 8.1 Porcelain veneers. Carillas de porcelana. *Courtesy Dr. Mohsen Taleghani.*

When you bring your teeth together, does the crown feel high?
Cuando junta los dientes, ¿la corona se siente alta? (Audio 8.14)

Now we will cement your crown onto your tooth.
Ahora cementaremos la corona sobre el diente. (Audio 8.15)

A crown is cemented permanently onto your tooth.
La corona se cementa permanentemente sobre el diente. (Audio 8.16)

We need to match the color for the crown.
Necesitamos hacer coincidir el color de la corona. (Audio 8.17)

Do you agree with this (shade/color)?
¿Está de acuerdo con este (tono/color)? (Audio 8.18)

A bridge can replace one or more missing teeth.
Un puente puede reemplazar uno o más dientes faltantes.
(Audio 8.19)

A bridge will connect to the teeth on both sides of the space left by a missing tooth.
Un puente se conectará a los dientes de ambos lados del espacio causado por un diente que falta. (Audio 8.20)

Gently bite down on this marking paper.
Muerda suavemente sobre este papel para marcar. (Audio 8.21)

TOOTH WHITENING (BLEACHING)
BLANQUEAMIENTO DENTAL (AUDIO 8.22)

Do you like the way your teeth look?
Le gusta cómo (lucen/se ven) sus dientes? (Audio 8.23)

Are you satisfied with the way your teeth look?
¿Está satisfecho(a) con la manera en que se ven sus dientes?
(Audio 8.24)

Would you like to (whiten/bleach) your teeth?
¿Le gustaría blanquear sus dientes? (Audio 8.25)

Bleaching (will/will not) remove the stains on your teeth.
El blanquear (le va/no le va) a eliminar las manchas de los dientes.
(Audio 8.26)

We recommend an (in-office/at-home) bleach procedure.
Le recomendamos un procedimiento para blanquear (de oficina/para usar en casa). (Audio 8.27)

We can bleach most external stains.
Podemos blanquear la mayoría de las manchas externas. (Audio 8.28)

Stains from medication are the most difficult to bleach.
Las manchas causadas por medicamentos son las más difíciles de blanquear. (Audio 8.29)

BLEACHING IN-OFFICE
BLANQUEAMIENTO EN LA OFICINA (AUDIO 8.30)

An in-office or chairside bleaching will take from 30 minutes to one hour to complete.
Un blanqueamiento en el consultorio tomará entre 30 minutos a una hora para completarse. (Audio 8.31)

We will place a protective coating over your gum tissues.
Colocaremos una capa protectora sobre los tejidos de sus encías. (Audio 8.32)

We will apply the bleaching agent to your teeth.
Aplicaremos el agente blanqueador a sus dientes. (Audio 8.33)

We will use a special light to activate the bleach while it is on your teeth.
Utilizaremos una luz especial para activar el blanqueador mientras está en sus dientes. (Audio 8.34)

BLEACHING AT HOME
BLANQUEAMIENTO CASERO (AUDIO 8.35)

Trays
Bandejas (Audio 8.36)

We will take impressions of your teeth and construct a custom-fitted tray to hold the bleach against your teeth.
Tomaremos impresiones de sus dientes y construiremos una bandeja a su medida para sostener el blanqueador contra sus dientes. (Audio 8.37)

You will take home the bleach material and trays in order to apply the whitening product to your teeth.
Usted se llevará a su casa el material para blanquear y las bandejas para aplicar el producto para blanquear sus dientes. (Audio 8.38)

Fill the tray with bleach this way.
Llene la bandeja con el blanqueador de esta manera. (Audio 8.39)

Wear the tray for _____ minutes a day, for _____ (days/weeks).
Use la bandeja por _____ minutos al día, por _____ (dias/semanas). (Audio 8.40)

Strips
Tiras (Audio 8.41)

Use these bleaching strips as instructed on the box.
Use estas tiras blanqueadoras según lo indicado en la caja.
(Audio 8.42)

They should be applied twice a day for _____ minutes until the supply is gone.
Debe aplicarse dos veces al día durante __ minutos hasta que se
acabe el producto. (Audio 8.43)

Do not eat, drink, or sleep while wearing the strip.
No coma, beba, o duerma mientras usa la tira. (Audio 8.44)

BLEACHING SIDE EFFECTS
EFECTOS SECUNDARIOS DEL BLANQUEAR
(AUDIO 8.45)

If you have any bothersome side effects, call the office to make an appointment.
Si usted tiene algún efecto secundario que le moleste, llame la
oficina para hacer una cita. (Audio 8.46)

Your gum tissue may become irritated.
El tejido de las encías puede irritarse. (Audio 8.47)

Gum irritation is temporary.
La irritación de las encías es is temporal. (Audio 8.48)

The tray may need to be trimmed down.
Puede ser necesario recortar la bandeja. (Audio 8.49)

You may need to put less bleaching gel into the tray.
Puede que necesite colocar menos gel blanqueador en la bandeja.
(Audio 8.50)

Your teeth may become sensitive.
Sus dientes pueden volverse sensibles. (Audio 8.51)

Sensitivity of the teeth is temporary.
La sensibilidad de los dientes es temporal. (Audio 8.52)

Stop bleaching for a day or two until the sensitivity subsides.
Pare de blanquear por un día o dos hasta que la sensibilidad se calme. (Audio 8.53)

Use a desensitizing toothpaste, such as this one.
Utilice una (pasta de dientes/pasta dental/crema dental) para desensibilizar como ésta. (Audio 8.54)

Bleaching will not (damage/weaken) your teeth.
El blanquear no (dañará/debilitará) sus dientes. (Audio 8.55)

Bleaching effects will last at least _____ months.
El efecto del blanqueador durará al menos ____meses. (Audio 8.56)

Chapter 9
Prosthodontics

Capítulo 9
Prostodoncia (Audio 9.1)

PROSTHODONTIC EXAMINATION
EXAMEN PROSTÉTICO (AUDIO 9.2)

Are you happy with your _____ denture? (See Box 9.1)
¿Está feliz con su dentadura _____? (Vea el Cuadro 9.1) (Audio 9.3)

Do you like your denture's appearance?
¿Le gusta la apariencia de su dentadura? (Audio 9.4)

How long have you had your denture?
¿Hace cuánto tiempo tiene su dentadura? (Audio 9.5)

Do you wear your denture every day?
¿Usa su dentadura todos los días? (Audio 9.6)

Do you remove your denture to let the tissue rest while you sleep?
¿Se quita la dentadura para que repose el tejido mientras duerme? (Audio 9.7)

Does your denture fit properly?
¿Le queda bien su dentadura? (Audio 9.8)

I will be checking the fit of your denture.
Examinaré cómo le queda su dentadura. (Audio 9.9)

Box 9.1 Types of removable dentures (Audio 9.227)	Cuadro 9.1 Tipos de dentaduras removibles (Audio 9.227)
• Full (Audio 9.228)	• Completa (Audio 9.228)
• Lower (Audio 9.229)	• Inferior (Audio 9.229)
• Partial (Audio 9.230)	• Parcial (Audio 9.230)
• Over (Audio 9.231)	• Sobre (Audio 9.231)
• Upper (Audio 9.232)	• Superior (Audio 9.232)

We will be using a white paste to check the fit of your denture.
Usaremos una pasta blanca para evaluar cómo le queda su dentadura. (Audio 9.10)

Take out your denture so I can examine it.
Quítese la dentadura para poder examinarla. (Audio 9.11)

Put in your denture so I can check its fit.
Póngase la dentadura para poder examinar cómo le queda. (Audio 9.12)

Can you (chew/eat/smile/talk) with your denture?
¿Puede (morder/comer/sonreír/hablar) con su dentadura? (Audio 9.13)

Repeat these words: six hundred, zero, Saturday.
Repita estas palabras: seiscientos, cero, sábado. (Audio 9.14)

Have you had your denture (relined/repaired)?
¿Le han (revestido/reparado) la dentadura? (Audio 9.15)

Does your denture seem loose?
¿Siente floja la dentadura? (Audio 9.16)

Do you use adhesive to hold your denture?
¿Usa pegamento para sostener su dentadura? (Audio 9.17)

Do you have any (sores/ulcers) with your denture?
¿Tiene (algún dolor/alguna úlcera) a causa de su dentadura? (Audio 9.18)

We will refer you to a prosthodontist for _____. (See Box 9.2)
Lo(a) referiremos a un(a) prostodoncista para _____. (Vea el Cuadro 9.2) (Audio 9.19)

CROWNS
CORONAS (AUDIO 9.20)

A crown is a(n) _____ covering cemented onto your tooth. (See Box 9.3 and Figure 9.1, A–C)
Una corona es una cobertura _____ cementada a su diente. (Vea el Cuadro 9.3 y la Imagen 9.1, A-C) (Audio 9.21)

**Box 9.2
Reasons to refer
a patient to a
prosthodontist
(Audio 9.233)**

- A second opinion
  (Audio 9.234)
- An evaluation (Audio 9.235)
- Treatment (Audio 9.236)

**Cuadro 9.2
Razones para referir
a un(a) paciente a
un(a) prostodoncista
(Audio 9.233)**

- Una segunda opinión
  (Audio 9.234)
- Una evaluación (Audio 9.235)
- Tratamiento (Audio 9.236)

**Box 9.3
Types of crowns and
bridges (Audio 9.237)**

- All-ceramic (Audio 9.238)
- All-metal (Audio 9.239)
- Ceramic-over-metal
  (Audio 9.240)

**Cuadro 9.3
Tipos de coronas y de
puentes (Audio 9.237)**

- De cerámica (Audio 9.238)
- De metal (Audio 9.239)
- De cerámica sobre metal
  (Audio 9.240)

A crown should be placed on this tooth to _____. (See Box 9. 4)
A este diente se le debe colocar una corona para _____. (Vea el
Cuadro 9.4) (Audio 9.22)

**A crown should be placed on a tooth that has been
weakened by decay or fracture.**
Se debe colocar una corona en un diente que ha sido debilitado por
caries o fractura. (Audio 9.23)

A root-canal tooth needs a crown for strength.
Un diente con un (tratamiento de conducto/endodoncia) necesita
una corona para fortalecerse. (Audio 9.24)

**This root-canal tooth will need a post and core before a
crown can be put in place. (See Figures 9.2 and 9.3)**
Este diente con (tratamiento de conducto/endodoncia) necesitará
un poste y una base antes de que podamos colocar la corona. (Vea
las Imagen 9.2 y 9.3) (Audio 9.25)

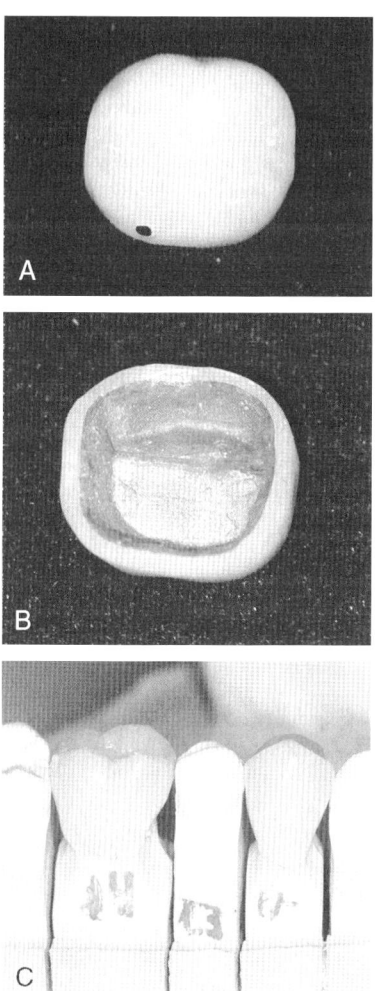

Fig. 9.1 A, Porcelain crown (view of the top). Corona de porcelana (vista superior). B, View of the inside of a porcelain crown. Vista del interior de una corona de porcelana. C, Porcelain crown in place. Corona de porcelana colocada. *(Courtesy Dr. Mohsen Taleghani.)*

Box 9.4
Reasons to place a crown (Audio 9.241)

- Fix the crack in the enamel (Audio 9.242)
- Improve the appearance of the tooth (Audio 9.243)
- Replace the fractured tooth (Audio 9.244)
- Replace the large filling (Audio 9.245)

- Restore the function of the tooth (Audio 9.246)

Cuadro 9.4
Razones para colocar una corona (Audio 9.241)

- Arreglar la grieta en el esmalte (Audio 9.242)
- Mejorar la apariencia del diente (Audio 9.243)
- Sustituir el diente fracturado (Audio 9.244)
- Reemplazar un/a (calza/ empastadura/empaste/ relleno) grande (Audio 9.245)
- Restaurar la función del diente (Audio 9.246)

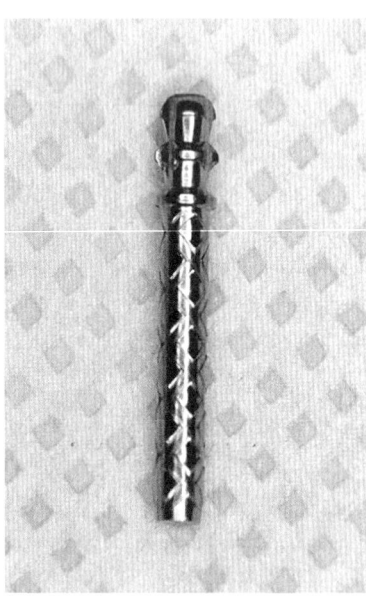

Fig. 9.2 Dental post. Poste dental. *(Courtesy Dr. Mohsen Taleghani.)*

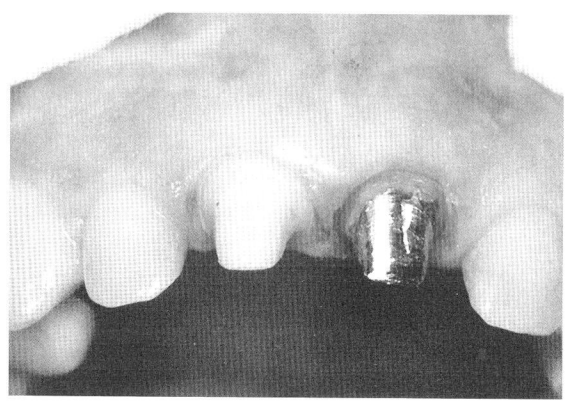

Fig. 9.3 Dental post and core. Poste y núcleo dental.
(Courtesy Dr. Mohsen Taleghani.)

We will place a prefabricated post into the tooth.
Pondremos un poste prefabricado en el diente. (Audio 9.26)

This tooth needs a core to replace missing tooth structure.
Este diente necesita una base para sustituir la estructura que le falta.
(Audio 9.27)

We will fortify this tooth with a core.
Vamos a fortalecer este diente con una base. (Audio 9.28)

A core replaces missing coronal tooth surface.
Una base reemplaza lo que falta de la superficie coronal del diente.
(Audio 9.29)

An impression will be taken to make a cast for the post and core.
Se tomará una impresión para hacer un molde para el poste y la
base. (Audio 9.30)

The lab will make the post and core and return them to the office.
El laboratorio hará el poste y la base y los devolverá a la oficina.
(Audio 9.31)

Box 9.5
Types of restorations
(Audio 9.247)

- Inlay/incrustación
  (Audio 9.248)
- Onlay
  (Audio 9.249)
- Partial veneer
  (Audio 9.250)
- Veneer
  (Audio 9.251)

Cuadro 9.5
Tipos de restauraciones
(Audio 9.247)

- Inlay/ incrustación
  (Audio 9.248)
- Onlay/ recubrimiento
  (Audio 9.249)
- Revestimiento/carilla parcial
  (Audio 9.250)
- Revestimiento/carilla
  (Audio 9.251)

You will need an appointment in ___ days to have the post and core placed.
Usted necesitará una cita en ___ días para reemplazar el poste y la base. (Audio 9.32)

I will take an impression after the post and core have been placed.
Tomaré una impresión después de que se hayan puesto el poste y la base. (Audio 9.33)

A crown will improve the (strength/function/appearance) of this tooth.
Una corona mejorará la (fuerza/función/apariencia) de este diente. (Audio 9.34)

This tooth can be restored with a(n) _____. (See Box 9.5)
Se puede restaurar este diente con un _____. (Vea el Cuadro 9.5) (Audio 9.35)

A veneer is a thin layer of porcelain bonded to the tooth.
Una carilla es una capa fina de porcelana pegada al diente. (Audio 9.36)

A veneer can _____ of a tooth. (See Box 9.6)
Una carilla puede _____ de un diente. (Vea el Cuadro 9.6) (Audio 9.37)

A partial veneer will leave uncovered some of the tooth surface.
Una carilla parcial dejará descubierta parte de la superficie del diente. (Audio 9.38)

Box 9.6
Improvements that
a veneer can make
(Audio 9.252)

- Correct the color
  (Audio 9.253)
- Correct the fractured part
  (Audio 9.254)
- Correct the shape
  (Audio 9.255)
- Restore the appearance
  (Audio 9.256)

Cuadro 9.6
Mejoramientos posibles
con una carilla
(Audio 9.252)

- Corregir el color
  (Audio 9.253)
- Corregir la parte fracturada
  (Audio 9.254)
- Corregir la forma
  (Audio 9.255)
- Restaurar la apariencia
  (Audio 9.256)

An inlay will be placed into the crown portion of the tooth.
Se pondrá una (incrustación/inlay) dentro de la corona del diente.
(Audio 9.39)

An onlay covers the biting surface of the tooth.
Un (recubrimiento/onlay) cubre la superficie del diente que se usa
para morder. (Audio 9.40)

BRIDGE (FIXED PARTIAL DENTURE)
PUENTE (DENTADURA PARCIAL FIJA) (AUDIO 9.41)

A bridge can replace (a missing tooth/missing teeth).
(See Figure 9.4)
Un puente puede reemplazar (un diente que falta/dientes que faltan).
(Vea la Imagen 9.4) (Audio 9.42)

A bridge is cemented to the teeth on each side of the
missing (tooth/teeth).
Un puente se cementa a los dientes a cada lado (del diente/de los
dientes) perdido(s). (Audio 9.43)

A bridge is permanently attached to the teeth.
Un puente se fija permanentemente a los dientes. (Audio 9.44)

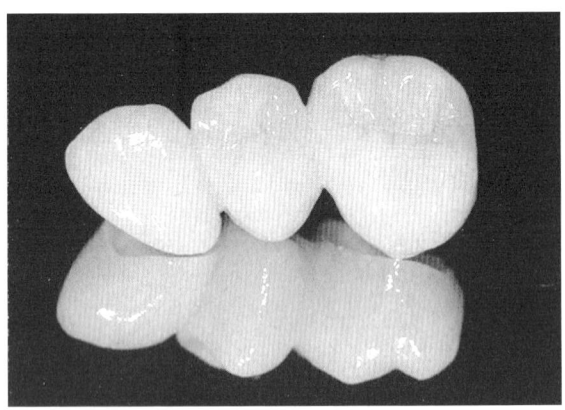

Fig. 9.4 Porcelain bridge. Puente de porcelana.
(Courtesy Dr. Mohsen Taleghani.)

A bridge cannot be removed once it has been cemented into place.
Un puente no puede quitarse una vez que ha sido cementado. (Audio 9.45)

The bridge will be _____. (See Box 9.3)
El puente será _____. (Vea el Cuadro 9.3) (Audio 9.46)

An all-ceramic bridge will look (the best/most natural).
Un puente completo en cerámica se verá (mejor/más natural). (Audio 9.47)

A bridge will feel natural when you bite down.
Un puente se sentirá natural cuando usted muerda. (Audio 9.48)

A bridge can be attached to implants.
Un puente se puede unir a implantes. (Audio 9.49)

You must use floss daily to clean under the bridge.
Debes usar hilo dental diariamente para limpiar debajo del puente. (Audio 9.50)

We will show you how to use the floss under your bridge.
Le enseñaremos a utilizar el hilo dental debajo de su puente. (Audio 9.51)

PREPARATION APPOINTMENT FOR CROWNS/BRIDGES
CITA PARA LA PREPARACIÓN DE CORONAS/ PUENTES (AUDIO 9.52)

(The term *crown* can be interchanged with *bridge* in the next two sections).
(El término corona se puede intercambiar con puente en las dos secciones siguientes). (Audio 9.53)

To make this crown I need to prepare the tooth and take an impression.
Para hacer esta corona necesito preparar el diente y tomar una impresión. (Audio 9.54)

The impression will be sent to a lab, where the crown will be fabricated.
La impresión será enviada a un laboratorio, donde se fabricará la corona. (Audio 9.55)

You will need another appointment in _____ (days/weeks).
Usted necesitará otra cita dentro de _____ (días/semanas). (Audio 9.56)

You will wear a temporary crown over this tooth until the lab returns the finished product.
Usted usará una corona temporal sobre este diente hasta que el laboratorio nos envíe el producto terminado. (Audio 9.57)

We will (anesthetize/numb) the area.
Le vamos a (anestesiar/adormecer) el área. (Audio 9.58)

We will prepare the tooth for the crown by removing a portion of the tooth on all sides.
Prepararemos el diente para la corona quitando una porción del diente en todos los lados. (Audio 9.59)

We will try this impression tray.
Le probaremos esta bandeja para impresión. (Audio 9.60)

Is this tray comfortable?
Esta comoda la bandeja. (Audio 9.61)

We will place this cord around the tooth to get a good impression of the margins.
Colocaremos esta (cuerda/cordon) alrededor del diente para conseguir una buena impresión de los márgenes. (Audio 9.62)

We will now take an impression of the prepared tooth.
Ahora tomaremos una impresión del diente preparado. (Audio 9.63)

The impression must stay in your mouth for ____ minutes.
La impresión debe permanecer en su boca por ____ minutos. (Audio 9.64)

Then we will take an impression of your bite.
Luego, tomaremos una impresión de su mordida. (Audio 9.65)

Keep your mouth (open/closed).
Mantenga la boca (abierta/cerrada). (Audio 9.66)

Bite down (on your back teeth).
Muerda (con los dientes traseros). (Audio 9.67)

We need to match the color of the crown with your teeth.
Necesitamos hacer coincidir el color de la corona con sus dientes. (Audio 9.68)

We will now make a temporary crown for you to wear until the lab returns the finished product.
Ahora haremos una corona temporal para que use hasta que el laboratorio nos devuelva el producto terminado. (Audio 9.69)

You will have a temporary crown on your tooth until the permanent crown is made.
Usted tendrá una corona temporal en su diente hasta que se haga la corona permanente. (Audio 9.70)

Do not eat anything hard or sticky with this temporary crown.
No coma nada duro o pegajoso con esta corona temporal. (Audio 9.71)

Chew on the opposite side of your mouth until we seat the final crown.
Mastique con el lado opuesto de la boca hasta que le coloquemos la corona final. (Audio 9.72)

If the temporary crown comes off, call our office right away.
Si la corona temporal se cae, llame nuestra oficina inmediato. (Audio 9.73)

SEATING APPOINTMENT FOR CROWNS/BRIDGES
CITA PARA COLOCAR LA CORONA/EL PUENTE (AUDIO 9.74)

We will now remove the temporary crown.
Ahora quitaremos la corona temporal. (Audio 9.75)

We will now try the final crown.
Ahora probaremos la corona final. (Audio 9.76)

Bite down on this blue marking paper.
Muerda en este papel azul para marcar. (Audio 9.77)

Does the crown feel normal when you bite?
¿La corona se siente normal al morder? (Audio 9.78)

We will polish the crown.
Puliremos la corona. (Audio 9.79)

We will now cement the crown onto your tooth.
Ahora cementaremos la corona sobre su diente. (Audio 9.80)

The crown will be cemented permanently onto your tooth.
La corona será cementada permanentemente sobre su diente. (Audio 9.81)

We will remove the excess cement from around your crown.
Quitaremos el exceso de cemento alrededor de su corona. (Audio 9.82)

REMOVABLE PARTIAL DENTURE
DENTADURA PARCIAL REMOVIBLE (AUDIO 9.83)

A partial denture consists of replacement teeth on a gum-colored base.
Una dentadura postiza parcial consiste en dientes de reemplazo sobre una base del color de la encías. (Audio 9.84)

A partial denture has a (wire/metal) framework for strength.
Una dentadura postiza parcial tiene una estructura (de alambre/metal) para solidez. (Audio 9.85)

A partial denture will attach to your natural teeth by (clasps/precision attachments).
Una dentadura postiza parcial se adherirá a sus dientes naturales mediante (broches/accesorios de precisión). (Audio 9.86)

A partial denture clasp needs to sit in a spoon-shaped area on your natural tooth.
Los (broches/gancho) de una dentadura parcial necesitan apoyarse sobre un área en forma de cuchara en su diente natural. (Audio 9.87)

We will now prepare on your tooth the spoon-shaped rests for the clasps.
Ahora prepararemos en su diente los apoyos en forma de cuchara para los (broches/ganchos). (Audio 9.88)

A precision attachment requires a crown on your tooth.
Un accesorio de precisión requiere de una corona en su diente. (Audio 9.89)

A lower partial denture will have a bar across the back of these teeth.
Una dentadura parcial inferior tendrá una barra a través de la parte posterior de estos dientes. (Audio 9.90)

An upper partial denture will have a connector across your palate.
Una dentadura parcial superior tendrá un conector a través del paladar. (Audio 9.91)

It will take _____ appointments to finish the partial denture.
Tomará _____ citas para terminar la dentadura parcial. (Audio 9.92)

PREPARATION APPOINTMENT FOR PARTIAL DENTURE
CITA PARA LA PREPARACIÓN DE LA DENTADURA PARCIAL (AUDIO 9.93)

I will now take an impression of the area.
Ahora tomaré una impresión del área. (Audio 9.94)

The impression must remain in your mouth for _____ minutes.
La impresión debe permanecer en su boca por _____ minutos. (Audio 9.95)

I will now take an impression of your bite.
Ahora tomaré una impresión de su mordida. (Audio 9.96)

Keep your mouth open.
Mantenga la boca abierta. (Audio 9.97)

Bite down.
Muerde. (Audio 9.98)

This (impression/framework/wax-up) will now be sent to the lab.
(Esta impresión/Este(armazón/estructura)/Esta matriz de cera) se enviará al laboratorio. (Audio 9.99)

(I/We) need to select a shade and shape for your new teeth.
(Necesito/Necesitamos) seleccionar un (matiz/color) y una forma para sus nuevos dientes. (Audio 9.100)

You will need another appointment in _____ (days/weeks).
Usted necesitará otra cita en _____ (días/semanas). (Audio 9.101)

SEATING APPOINTMENT FOR PARTIAL DENTURE
CITA PARA COLOCAR LA DENTADURA PARCIAL (AUDIO 9.102)

This is your finished partial denture.
Ésta es su dentadura parcial terminada. (Audio 9.103)

Let's check the bite.
Vamos a examinar la mordida. (Audio 9.104)

Bite down on this marking paper.
Muerda sobre este papel de marcar. (Audio 9.105)

It may take a few weeks for your partial denture to become comfortable.
Puede tomar algunas semanas antes de que su dentadura postiza parcial se sienta cómoda. (Audio 9.106)

Remove the partial denture like so.
Quítese la dentadura parcial así. (Audio 9.107)

Place your fingers on the clasps to remove the partial denture.
Coloque los dedos sobre los ganchos para quitarse la dentadura parcial. (Audio 9.108)

When inserting it, don't force the partial denture into place.
Al insertarla, no fuerce la prótesis parcial en su lugar. (Audio 9.109)

Wear your partial denture all day and all night for the next _____ days.
Use su dentadura parcial todo el día y toda la noche por los próximos _____ días. (Audio 9.110)

Wear your partial denture only when you are awake.
Use la dentadura parcial sólo cuando está despierto(a). (Audio 9.111)

Remove your partial denture before going to sleep.
Quítese la dentadura parcial antes de irse a dormir. (Audio 9.112)

Do not sleep while wearing your partial denture.
No duerma con la dentadura parcial puesta. (Audio 9.113)

Sore spots may develop on your (gum/gingival) tissue.
Pueden surgir áreas adoloridas en el tejido de la encía. (Audio 9.114)

If (a sore spot/an irritation) develops, call the office for an appointment.
Si (un área adolorida/una irritación) se desarrolla, llame la oficina para una cita. (Audio 9.115)

Leave the partial denture in your mouth on the day (of/ before) your appointment so we are able to identify the sore spot.
Deje la dentadura postiza parcial en su boca el día (de/antes) de su cita para que podamos identificar el punto dolorido. (Audio 9.116)

To find the sore spot we will _____. (See Box 9.7)
Para encontrar el área adolorida vamos a
_____. (Vea el Cuadro 9.7) (Audio 9.117)

**Box 9.7
Methods for
finding sore spots
(Audio 9.257)**

- Paint the denture with white cream (Audio 9.258)
- Spray the partial denture with this marking medium (Audio 9.259)
- Touch this blue stick to the sore area in your mouth (Audio 9.260)

**Cuadro 9.7
Métodos para encontrar
áreas adoloridas
(Audio 9.257)**

- Pintar la dentadura con una crema blanca (Audio 9.258)
- Rociar la dentadura parcial con este medio de marcado (Audio 9.259)
- Tocar el área adolorida en su boca con esta varilla azul (Audio 9.260)

When not wearing your partial denture, clean it and store it in clean, fresh water.
Cuando no esté usando su dentadura parcial, límpiela y guárdela en agua limpia y fresca. (Audio 9.118)

Use this container to store your denture when you are not wearing it.
Use este contenedor para guardar su dentadura cuando no la esté usando. (Audio 9.119)

(Brush/Clean) your partial denture every (day/night).
(Cepille/Limpie) su dentadura parcial (todos los días/todas las noches). (Audio 9.120)

Use this special denture brush to clean your partial denture.
Utilice este cepillo especial para dentaduras para limpiar su dentadura parcial. (Audio 9.121)

Eating with your new partial denture may take some practice.
El comer con su nueva dentadura parcial puede requerir práctica. (Audio 9.122)

Start by eating soft food that has been cut into small pieces.
(Comience/empiece) por comer (comida/alimentos) blandas cortada(s) en pedazos pequeños. (Audio 9.123)

Chew on both sides of your mouth to balance the pressure.
Mastique en los dos lados de su boca para balancear la presión.
(Audio 9.124)

Don't eat foods that are very sticky or hard.
No coma (comidas/alimentos) que sean muy (pegajosas/pegajosos) o
(duras/duros). (Audio 9.125)

Pronouncing certain words may be difficult at first.
Al principio, puede ser difícil pronunciar ciertas palabras. (Audio 9.126)

Read out loud and repeat the difficult words.
Lea en voz alta y repita las palabras difíciles. (Audio 9.127)

Speak more slowly.
Hable más lentamente. (Audio 9.128)

Practice makes perfect.
Con la práctica se llega a la perfección. (Audio 9.129)

COMPLETE DENTURES
DENTADURAS COMPLETAS (AUDIO 9.130)

**A complete denture consists of replacement teeth on a
gum-colored base**.
Una dentadura postiza completa consiste de dientes de reemplazo
en una base del color de la encía. (Audio 9.131)

**An upper denture will be held in place by the natural
suction in your mouth**.
La dentadura superior se mantiene en su lugar con la succión
natural de su boca. (Audio 9.132)

A lower denture is held in place by your muscles.
La dentadura inferior se mantiene en su lugar con sus músculos.
(Audio 9.133)

The fit of the denture will depend on your saliva and bone.
El ajuste de la dentadura dependerá de su saliva y hueso. (Audio 9.134)

A complete denture rests on the tissues in your mouth.
Una dentadura completa descansa en los tejidos de su boca.
(Audio 9.135)

It will take _____ appointments to finish the complete denture.

Tomará_____ citas para terminar la dentadura completa. (Audio 9.136)

PREPARATION APPOINTMENT FOR COMPLETE DENTURE
CITA PARA LA PREPARACIÓN DE LA DENTADURA COMPLETA (AUDIO 9.137)

I will now take an impression of the entire area.
Ahora tomaré una impresión del área completa. (Audio 9.138)

The impression must remain in your mouth for _____ minutes.
La impresión debe permanecer en su boca por _____ minutos. (Audio 9.139)

This is called a face bow.
Esto se llama un arco de la cara. (Audio 9.140)

A face bow helps me get your teeth biting together properly.
Un arco de la cara me ayuda a conseguir que sus dientes muerdan correctamente. (Audio 9.141)

I will now take an impression of your bite.
Ahora tomaré una impresión de su mordida. (Audio 9.142)

Keep your mouth (open/closed).
Mantenga la boca (abierta/cerrada). (Audio 9.143)

Bite down.
Muerda. (Audio 9.144)

This (impression/framework/wax-up) will now be sent to the lab.
(Esta impresión/Este armazón/Esta matriz de cera) se enviará al laboratorio. (Audio 9.145)

(I/We) need to select a shade and shape for your new teeth.
(Necesito/Necesitamos) escoger un matiz y una forma para sus nuevos dientes. (Audio 9.146)

You will need another appointment in ____ (days/weeks).
Usted necesitará otra cita en ____ (días/semanas). (Audio 9.147)

This is your denture with the teeth set in wax.
Ésta es su dentadura con los dientes hechos en cera. (Audio 9.148)

Bite down gently on this marking paper.
Muerda suavemente sobre este papel para marcar. (Audio 9.149)

How do you like the color and shape of the teeth?
¿Le gustan el color y la forma de los dientes? (Audio 9.150)

SEATING APPOINTMENT FOR COMPLETE DENTURE
CITA PARA COLOCAR LA DENTADURA COMPLETA (AUDIO 9.151)

This is your finished complete denture.
Ésta es su dentadura completa (acabada/terminada). (Audio 9.152)

Let's check your bite.
Vamos a examinar su mordida. (Audio 9.153)

Bite down on this blue marking paper.
Muerda sobre este papel azul para marcar. (Audio 9.154)

It may take a few weeks for your denture to become comfortable.
. Es posible que pasen algunas semanas hasta que su dentadura se sienta cómoda. (Audio 9.155)

Remove the denture like so.
Quítese la dentadura así. (Audio 9.156)

Wear your denture all day and all night for the next ____ days.
Use su dentadura todo el día y toda la noche por los próximos ____ días. (Audio 9.157)

Wear your denture only while you are awake.
Use su dentadura sólo cuando esté despierto(a). (Audio 9.158)

Remove your denture before going to sleep.
Quítese la dentadura antes de irse a dormir. (Audio 9.159)

Sore spots may develop on your gum tissue.
Es ossible que se desarrollen puntos dolorosos en el tejido de las encías. (Audio 9.160)

If (a sore spot/an irritation) develops, call the office for an appointment.
Si (un área adolorida/una irritación) se desarrolla, llame la oficina para una cita. (Audio 9.161)

Leave the denture in your mouth on the day (of/before) your sore-spot appointment.
Use la dentadura el día (de/antes de) la cita para el área adolorida. (Audio 9.162)

To find the sore spot I will _____. (See Box 9.7)
Para encontrar el área adolorida voy a _____. (Vea el Cuadro 9.7) (Audio 9.163)

When not wearing your denture, clean it and store it in clean, fresh water.
Cuando no esté usando su dentadura, límpiela y guárdela en agua limpia y fresca. (Audio 9.164)

Use this container to store your denture when you are not wearing it.
Use este contenedor para guardar su dentadura cuando no la esté usando. (Audio 9.165)

(Brush/Clean) your denture every (day/night).
(Cepille/Limpie) su dentadura (todos los días/todas las noches). (Audio 9.166)

Use this special denture brush to clean your denture.
Utilice este cepillo especial para dentaduras postizas para limpiar su dentadura postiza. (Audio 9.167)

Eating with your new denture may take some practice.
El comer con su nueva dentadura puede requerir práctica. (Audio 9.168)

Start by eating soft food that has been cut into small pieces.
(Comience/empiece) por comer (comida/alimentos) blandas cortada(s) en pedazos pequeños. (Audio 9.169)

Chew on both sides of your mouth to balance the pressure.
Mastique en los dos lados de la boca para balancear la presión.
(Audio 9.170)

Don't eat foods that are very sticky or hard.
No coma (comidas/alimentos) que son muy (pegajosas/pegajosos) o
(duras/duros). (Audio 9.171)

Pronouncing certain words may be difficult at first.
Al principio, puede ser difícil pronunciar ciertas palabras.
(Audio 9.172)

Read out loud and repeat the bothersome words.
Lea en voz alta y repita las palabras difíciles. (Audio 9.173)

Speak more slowly.
Hable más lentamente. (Audio 9.174)

**Occasionally the denture may slip when you laugh, cough,
or smile**.
A veces la dentadura puede deslizarse cuando usted se ríe, tose o
sonríe. (Audio 9.175)

Reposition it by putting your teeth together and swallowing.
Para reposicionarla, cierre bien los dientes y trague. (Audio 9.176)

Practice makes perfect.
Con la práctica se llega a la perfección. (Audio 9.177)

**Should you become ill and need to vomit, remove your
denture(s) first if possible**.
Si se enferma y necesita vomitar, quítese su(s) dentadura(s) primero
si es posible. (Audio 9.178)

REPAIR OF PROSTHODONTIC APPLIANCES
REPARACIÓN DE LOS APARATOS PROSTÉTICOS
(AUDIO 9.179)

**I suggest that you have your denture (replicated/copied) for
a spare**.
Sugiero que (copie/duplique) su dentadura para tener una de
recambio. (Audio 9.180)

You need to have your denture relined.
Es necesario revestir su dentadura. (Audio 9.181)

Relining your denture will help it fit properly.
Revestir su dentadura ayudará a que se encaje apropiadamente.
(Audio 9.182)

A reline can improve the retention of your denture.
Un revestido puede mejorar la retención de su dentadura.
(Audio 9.183)

I will place a soft reline in your denture.
Colocaré un revestido suave en su dentadura. (Audio 9.184)

I can do an in-office reline.
Puedo hacer un cambio de revestimiento en la oficina. (Audio 9.185)

To have your denture relined, we will have to send it to the lab.
Para revestir su dentadura, tendremos que enviarla al laboratorio.
(Audio 9.186)

You have a broken (clasp/tooth) on your (partial/complete) denture.
Usted tiene (un broche/un diente) roto(a) en su dentadura (parcial/completa). (Audio 9.187)

You have cracked your denture.
Usted ha fracturado su dentadura. (Audio 9.188)

You have worn down the teeth on your denture.
Usted ha desgastado los dientes de su dentadura. (Audio 9.189)

Your denture teeth need to be replaced.
Los dientes de su dentadura necesitan reemplazarse. (Audio 9.190)

Your denture is beyond repair.
Su dentadura es irreparable. (Audio 9.191)

You need a new denture.
Usted necesita una dentadura nueva. (Audio 9.192)

I will be able to fix your denture today.
Puedo reparar su dentadura hoy. (Audio 9.193)

Will you wait for it?
¿Usted esperaría por ella? (Audio 9.194)

Can you come back later today for the repaired denture?
¿Puede regresar hoy más tarde para recoger la dentadura reparada?
(Audio 9.195)

To have this denture repaired, I will have to send it to the dental laboratory.
Para reparar esta dentadura, tendré que enviarla al laboratorio dental. (Audio 9.196)

You will be without your denture for _____ days.
Usted estará sin su dentadura por _____ días. (Audio 9.197)

We can place your name on your denture. The text will not be visible but can help you recover your denture if it becomes lost.
Podemos poner su nombre en la dentadura. El texto no será visible, pero puede ayudarle a recuperar su dentadura si la pierde. (Audio 9.198)

DENTURE/PARTIAL DENTURE CARE
CUIDADO DE LA DENTADURA/DENTADURA PARCIAL (AUDIO 9.199)

Brush your (denture/partial denture) twice daily with a firm brush.
Cepille su (dentadura postiza /dentadura parcial) dos veces al día con un cepillo firme. (Audio 9.200)

Brushing plaque from your (denture/partial denture) will remove plaque from your mouth and freshen your breath.
El cepillar la placa de su (dentadura/dentadura parcial) removerá la placa de su boca y refrescará su aliento. (Audio 9.201)

Rinsing your (denture/partial denture) alone does not remove plaque.
El sólo enjuagar su (dentadura/dentadura parcial) no remueve la placa. (Audio 9.202)

Plaque can harm the gum ridges under your (denture/ partial denture).
La placa puede dañar el borde de las encías debajo de su (dentadura/dentadura parcial). (Audio 9.203)

You can use denture powder or paste when brushing your (denture/partial denture).
Usted puede usar un polvo o pasta para dentaduras cuando cepilla su (dentadura/dentadura parcial). (Audio 9.204)

Wire brushes should never be used on your (denture/ partial denture).
Nunca use cepillos de alambres en su (dentadura/dentadura parcial). (Audio 9.205)

Household cleaners should never be used on your (denture/ partial denture).
Nunca se deben utilizar limpiadores domésticos en su (dentadura postiza/dentadura postiza parcial). (Audio 9.206)

Don't use bleach on your denture since it is plastic and will absorb bleach molecules.
No use (lejía/blanqueador/cloro) en su dentadura postiza, ya que es plástico y absorberá las moléculas de lejía. (Audio 9.207)

Don't use (bleach/whitening/chlorine) on your removable partial denture since it has metal parts and will corrode.
No use (lejía/blanqueador/cloro) en su dentadura parcial removible, ya que tiene partes de metal y se corroerá. (Audio 9.208)

Don't use any glues to fix your (denture/partial denture).
No utilice pegamentos para arreglar su (dentadura postiza/ dentadura parcial). (Audio 9.209)

Don't use any type of file to fix your (denture/partial denture).
No use ningún tipo de lima para arreglar su (dentadura/dentadura parcial). (Audio 9.210)

Don't repair your (denture/partial denture) yourself.
No repare su (dentadura/dentadura parcial) usted mismo(a). (Audio 9.211)

Contact our (office/clinic) if your (denture/partial denture) is broken.
Llame a nuestra (oficina/clínica) si su (dentadura/dentadura parcial) se (rompe/quebra). (Audio 9.212)

The dentist recommends that you take out your (denture/ partial denture) during sleep.
El/La dentista recomienda que usted se quite la (dentadura/ dentadura parcial) mientras duerme. (Audio 9.213)

A poorly fitting (denture/partial denture) can result in _____. (See Box 9.8)
Una (dentadura/dentadura parcial) que no ajusta bien puede resultar en _____. (Vea el Cuadro 9.8) (Audio 9.214)

IMPLANTS
IMPLANTES (AUDIO 9.215)

We will refer you to a(n) _____ for an implant evaluation. (See Box 9.9)
Lo(a) referiremos a un(a) _____ para una evaluación de implante. (Vea el Cuadro 9.9) (Audio 9.216)

Box 9.8 **Results of a poorly fitting denture/partial denture (Audio 9.261)**	**Cuadro 9.8** **Resultados de una dentadura/dentadura parcial que no encaja bien (Audio 9.261)**
• A poor bite (Audio 9.262) • A poor diet (Audio 9.263) • Mouth sores (Audio 9.264) • Infection (Audio 9.265)	• Una mala mordida (Audio 9.262) • Una mala dieta (Audio 9.263) • Úlceras bucales/orales (Audio 9.264) • Infección (Audio 9.265)

**Box 9.9
Types of specialists that may perform implant surgery (Audio 9.266)**

- Implant specialist (Audio 9.267)
- Oral surgeon (Audio 9.268)
- Periodontist (Audio 9.269)

**Cuadro 9.9
Tipos de especialistas que podrían llevar a cabo una cirugía de implantes (Audio 9.266)**

- Especialista de implantes (Audio 9.267)
- Cirujano(a) oral (Audio 9.268)
- Periodoncista (Audio 9.269)

Have you considered a dental implant to replace your missing (tooth/teeth)?
¿Ha considerado la posibilidad de reemplazar (el diente/los dientes) que falta(n) con un implante? (Audio 9.217)

Would you like to replace the missing (tooth/teeth)?
¿Le gustaría reemplazar (el diente/los dientes) que falta(n)? (Audio 9.218)

An implant can replace (a missing tooth/missing teeth).
Un implante puede reemplazar (un diente/los dientes) que falta(n). (Audio 9.219)

This baby tooth can be replaced with an implant.
Este diente de leche se puede reemplazar con un implante. (Audio 9.220)

Implants can give a denture greater stability.
Los implantes pueden dar mejor (solidez/estabilidad) a la dentadura. (Audio 9.221)

An implant can be used to support a (crown/bridge/ denture).
Se puede usar un implante para sostener (una corona/un puente/una dentadura). (Audio 9.222)

The fee for the implant does not include the fee for the (crown/bridge/denture).
El costo del implante no incluye el costo de (la corona/el puente/la dentadura). (Audio 9.223)

We need to evaluate the bone to determine whether an implant can be placed into the area.

Necesitamos evaluar el hueso para determinar si se puede colocar un implante en el área. (Audio 9.224)

We need to take radiographs to look at the bone.

Necesitamos tomar radiografías para examinar el hueso. (Audio 9.225)

An implant is set into the bone.

Un implante se coloca en el hueso. (Audio 9.226)

Chapter 10
Dental Implants

Capítulo 10
Implantes Dentales (Audio 10.1)

IMPLANT PLACEMENT
COLOCACIÓN DEL IMPLANTE (AUDIO 10.2)

Today we will be placing the implant fixture (root) in your bone.
Hoy vamos a colocar el implante (la raíz) en su hueso. (Audio 10.3)

First we will apply a dental anesthetic so that you will not experience any discomfort. (See Figure 10.1)

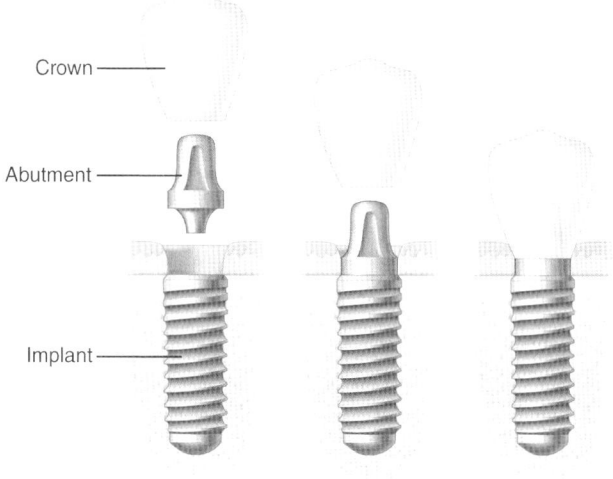

Crown

Abutment

Implant

Fig. 10.1 An illustration of components of a dental implant with parts labeled, crown, abutment, and implant. Una ilustración de los componentes de un implante dental con piezas etiquetadas, corona, pilares y implante. From Darby and Walsh Dental Hygiene: Theory and Practice, Sixth Edition; Fig. 31.1; ISBN: 9780323877824.

Primero le aplicaremos anestésico dental para que no experimente ninguna molestia. (Vea la Imagen 10.1) (Audio 10.4)

We will use a special drill to make a space for your implant slowly, gently, and safely.
Usaremos un taladro especial para hacer un espacio para su implante de manera lenta, suave, y segura. (Audio 10.5)

Here is what it will sound like.
Así es como sonará. (Audio 10.6)

Let us know if you have any questions or if you experience any discomfort.
Háganos saber si tiene preguntas o si siente algúna molestia. (Audio 10.7)

You will have sutures over the surgical site.
Le suturarán en el sitio de la cirugía. (Audio 10.8)

The sutures will be removed in _____ days.
Le quitaremos los puntos en _____ días. (Audio 10.9)

You may have some _____ at this site. (See Box 10.1)
Es posible que tenga _____ en este sitio. (Vea el Cuadro 10.1) (Audio 10.10)

You may take (an antiinflammatory/ibuprofen) to relieve any pain.

Box 10.1
Problems that patients may experience
(Audio 10.29)

- Bleeding (Audio 10.30)
- Discomfort (Audio 10.31)
- Foul taste (Audio 10.32)
- Mobility (Audio 10.33)
- Pain (Audio 10.34)
- Swelling (Audio 10.35)

Cuadro 10.1
Problemas que pueden tener los pacientes
(Audio 10.29)

- Sangrado (Audio 10.30)
- Molestia/incomodidad (Audio 10.31)
- Mal sabor (Audio 10.32)
- Movilidad (Audio 10.33)
- Dolor (Audio 10.34)
- Hinchazón (Audio 10.35)

Usted puede tomar un (anti-inflamatorio/ibuprofeno) para aliviar cualquier dolor. (Audio 10.11)

You may gently rinse with (warm salt water/chlorhexidine) for the next _____ days.
Puede enjuagarse suavemente con (agua salada tibia/clorohexidina) durante los próximos _____ días. (Audio 10.12)

You will return for reevaluation in _____ days.
Debe regresar para una reevaluación en _____ días. (Audio 10.13)

Once the implant has been set into the bone, it is left to heal for _____ (weeks/months).
Después de que se ha colocado el implante en el hueso, se deja sanar por _____(semanas/meses). (Audio 10.14)

The implant will be uncovered in _____ (weeks/months).
Destaparemos el implante dentro de _____ (semanas/meses). (Audio 10.15)

A healing collar will be placed on the healed implant site.
Cuando el sitio del impalante este sandado colocaremos un collar cicatrizacion. (Audio 10.16)

A clip bar will be attached to the implants after they have healed.
Le agregaremos una barra sujetadora a los implantes después de que éstos hayan sanado. (Audio 10.17)

A ball attachment device will be attached to the implants after they have healed.
Le agregaremos un pilar de bola a los implantes una vez que se hayan sanado. (Audio 10.18)

Sutures will be placed over the site after the (healing collar/clip bar/ball attachment) has been put in place.
Las suturas se colocarán sobre el sitio después de que se haya colocado (el collar de cicatrización/la barra sujetadora/el pilar de bola). (Audio 10.19)

Let us know if after the first day you experience any bleeding, swelling, or pain.
Háganos saber si después del primer día experimenta algún sangrado, hinchazón o dolor. (Audio 10.20)

In _____months, after the bone has healed around the implant, the (crown/bridge/denture) can be made.
En _____ meses, después de que el hueso haya sanado alrededor del implante, se puede hacer (la corona/el puente/la dentadura). (Audio 10.21)

IMPLANT RESTORATION
RESTAURACIÓN DE IMPLANTES (AUDIO 10.22)

Now that your implant has fused to the bone, it is time to restore the implant with a (crown/bridge).
Ahora que su implante se ha fusionado con el hueso, es el momento de restaurar el implante con una (corona/puente). (Audio 10.23)

After we remove the healing abutment, we will make an impression of the implant.
Después de quitar el pilar de cicatrización, haremos una impresión del implante. (Audio 10.24)

We are going to take an impression of the implant now.
Ahora vamos a tomar una impresión del implante. (Audio 10.25)

We need to remove a small area of gingiva next to the implant, in order to make a good impression.
Necesitamos eliminar una pequeña zona de la encía al lado del implante, para poder tomar una buena impresión. (Audio 10.26)

We are going to cement a temporary crown on this implant, until the final crown is returned from the lab.
Vamos a colocar una corona temporal en este implante, hasta que nos llegue la corona final del laboratorio. (Audio 10.27)

I think you are going to be very pleased with this implant.
Creo que va a estar muy contento(a) con este implante. (Audio 10.28)

Chapter 11
Oral Surgery

Capítulo 11
Cirugía Oral (Audio 11.1)

EXTRACTIONS AND ORAL SURGERY
EXTRACCIONES Y CIRUGÍA ORAL (AUDIO 11.2)

**We will refer you to an oral surgeon for _____.
(See Box 11.1)**
Lo(a/e) enviaremos a un(a) cirujano(a) oral para _____.
(Vea el Cuadro 11.1) (Audio 11.3)

You need to have (a tooth_____ teeth) extracted.
Usted necesita que le extraigan (un diente_____dientes).
(Audio 11.4)

You need to have _____ wisdom teeth extracted. (See Figure 11.1)
Usted necesita que le extraigan _____ (muelas cordales/muelas del juicio). (Vea el Cuadro 11.1) (Audio 11.5)

Box 11.1
Reasons to refer a patient to an oral surgeon
(Audio 11.57)

- Treatment (Audio 11.58)
- A biopsy (Audio 11.59)
- An evaluation (Audio 11.60)
- An extraction (Audio 11.61)
- A second opinion (Audio 11.62)
- An implant evaluation (Audio 11.63)

Cuadro 11.1
Razones para referir a un(a) paciente a un(a) cirujano(a) oral
(Audio 11.57)

- Tratamiento (Audio 11.58)
- Una biopsia (Audio 11.59)
- Una evaluación (Audio 11.60)
- Una extracción (Audio 11.61)
- Una segunda opinión (Audio 11.62)
- Una evaluación para un implante (Audio 11.63)

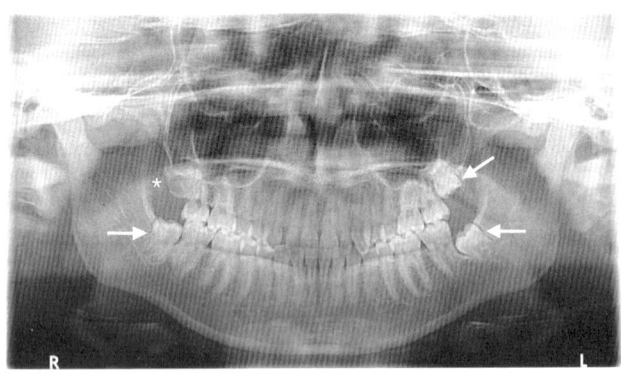

Fig. 11-1 Dental x-ray in an older adolescent demonstrating three erupting/ impacted wisdom teeth with some malalignments (*arrows*). Note that the patient lacks a fourth wisdom tooth (*asterisk*). Radiografía dental en un adolescente mayor que muestra tres muelas del juicio impactadas o en erupción con algunas desalineaciones (*flechas*). Nótese que al paciente le falta una cuarta muela del juicio (*asterisco*). *(From Pediatric Secrets, Seventh Edition; Fig. 2.5; ISBN: 9780323636650; Photo courtesy Mark F. Ditmar.)*

You need to have (an area/this area) biopsied.
Es necesario que le hagan una biopsia de (una zona/esta zona). (Audio 11.6)

During a biopsy a small piece of tissue is removed and examined under a microscope to aid in your diagnosis.
Durante una biopsia, se extrae una pequeña porción de tejido y se examina bajo un microscopio para ayudar en el diagnóstico. (Audio 11.7)

The tissue I removed will be sent to a laboratory for examination.
El tejido que saqué se enviará a un laboratorio para un examen. (Audio 11.8)

The laboratory will return a diagnosis in _____ days.
El laboratorio nos presentará un diagnóstico en _____ días. (Audio 11.9)

We will place a mouth prop in your mouth so that you will be more comfortable during the procedure.
Le pondremos un apoyo bucal en la boca para que esté más cómodo(a) durante el procedimiento. (Audio 11.10)

Before starting we will (numb/anesthetize/put to sleep) the area.
Antes de comenzar vamos a (adormecer/anestesiar/dormir) el área.
(Audio 11.11)

First, I will apply a topical anesthetic to numb the gum.
Primero, aplicaré un anestésico tópico para adormecer la encía.
(Audio 11.12)

You will hear sounds when I extract the tooth.
Usted oirá sonidos cuando le extraiga el diente. (Audio 11.13)

You may feel some pressure while I extract the tooth.
Es posible que sienta algo de presión mientras extraigo el diente.
(Audio 11.14)

If you experience pain or discomfort, raise your (right/left) hand and I will stop.
Si siente dolor o malestar, levante la mano (derecha/izquierda) y
pararé. (Audio 11.15)

You will need a (suture/stitch) to close the space.
Usted necesitará (un punto/puntadas/una sutura) para cerrar el
espacio. (Audio 11.16)

We have placed _____ sutures in the area.
Le hemos puesto _____ (puntos/puntadas) en el área. (Audio 11.17)

The sutures will dissolve on their own.
(Los puntos/las puntadas/las suturas) se disolverán por su cuenta.
(Audio 11.18)

We will need to remove the sutures in _____ days.
Necesitaremos sacar (los puntos/las puntadas/las suturas) en _____
días. (Audio 11.19)

A small amount of bleeding is normal.
Un poco de sangrado es normal. (Audio 11.20)

Bite down on this gauze.
Muerda esta gaza. (Audio 11.21)

Smokers are slower to heal after (surgery/extraction).
Los fumadores tardan más en sanar después (de cirugía/una
extracción). (Audio 11.22)

Rinse your mouth gently.
Enjuáguese la boca con cuidado. (Audio 11.23)

You may experience some (pain/discomfort) when the anesthetic wears off.
Es posible que sienta (dolor/molestias) cuando se disipe la anestesia. (Audio 11.24)

You will feel some pressure, but it should not hurt.
Sentirás algo de presión, pero no debería doler. (Audio 11.25)

You should not feel sharp pain or pain in general, just pressure.
No debes sentir dolores agudos ni dolor en general, sólo presión. (Audio 11.26)

Do you feel pressure or pain?

¿Sientes presión o dolor? (Audio 11.27)

ORTHOGNATHIC SURGERY
CIRUGÍA ORTOGNÁTICA (AUDIO 11.28)

Orthognathic surgery is jaw surgery performed to align your jaws and teeth.
La cirugía ortognática es la cirugía de la mandíbula que se realiza para alinear las mandíbulas y dientes. (Audio 11.29)

This surgery must be performed in conjunction with orthodontics.
Esta cirugía debe realizarse en conjunto con la ortodoncia. (Audio 11.30)

You must wear braces for _____ months prior to the surgery, and for _____months afterward.
Tiene que usar (frenillos/frenos/brackets) por _____ meses antes de la cirugía, y durante _____ meses después. (Audio 11.31)

During the surgery, we will reposition your (lower/upper) jaw in order to correct the alignment.
Durante la cirugía, vamos a cambiar la posición de la mandíbula (inferior/superior), para corregir la alineación. (Audio 11.32)

I will use titanium plates and screws to fuse your jaw together.

Voy a usar placas de titanio y tornillos para fusionar su mandíbula. (Audio 11.33)

Your surgery will be performed in a hospital, under general anesthesia.

La cirugía se llevará a cabo en un hospital, bajo anestesia general. (Audio 11.34)

We will need to wire your teeth and your jaws shut for _____ weeks.

Tendremos que alambrar y cerrar sus dientes y mandíbulas por _____ semanas. (Audio 11.35)

POSTOPERATIVE CARE
CUIDADO POSTOPERATORIO (AUDIO 11.36)

Rinse gently with warm salt water _____ times a day for _____ days.

Enjuáguese suavemente con agua salada tibia _____ veces al día por _____ días. (Audio 11.37)

As a rinse use a small glass of warm water with a few shakes of salt in it.

Como enjuague, utilice un vaso pequeño de agua tibia con un poco de sal. (Audio 11.38)

You may experience some bruising.

Puede que usted tenga algunos (hematomas/moretones). (Audio 11.39)

You may experience some swelling.

Puede que usted tenga algo de hinchazón. (Audio 11.40)

Replace the gauze every _____minutes for the next hour.

Reemplace la gasa cada _____ minutos durante la próxima hora. (Audio 11.41)

Some bleeding is normal.

Es normal tener algo de sangrado. (Audio 11.42)

Don't (smoke/rinse/spit) for the next _____ (hours/days).
No (fume/se enjuague/escupa) por las/los próximas(os) _____
(horas/días). (Audio 11.43)

Avoid tobacco products for the next _____ days.
Evite los productos de tabaco por los próximos _____; días. (Audio
11.44)

**To reduce swelling apply (a cold cloth/an ice pack) to this
area**.
Para reducir la hinchazón, aplique (un paño frío/una compresa de
hielo) en esta área. (Audio 11.45)

Brush and floss your other teeth as usual.
Cepíllese los demás dientes y use hilo dental normalmente.
(Audio 11.46)

**Don't (clean the teeth/use your toothbrush) next to the
tooth socket**.
No (limpie los dientes/use su cepillo de dientes) cerca de la cavidad.
(Audio 11.47)

Don't disturb the blood clot in the socket.
No se toque el coágulo de sangre en la cavidad. (Audio 11.48)

Don't use a straw to drink liquids for _____ days.
No use un/a (_____) para beber líquidos por _____ días.
(See Box 11.2)(Audio 11.49)

This is a prescription for _____ medication. (See Box 11.3)
Esta receta es para el medicamento _____. (Vea el Cuadro 11.3)
(Audio 11.50)

Have you ever had a reaction to any medication?
Ha tenido alguna reacción a algún medicamento? (Audio 11.51)

**It is important that you finish the entire prescription of
antibiotic medication, even if you begin to feel better**.
Es importante que termine de usar todo el medicamento antibiótico
recetado, aun cuando comience a sentirse mejor. (Audio 11.52)

Take all of the medication as prescribed.
Tome todo el medicamento tal como se ha recetado. (Audio 11.53)

Box 11.2
Straw in Spanish by country (Audio 11.70)

- Argentina: Sorbete, pajita (Audio 11.71)
- Bolivia: Bombilla (Audio 11.72)
- Chile: Bombilla, pajita (Audio 11.73)
- Colombia: Pitillo (Audio 11.74)
- Costa Rica: Pajilla (Audio 11.75)
- Cuba: Absorbente (Audio 11.76)
- Dominican Republic: Calimete (Audio 11.77)
- Ecuador: Sorbete (Audio 11.78)
- El Salvador: Pajilla (Audio 11.79)
- Guatemala: Pajilla (Audio 11.80)
- Honduras: Pajilla (Audio 11.81)
- Mexico: Popote (Audio 11.82)
- Nicaragua: Pajilla (Audio 11.83)
- Panama: Carrizo (Audio 11.84)
- Peru: Sorbete, cañita (Audio 11.85)
- Puerto Rico: Sorbeto (Audio 11.86)
- Spain: Caña, pajita (Audio 11.87)
- Uruguay: Pajita (Audio 11.88)
- Venezuela: Pitillo (Audio 11.89)

Box 11.3
Types of prescriptions
(Audio 11.64)

- Pain (Audio 11.65)
- Antibiotic (Audio 11.66)
- Narcotic (Audio 11.67)
- Nonnarcotic (Audio 11.68)
- Anti-fungal (Audio 11.69)

Cuadro 11.3
Tipos de recetas
(Audio 11.64)

- Para el dolor (Audio 11.65)
- Antibiótico (Audio 11.66)
- Narcótico (Audio 11.67)
- No-narcótico (Audio 11.68)
- Antifúngico (Audio 11.69)

Make an appointment to have that area examined in _____ days.
Haga una cita para examinar esa área en _____; días. (Audio 11.54)

If you have bleeding that does not subside, you can bite on a tea bag to help reduce bleeding. If this happens, please also contact us.

Si tienes sangrado que no cede, puedes morder una bolsita de té para ayudar a reducir el sangrado. Si esto sucede por favor contáctenos. (Audio 11.55)

If after _____ days, you are experiencing pain that has intensified or not subsided please call the dental office.

Si después de _____ días siente un dolor intenso o que no ha disminuido, llame al consultorio dental. (Audio 11.56)

Chapter 12
Laser Surgery and Radiosurgery

Capítulo 12
Cirugía Láser y Radiocirugía (Audio 12.1)

GENERAL
GENERAL (AUDIO 12.2)

We need to remove a small amount of tissue from around this crown preparation in order to make an accurate impression.
Necesitamos eliminar una pequeña cantidad de tejido alrededor de esta preparación de corona para poder tomar una impresión precisa. (Audio 12.3)

Because you are numb, you should not feel any of this.
Ya que está anestesiado, no deberías sentir nada de esto.
(Audio 12.4)

In order to control the bleeding in this area, we would like to use a device called a (laser/radiosurgery).
Para controlar el sangrado en esta área, nos gustaría utilizar un dispositivo llamado (láser/radiocirugía). (Audio 12.5)

LASER SURGERY
CIRUGÍA LÁSER (AUDIO 12.6)

A laser unit uses high-energy lightwaves to vaporize tissue. They can be used to cut tissue, treat ulcers, stop bleeding, and for a number of other medical uses.
Un dispositivo láser utiliza ondas de luz de alta energía para vaporizar los tejidos. Pueden utilizarse para cortar el tejido, tratar úlceras, detener el sangrado, y un número de otros usos médicos.
(Audio 12.7)

It is very important that you use these special glasses while we are using the laser.
Es muy importante que usted use estos (lentes/gafas) especiales mientras estamos utilizando el láser. (Audio 12.8)

It is very uncommon to have any discomfort following laser surgery. However, if you should experience any discomfort, please call our office right away.
Es muy raro sentir alguna molestia después de la cirugía con láser. Sin embargo, si siente alguna molestia, por favor llame a nuestra oficina inmediatamente. (Audio 12.9)

Viral ulcers treated with lasers oftentimes do not recur.
Las úlceras (virales/fuegos) que se tratan con láser no suelen repetirse. (Audio 12.10)

Unlike incisions made with a scalpel, incisions made with a laser do not bleed as much and heal much faster.
A diferencia de las incisiones hechas con bisturí, las incisiones hechas con láser no sangran tanto y sanan mucho más rápido. (Audio 12.11)

Let me know if you feel a burning sensation while we are using the laser.
Déjame saber si sientes una sensación de ardor mientras usamos el láser. (Audio 12.12)

Laser therapy can be used to treat (labial herpes/cold sores/ulcers) to help them heal faster.
La terapia con láser se puede utilizar para tratar (herpes labial/fuegos/úlceras) para ayudar a que se sanen más rápido. (Audio 12.13)

Laser therapy can be used in combination with periodontal therapy to combat gum disease.
La terapia con láser se puede utilizar en combinación con la terapia periodontal para combatir la enfermedad de las encías. (Audio 12.14)

Does it feel warm and tingly? Let me know if it starts to feel hot.
¿Se siente cálido y con hormigueo? Avíseme si se empieza a sentir caliente. (Audio 12.15)

I am going to press a cotton tip applicator on the cold sore, tell me if it feels numb.
Voy a presionar un aplicador con punta de algodón sobre el (herpes labial/fuego), dime si se siente entumecido. (Audio 12.16)

RADIOSURGERY
RADIOCIRUGÍA (AUDIO 12.17)

Similar to a laser, radiosurgery vaporizes tissue; however, it uses radiowaves rather than lightwaves to do so.
Al igual que un láser, la radiocirugía vaporiza el tejido, sin embargo, utiliza ondas de radio en vez de ondas de luz. (Audio 12.18)

Radiosurgery sometimes produces a slight burning smell while in use. This is nothing to worry about, and we will do our best to minimize this effect.
A veces, la radiocirugía produce un ligero olor a quemado mientras está en uso. No hay nada de que preocuparse, y haremos nuestro mejor esfuerzo para minimizar este efecto. (Audio 12.19)

This flat plate is an antenna for the radiosurgery unit and needs to be placed behind your back.
Esta placa plana es una antena para la unidad de radiocirugía y debe colocarse detrás de su espalda. (Audio 12.20)

Radiosurgery will be used to cauterize the small bleeding points.
Usaremos la radiocirugía para cauterizar las pequeñas áreas sangrantes. (Audio 12.21)

No sutures will be required with this procedure.
No se requerirá suturas con este procedimiento. (Audio 12.22)

Chapter 13
Periodontics

Capítulo 13
Periodoncia (Audio 13.1)

PERIODONTAL EXAMINATION
EXAMEN PERIODONTAL (AUDIO 13.2)

Periodontal disease is an infection of the (tissues/bone and gum) surrounding the tooth.
La enfermedad periodontal es una infección (de los tejidos/del hueso y de la encía) que rodean el diente. (Audio 13.3)

Periodontal disease is caused by plaque.
La enfermedad periodontal es causada por placa bacteriana (Audio 13.4)

We will refer you to a periodontist for _____. (See Box 13.1)
Le enviaremos a un(a) periodoncista para _____ (Vea el Cuadro 13.1) (Audio 13.5)

You have (gum disease/gingivitis/periodontitis). (See Box 13.2 and Figure 13.1)
Usted tiene enfermedad en las (encías/gingivitis/periodontitis). (Vea el Cuadro 13.2 y la Imagen 13.1) (Audio 13.6)

If gingivitis is not treated, it can infect deeper tissues and damage the bone and structures that support the teeth.
Si la gingivitis no se trata, puede infectar tejidos más profundos y dañar el hueso y las estructuras que sostienen los dientes. (Audio 13.7)

If periodontal disease is left untreated, it can result in the loss of your (tooth/teeth).
Si la enfermedad periodontal no se trata, puede resultar en la pérdida de (su diente/sus dientes). (Audio 13.8)

Plaque on the tooth surface can cause your (gum/gingival) tissues to become red and swollen and to bleed.
La placa en la superficie del diente puede causar que los tejidos (de las encías/gingival) se pongan rojos, se hinchen y sangren. (Audio 13.9)

Box 13.1
**Reasons to refer
a patient to a
periodontist
(Audio 13.63)**

- Periodontal surgery
(Audio 13.64)
- A biopsy (Audio 13.65)
- An evaluation (Audio 13.66)
- A second opinion
(Audio 13.67)
- An implant evaluation
(Audio 13.68)
- Crown lengthening
(Audio 13.69)
- Grafting (Audio 13.70)

- Correction of a bony defect
(Audio 13.71)

Cuadro 13.1
**Razones para referir
a un paciente a
un(a) periodoncista
(Audio 13.63)**

- Cirugía periodontal
(Audio 13.64)
- Una biopsia (Audio 13.65)
- Una evaluación (Audio 13.66)
- Una segunda opinión
(Audio 13.67)
- Una evaluación de un
implante (Audio 13.68)
- Alargar una corona
(Audio 13.69)
- Aplicar un injerto
(Audio 13.70)
- Corregir un defecto del
hueso (Audio 13.71)

Box 13.2
**Descriptions of
periodontal disease
(Audio 13.72)**

- Mild (Audio 13.73)
- Moderate (Audio 13.74)
- Extensive (Audio 13.75)
- Severe (Audio 13.76)
- Localized (Audio 13.77)
- Generalized (Audio 13.78)

Cuadro 13.2
**Descripciones de
enfermedades
periodontales
(Audio 13.72)**

- Poco severa (Audio 13.73)
- Moderada (Audio 13.74)
- Extensa (Audio 13.75)
- Severa (Audio 13.76)
- Localizada (Audio 13.77)
- Generalizada (Audio 13.78)

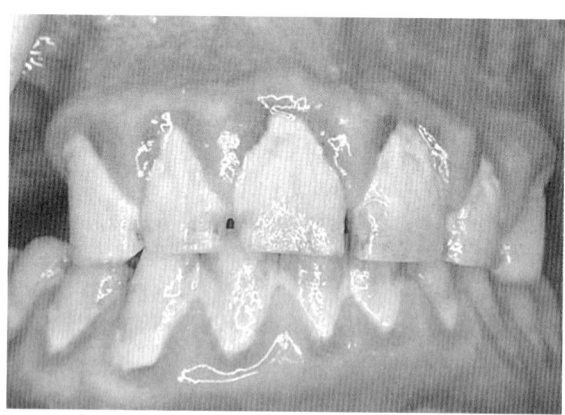

Fig. 13.1 Gingivitis.

Plaque buildup causes the (gums/gingiva) to pull away from the teeth.
La acumulación de placa causa que las encías se separen del diente. (Audio 13.10)

Plaque has caused your (gum/gingival) tissues to recede.
La placa ha causado el retiro de sus tejidos (de las encías/gingivales). (Audio 13.11)

I am going to check your teeth for periodontal disease.
Voy a examinar sus dientes para enfermedad periodontal. (Audio 13.12)

I will use a periodontal probe to measure the area around each tooth.
Usaré una sonda periodontal para medir el área alrededor de cada diente. (Audio 13.13)

This probe will help determine whether there is any breakdown in the connective tissue between your tooth and (gum/gingiva). If there is, it is called a pocket.
Esta sonda ayudará a determinar si hay algún deterioro en el tejido conectivo entre su diente y la encía. Si lo hay, se le llama un bolsillo periodontal. (Audio 13.14)

A periodontal pocket is a sign that the tissue is not healthy.
Una bolsa periodontal es una señal de que el tejido no está sano.
(Audio 13.15)

**The normal (space/sulcus) or measurement in healthy
areas is 3 millimeters or less**.
El (espacio normal/surco) o medida en las áreas sanas es de
3 milímetros o menos. (Audio 13.16)

**Any measurement greater than 3 millimeters indicates an
area that will need treatment**.
Cualquier medida mayor de 3 milímetros indica un área que
necesitará tratamiento. (Audio 13.17)

We will be recording these measurements in your chart.
Registraremos estas medidas en su hoja clínica. (Audio 13.18)

**We will routinely check your gums for signs of periodontal
disease**.
Revisaremos sus encías rutinariamente por signos de enfermedad
periodontal. (Audio 13.19)

**We will routinely check these readings (to be sure that
your periodontal disease has not progressed/to monitor the
health of your (gums/gingiva))**.
Revisaremos estas medidas rutinariamente (para asegurarnos de que
su enfermedad periodontal no haya (progresado/para observar la
salud de sus encías). (Audio 13.20)

**I will be checking your (gums/gingiva) for _____. (See
Box 13.3)**
Le examinaré las encías para buscar _____. (Vea el Cuadro 13.3)
(Audio 13.21)

(Gum/Gingival) tissues should not bleed when touched.
Los tejidos (de las encías/gingivales) no deben sangrar cuando se
tocan. (Audio 13.22)

(Gums/Gingiva) should not bleed when brushed and flossed.
Las encías no deben sangrar cuando se cepilla y usa hilo dental.
(Audio 13.23)

Do your gums bleed when you brush, floss, or eat?
¿Le sangran las encías cuando se cepilla, se limpia con hilo dental,
o come? (Audio 13.24)

Box 13.3
Common periodontal findings (Audio 13.79)

- Attrition (Audio 13.80)
- Bleeding (Audio 13.81)
- Cleft (Audio 13.82)
- Deposits (Audio 13.83)
- Exposed roots (Audio 13.84)
- Gingivitis (Audio 13.85)
- Gum boil (abscess) (Audio 13.86)
- Gum defect (Audio 13.87)
- Horizontal bone loss (Audio 13.88)
- Infection (Audio 13.89)
- Inflammation (Audio 13.90)
- Periodontal disease (Audio 13.91)
- Plaque (Audio 13.92)
- Pockets (Audio 13.93)
- Pus (suppuration) (Audio 13.94)
- Recession (Audio 13.95)
- Staining (Audio 13.96)
- Tartar (calculus) (Audio 13.97)
- Vertical bone loss (Audio 13.98)

Cuadro 13.3
Resultados periodontales comunes (Audio 13.79)

- Desgaste (Audio 13.80)
- Sangrado (Audio 13.81)
- Hendidura (Audio 13.82)
- Depósitos (Audio 13.83)
- Raíces expuestas (Audio 13.84)
- Gingivitis (Audio 13.85)
- Flemón (absceso) (Audio 13.86)
- Defectos de las encías (Audio 13.87)
- Pérdida de hueso horizontal (Audio 13.88)
- Infección (Audio 13.89)
- Inflamación (Audio 13.90)
- Enfermedad periodontal (Audio 13.91)
- Placa bacteriana (Audio 13.92)
- Bolsillos/bolsa periodontal (Audio 13.93)
- Pus (supuración) (Audio 13.94)
- Recesión (Audio 13.95)
- Mancha (Audio 13.96)
- Sarro (cálculo) (Audio 13.97)
- Pérdida de hueso vertical (Audio 13.98)

This is a sign of disease.
Esto es un síntoma de enfermedad. (Audio 13.25)

Are you happy with the way your (gums/gingiva) look?
¿Le gusta como lucen sus encías? (Audio 13.26)

Are you comfortable while I (examine/probe) your (gums/gingiva)?

¿Se siente cómodo(a) mientras le (examino/exploro) las encías? (Audio 13.27)

Let me know if you are uncomfortable while I (examine/probe) your (gums/gingiva).

Hágame saber si está incómodo(a) mientras le (examino/exploro) las encías. (Audio 13.28)

I will be gentle in examining your (gums/gingiva).

Seré cuidadoso(a) mientras le examino las encías. (Audio 13.29)

Along with the exam, we will be taking radiographs in order to determine your (gum/gingival) health.

Junto con el examen, le tomaremos radiografías para determinar la salud (de sus encías/gingival). (Audio 13.30)

I will be using a special probe to check around your implant.

Usaré una sonda especial para examinar alrededor del implante. (Audio 13.31)

Do your gums (bleed/have pus)? Here?

¿Sus encías (sangran/tienen pus)? ¿Aquí? (Audio 13.32)

Do you have (tartar/calculus) buildup? Where?

¿Tiene acumulación de (sarro/cálculo)? ¿Dónde? (Audio 13.33)

Do you have a bad taste in your mouth? Where?

¿Tiene mal sabor en la boca? ¿Dónde? (Audio 13.34)

I will be checking your teeth for movement.

Le examinaré los dientes para ver si se mueven. (Audio 13.35)

Do any of your teeth move when you use them?

¿Alguno de sus dientes se mueve cuando los usa? (Audio 13.36)

Do you feel movement with your implant?

¿Siente movimiento con su implante? (Audio 13.37)

Have you had (an abscess/a gum boil) here?

¿Ha tenido un (absceso/flemón) aquí? (Audio 13.38)

Have you had (gum/gingival) surgery? (Where/When)?

¿Ha tenido cirugía en las encías? ¿(Dónde/Cuándo)? (Audio 13.39)

Have you ever had a (scaling/root planning/deep cleaning)? (Where/When)?
¿Ha tenido alguna vez un (raspado/alisado radicular/limpieza profunda)? ¿(Dónde/Cuándo)? (Audio 13.40)

Your (gum/periodontal) charting will be stored in our computer.
Guardaremos su hoja clínica (para sus encías/periodontal) en nuestra computadora. (Audio 13.41)

Here's a (mirror/camera); let's look at your (gums/gingiva).
Aquí tiene (un espejo/una cámara); miremos sus encías. (Audio 13.42)

DISCUSSION OF FINDINGS
DISCUSIÓN DE LOS RESULTADOS (AUDIO 13.43)

I found _____ when I examined your (gums/gingiva). (See Box 13.3)
Encontré _____ cuando le examiné las encías. (Vea el Cuadro 13.3) (Audio 13.44)

Do you know you have _____? (See Box 13.3)
¿Usted sabe que tiene _____? (Vea el Cuadro 13.3) (Audio 13.45)

You have a pocket between the tooth and (gums/gingiva).
Usted tiene un bolsillo entre el diente y las encías. (Audio 13.46)

Your gum tissues bleed easily when I touch them with my instrument.
Los tejidos de sus encías sangran fácilmente cuando los toco con mi instrumento. (Audio 13.47)

You have a bone defect caused by periodontal disease.
Usted tiene un defecto al hueso causado por la enfermedad periodontal. (Audio 13.48)

You have _____ (tartar/calculus). (See Box 13.4)
Usted tiene (sarro/cálculo) _____. (Vea el Cuadro 13.4) (Audio 13.49)

You have _____ staining. (See Box 13.4)
Usted tiene manchas _____. (Vea el Cuadro 13.4) (Audio 13.50)

Box 13.4
Common descriptions of (tartar/staining/bone loss) (Audio 13.99)

- Slight (Audio 13.100)
- Moderate (Audio 13.101)
- Heavy (Audio 13.102)
- Localized (Audio 13.103)
- Generalized (Audio 13.104)

- Horizontal (Audio 13.105)
- Vertical (Audio 13.106)

Cuadro 13.4
Descripciones comunes de (sarro/manchas/ pérdida de hueso) (Audio 13.99)

- Leve (Audio 13.100)
- Moderado (Audio 13.101)
- Severo(a) (Audio 13.102)
- Localizado(a) (Audio 13.103)
- Generalizado(a) (Audio 13.104)

- Horizontal (Audio 13.105)
- Vertical (Audio 13.106)

You have _____ bone loss. (See Box 13.4)
Usted tiene pérdida de hueso _____. (Vea el Cuadro 13.4) (Audio 13.51)

You have _____ areas of bone loss. (See Box 13.4)
Usted tiene áreas de pérdida de hueso _____. (Vea el Cuadro 13.4) (Audio 13.52)

PERIODONTAL TREATMENT PLANNING
PLANIFICACIÓN DEL TRATAMIENTO PERIODONTAL (AUDIO 13.53)

We have determined that you have periodontal disease, and we need to treat it now.
Hemos determinado que usted tiene enfermedad periodontal, y necesitamos tratarla ahora. (Audio 13.54)

We will schedule you for a special procedure called scaling and root planing.
Le programaremos una cita para un procedimiento especial llamado raspado y alisado radicular. (Audio 13.55)

We can use an anesthetic to make you comfortable during this procedure.
Podemos utilizar un anestésico para que se sienta cómodo(a) durante este procedimiento. (Audio 13.56)

We will use (scalers/an ultrasonic scaler/special dental cleaning instruments) for scaling and root planing.
Utilizaremos (una cureta/una cureta ultrasónica/instrumentos de limpieza dental especiales) para el raspado y alisado radicular. (Audio 13.57)

After scaling and root planing, the (gum/gingival) tissue will heal and tightly fit itself to the tooth surface.
Después del raspado y alisado radicular, el tejido (de las encía/gingival) se sanará y se ajustará firmemente a la superficie del diente. (Audio 13.58)

You will need to come in more frequently for your dental cleanings.
Usted necesitará venir con más frecuencia para sus limpiezas dentales. (Audio 13.59)

We will monitor your healing (to/to try to) prevent further bone destruction.
Supervisaremos su curación (para/para intentar) prevenir la destrucción adicional del hueso. (Audio 13.60)

You need to have periodontal surgery.
Usted necesita cirugía periodontal. (Audio 13.61)

You need to brush and floss (as we have shown you/every day/to prevent periodontal disease).
Necesita cepillarse los dientes y usar hilo dental (como le hemos mostrado/todos los días/para prevenir la enfermedad periodontal). (Audio 13.62)

Chapter 14
Endodontics

Capítulo 14
Endodoncia (Audio 14.1)

ENDODONTIC EXAMINATION
EXAMEN DE ENDODONCIA (AUDIO 14.2)

**We will refer you to an endodontist for _____. (See
Box 14.1)**
Lo(a) referiremos a un(a) endodoncista para _____. (Vea el Cuadro
14.1) (Audio 14.3 new)

I will be checking the vitality of your tooth.
Examinaré la vitalidad de su diente. (Audio 14.4)

I will check your tooth to see if it is alive.
Revisaré su diente para ver si está vivo. (Audio 14.5)

I will be using a machine to check the vitality of your tooth.
Usaré una máquina para examinar la vitalidad de su diente.
(Audio 14.6)

Are you in pain?
¿Tiene dolor? (Audio 14.7)

Box 14.1 **Reasons to refer** **a patient to** **an endodontist** **(Audio 14.49)**	**Cuadro 14.1** **Razones para referir** **a un(a) paciente a** **un(a) endodoncista** **(Audio 14.49)**

• Treatment (Audio 14.50)
• A root canal
  (Audio 14.51)
• An evaluation (Audio 14.52)
• A second opinion
  (Audio 14.53)
• Apicoectomy (Audio 14.54)
	• Tratamiento (Audio 14.50)
	• Un tratamiento de conducto/
	  endodoncia (Audio 14.51)
	• Una evaluación (Audio 14.52)
	• Una segunda opinión
	  (Audio 14.53)
	• Apicectomía (Audio 14.54)

How would you describe your pain? Rate your pain on a scale of 1 to 10, with 1 being the least painful.
¿Cómo describiría su dolor? Clasifique su dolor en una escala del uno al diez, el uno siendo el 1 el nivel más bajo de dolor. (Audio 14.8)

Do you have pain when you bite on this tooth?
¿Siente dolor cuando muerde con este diente? (Audio 14.9)

Do you have pain when I tap here? Here?
¿Le duele cuando le doy golpecitos aquí? ¿Aquí? (Audio 14.10)
Do you have pain in the tooth with _____? (See Box 14.2)
¿Siente dolor en el diente con _____? (Vea el Cuadro 14.2)
(Audio 14.11)

Do you have pain when I place ice here? Here?
¿Siente dolor cuando le coloco hielo aquí? ¿Aquí? (Audio 14.12)

I am going to perform an ice test on your tooth. Raise your left hand when you feel cold. Then lower your hand once the cold goes away.
Voy a realizar una prueba de hielo en su diente. Levanta la mano izquierda cuando sientas frío. Luego baja la mano una vez que el frío desaparezca. (Audio 14.13)

Do you have pain when I place heat here? Here?
¿Siente dolor cuando le pongo algo caliente aquí? ¿Aquí? (Audio 14.14)

Box 14.2 Things that teeth can be sensitive to (Audio 14.55)	**Cuadro 14.2 Cosas a las que los dientes pueden ser sensibles (Audio 14.55)**
• Air (Audio 14.56)	• Aire (Audio 14.56)
• Biting (Audio 14.57)	• Morder (Audio 14.57)
• Cold (Audio 14.58)	• Frío (Audio 14.58)
• Drinking (Audio 14.59)	• Beber (Audio 14.59)
• Hot (Audio 14.60)	• Caliente (Audio 14.60)
• Sweets (Audio 14.61)	• Dulces (Audio 14.61)
• Sour things (Audio 14.62)	• Cosas amargas (Audio 14.62)

Where does it hurt? Show me. Point to it.
¿Dónde le duele? Enséñeme. Señálelo. (Audio 14.15)

Is that the only place it hurts?
¿Es ése el único lugar que le duele? (Audio 14.16)

Where else does it hurt? Show me. Point to it.
¿Dónde más le duele? Enséñeme. Señálelo. (Audio 14.17)

Where does it hurt the most? Here?
¿Dónde le duele más? ¿Aquí? (Audio 14.18)

I will need to take radiographs of your mouth.
Necesitaré tomar radiografías de su boca. (Audio 14.19)

DISCUSSION OF FINDINGS
DISCUSIÓN DE LOS RESULTADOS (AUDIO 14.20)

You have an abscess of this tooth.
Usted tiene un absceso en este diente. (Audio 14.21)

You have an infection in this tooth.
Usted tiene una infección en este diente. (Audio 14.22)

The cavity has infected the pulp of this tooth.
La caries dental ha infectado la pulpa de este diente. (Audio 14.23)

The crack on this tooth has let bacteria infect the pulp of the tooth.
La grieta en este diente ha dejado que las bacterias infecten la pulpa del diente. (Audio 14.24)

ENDODONTIC TREATMENT PLANNING
PLANIFICACIÓN DEL TRATAMIENTO DE ENDODONCIA (AUDIO 14.25)

You need to have a root canal. (See Figure 14.1)
Es necesario que le hagamos un (endodoncia/conducto radicular). (Vea la Imagen 14.1) (Audio 14.26)

A root canal will treat the (infection/abscess).
Un(a) (endodoncia/conducto radicular) tratará (la infección/el absceso). (Audio 14.27)

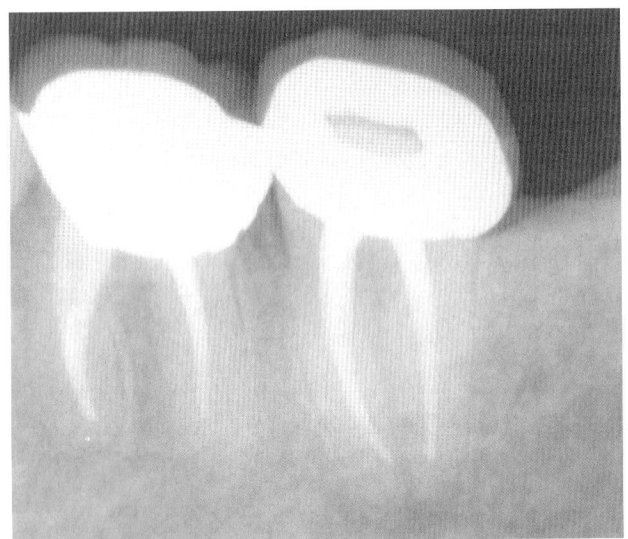

Fig. 14.1 (Imagen 14.1) Root canal. Endodoncia. *(From Torabinejad: Endodontics, 6e, Elsevier.)*

Without treatment you may (lose/have to extract) this tooth.
Sin el tratamiento quizás (pierda/tengamos que extraer) este diente. (Audio 14.28)

This infection will not go away without treatment.
Esta infección no se irá sin tratamiento. (Audio 14.29)

ENDODONTIC TREATMENT
TERAPIA DE ENDODONCIA (AUDIO 14.30)

Within the tooth is a chamber (pulp chamber) containing nerves, blood vessels, and other tissues.
Dentro del diente hay una cámara (cámara pulpar) que contiene nervios, vasos sanguíneos, y otros tejidos. (Audio 14.31)

Here is a picture of the interior of the tooth.
Esta es una ilustración del interior del diente. (Audio 14.32)

This is called the pulp.
Esto se llama pulpa. (Audio 14.33)

The pulp will be removed, and the inside of the tooth will be cleaned.
La pulpa será eliminada, y limpiaremos el interior del diente. (Audio 14.34)

To do this, we will use specialized instruments called files.
Para hacer esto, usaremos instrumentos especializados llamados limas. (Audio 14.35)

This procedure will take _____ appointments.
Este procedimiento tomará _____ citas. (Audio 14.36)

We will (anesthetize/numb) the tooth before starting.
(Anestesiaremos/Adormeceremos) el diente antes de comenzar. (Audio 14.37)

We need to (isolate/protect) the tooth from saliva by using a rubber sheet called a dam.
Necesitamos (aislar/proteger) el diente de la saliva con una hoja de hule llamada dique. (Audio 14.38)

Medication will be placed into this tooth for _____ days.
Se colocará medicamento en este diente por _____ días. (Audio 14.39)

I will need to take a radiograph of this tooth.
Necesitaré tomar una radiografía de este diente. (Audio 14.40)

This is a temporary filling in the tooth.
Ésta es una (empaste/relleno/calza) temporal para el diente. (Audio 14.41)

You need to see your dentist for a permanent filling.
Usted necesita ver a su dentista para un(a) (empaste/relleno/calza) permanente. (Audio 14.42)

A tooth that has had a root canal can become brittle and will require a crown to strengthen it.

Un diente que ha tenido (tratamiento de conducto/una endodoncia) puede volverse frágil y requerirá una corona para fortalecerlo. (Audio 14.43)

This root-canalled tooth will need a post and core before we can place a crown on it.
Este diente con (endodoncia/tratamiento de conducto) necesitará un poste y una base antes que podamos colocarle una corona. (Audio 14.44)

Be careful not to bite hard things with this tooth until a crown has been placed on it.
No muerda cosas duras con este diente hasta que se le coloque una corona. (Audio 14.45)

The fee for the root canal does not include the fee for the crown.
El costo de(l) la (endodoncia/tratamiento de conducto radicular) no incluye el costo de la corona. (Audio 14.46)

It is not unusual for a tooth to remain slightly sensitive for a few days following root canal treatment.
No es inusual que un diente quede levemente sensible por algunos días después (del tratamiento de conducto /de una endodoncia). (Audio 14.47)

You should not experience any looseness, swelling, drainage, or throbbing pain in this tooth. If you do, call our office right away.
Usted no debería experimentar ninguna flojedad, hinchazón, drenaje o dolor punzante en este diente. Si esto ocurriera, llame a nuestra oficina inmediatamente. (Audio 14.48)

Chapter 15
Pediatric Dentistry (Pedodontics)

Capítulo 15
Odontología Pediátrica (Odontopediatría) (Audio 15.1)

CONVERSING WITH CHILDREN
CONVERSANDO CON LOS NIÑOS (AUDIO 15.2)

Come with me.
Ven conmigo. (Audio 15.3)

Hold my hand.
Dame la mano. (Audio 15.4)

How old are you?
¿Cuántos años tienes? (Audio 15.5)

You look so nice today.
Te ves muy lindo(a) hoy. (Audio 15.6)

I like your (dress/shirt/shoes).
Me gusta(n) (tu traje/tu camisa/tus zapatos). (Audio 15.7)

(Climb/jump) into the chair.
Súbete a la silla. (Audio 15.8)

Let me show you how this chair works.
Déjame enseñarte cómo funciona esta silla. (Audio 15.9)

The chair goes up and down, like this.
Esta silla se sube y se baja, así. (Audio 15.10)

Let me tell you what we will be doing today.
Déjame contarte qué haremos hoy. (Audio 15.11)

Open (wide/wider).
Abre (grande/más grande). (Audio 15.12)

Do you know how many teeth you have? Let's count them. Hold this mirror.
¿Sabes cuántos dientes tienes? Vamos a contarlos. Aguanta este espejo. (Audio 15.13)

This is a little water fountain. It sprays water on your tooth.
Ésta es una pequeña fuente de agua. Rocía agua en tu diente.
(Audio 15.14)

This is air. I am going to spray some on your tooth to dry it.
Esto es aire. Voy a rociar aire en tu diente para secarlo. (Audio 15.15)

This is a bright light. It will help us to see better. Would you like to wear special sunglasses?
Ésta es una luz brillante. Nos ayudará a ver mejor. ¿Te gustaría usar unas (gafas/lentes de sol) especiales? (Audio 15.16)

Let me show you how this works.
Déjame mostrarte cómo funciona esto. (Audio 15.17)

This is a piece of cotton. It is soft and will keep your teeth dry.
Éste es un pedazo de algodón. Es suave y mantendrá tus dientes secos. (Audio 15.18)

This is a tooth pillow (bite block). It is soft and helps our mouth rest.
Esta es una almohada para los dientes. Es suave y ayuda a que nuestra boca descanse. (Audio 15.18b)

I am going to use this little toothpick to count your teeth.
Voy a usar este palillo pequeño para contar tus dientes.
(Audio 15.19)

Sugar bugs form on your teeth every day.
Los gusanos de azucar se forman en tus dientes todos los días.
(Audio 15.20)

Let's look at the plaque bugs I stained on your teeth!
Miremos a los microbios de placa que teñí en tus dientes!
(Audio 15.21)

Plaque bugs can cause holes in your teeth.
Los microbios de la placa pueden causar hoyos en tus dientes.
(Audio 15.22)

These holes in your teeth need to be repaired by the dentist.
Estos hoyos en tus dientes necesitan ser reparados por (el/la) dentista. (Audio 15.23)

Let's put a cover on your teeth to protect them.
Coloquemos una cubierta sobre tus dientes para protegerlos.
(Audio 15.24)

Let's paint vitamins on your teeth to make them strong.
Pintemos vitaminas en tus dientes para hacerlos fuertes.
(Audio 15.25)

We are going to put your tooth to sleep with some sleepy juice. Your tooth will feel tingly just like when your foot or leg falls asleep.
Vamos a poner tu diente a dormir con un poco de jugo para adormecer. Vas a sentir un hormigueo en el diente igual a cuando se te duerme el pie o la pierna. (Audio 15.26)

We are going to take this little piece of rubber and put it over your tooth.
Vamos a tomar este pedacito de goma y colocarlo sobre tu diente.
(Audio 15.27)

It is called a rubber dam. It is like a raincoat for your tooth.
Se llama dique de goma. Es como un impermeable para tu diente.
(Audio 15.28)

You are a good helper.
Qué buen ayudante eres. (Audio 15.29)

Thank you for being so good.
Gracias por ser tan bueno(a). (Audio 15.30)

CONVERSING WITH PARENTS
CONVERSANDO CON LOS PADRES (AUDIO 15.31)

Habits started young are important for keeping good dental health throughout life.
Los hábitos que se inician en la juventud son importantes para mantener una buena salud dental a lo largo de la vida. (Audio 15.32)

Thumb sucking can cause changes in your child's biting pattern.
El chuparse el dedo puede causar cambios en la mordedura de su niño(a). (Audio 15.33)

Long-term use of a pacifier can cause changes in your child's biting pattern.
El uso prolongado del chupete puede causar cambios en la mordedura de su niño(a). (Audio 15.34)

Here are some tablets for your child to chew that will stain the plaque. Be sure that he/she spits them out after chewing them.
Aquí tiene algunas tabletas para que su niño(a) mastique que van a teñir la placa. Asegúrese de que él/ella las escupa después de masticarlas. (Audio 15.35)

(Baby/Primary) teeth begin to erupt by the age of 6 to 8 months.
Los dientes (de leche/primarios) comienzan a salir a la edad de 6 a 8 meses. (Audio 15.36)

All the primary teeth have erupted by the age of 29 months.
Todos los dientes primarios ya han salido para la edad de 29 meses. (Audio 15.37)

(Baby/Primary) teeth are important to the health of the (adult/permanent) teeth.
Los dientes (de leche/primarios) son importantes para mantener la salud de los dientes (de adulto/permanentes). (Audio 15.38)

Early loss of (baby/primary) teeth can cause crowding of (adult/permanent) teeth.
La pérdida prematura de los dientes (de leche/primarios) puede causar que se apilen los dientes (de adulto/permanentes). (Audio 15.39)

At six years old, your child's first adult tooth comes in behind their baby teeth.
A los seis años, el primer diente adulto de su niño(a) sale detrás de los dientes (de leche/primarios). (Audio 15.40)

A child should first visit the dentist as an infant. We will let you know how to care for your baby's mouth and teeth. We will tell you what to expect as the child grows.
La primera visita al dentista de un(a) niño(a) debe ser de infante. Le diremos cómo cuidar la boca y dientes de su bebé. Le diremos qué esperar a medida que (el niño/la niña) crece. (Audio 15.41)

Until a child is _____ years old, it is the parents' job to brush and floss the child's teeth.
Hasta que un(a) niño(a) tiene _____ años de edad, es el trabajo de los padres cepillarle y limpiarle los dientes con hilo dental. (Audio 15.42)

Do not use threats as a way of getting your child to brush: for example, "If you don't brush, you'll have to go to the dentist."
No use amenazas como una manera de hacer que su niño(a) se cepille, por ejemplo: "Si no te cepillas, tendrás que ir al dentista." (Audio 15.43)

We see children for their first dental experience when they are around _____ years of age. It depends on when the child is ready.
Nosotros vemos a los niños para su primera experiencia dental alrededor de los _____ años de edad. Depende de cuando el niño esté listo. (Audio 15.44)

On the child's first visit, the dentist will check for cavities and growth problems.
En la primera visita (del niño/de la niña), el/la dentista le examinará para buscar caries y problemas de crecimiento. (Audio 15.45)

Speak positively about dentistry and dental experiences around your child.
Hable positivamente acerca de la odontología y las experiencias dentales alrededor de su niño(a). (Audio 15.46)

(I/The dentist/The office) will help you keep your healthy smile! Smile!
(Yo le ayudaré/(El/La dentista/La oficina) le ayudará) a mantener su sonrisa saludable! Sonría! (Audio 15.47)

TEETHING
DENTICIÓN (AUDIO 15.48)

When babies are teething, they can have sore gums.
Cuando los bebés les están saliendo los dientes, pueden tener dolor de encías. (Audio 15.49)

Keeping the gums and teeth free of plaque can reduce teething discomfort.
El mantener las encías y los dientes limpios de placa puede reducir el malestar de la dentición. (Audio 15.50)

The teething pain can be soothed by rubbing your baby's gums with a clean finger; a small, cool spoon; or a wet cloth.
El dolor de la dentición se puede aliviar frotando las encías de su bebé con un dedo limpio; una cuchara pequeña y fría; o un paño mojado. (Audio 15.51)

A clean teething ring for your baby to chew on may help.
Un anillo de dentición para que su bebé muerda puede ayudar. (Audio 15.52)

BRUSHING AND CHILDREN
EL CEPILLADO Y LOS NIÑOS (AUDIO 15.53)

Before your child has teeth, gently wipe the gum area with a soft, wet cloth wrapped over your finger.
Antes de que su niño(a) tenga dientes, limpie suavemente el área de la encía con un paño suave y mojado enrollado alrededor de su dedo. (Audio 15.54)

Start brushing your child's teeth with water as soon as the first tooth appears.
Comience a cepillar los dientes de su niño(a) con agua tan pronto como aparezca el primer diente.(Audio 15.55)

Brush your child's teeth twice daily until the child can thoroughly remove plaque.
Cepille los dientes de su niño(a) dos veces al día hasta que el/la niño(a) pueda remover la placa completamente. (Audio 15.56)

Your child can use toothpaste when the dentist recommends it.
Su niño(a) puede usar pasta dental cuando el/la dentista lo recomiende. (Audio 15.57)

Your child is too young for toothpaste.
Su niño(a) es demasiado pequeño(a) para usar pasta dental. (Audio 15.58)

For safety, monitor your child's use of toothpaste.
Por seguridad, vigile cuando su niño(a) usa pasta dental.
(Audio 15.59)

If ingested in large amounts, toothpaste can harm your child.
Si se ingiere en cantidades grandes, la pasta dental puede hacerle daño a su niño(a). (Audio 15.60)

If you show your child that you brush, it is more likely that he/she will brush too.
Si usted le muestra a su niño(a) que usted se cepilla, es más probable que él/ella también se cepille. (Audio 15.61)

You will need to show your child how to brush his/her teeth.
Usted necesitará mostrarle a su niño(a) cómo cepillarse los dientes. (Audio 15.62)

Watch your child's brushing until you're certain that he/she is doing it correctly.
Observe el cepillado de su niño(a) hasta que usted esté seguro(a) de que él/ella lo está haciendo correctamente. (Audio 15.63)

I will be showing your child how to brush his/her teeth.
Le mostraré a su niño(a) cómo cepillarse los dientes. (Audio 15.64)

We need to brush the plaque bugs off your teeth.
Nos cepillamos para sacar a los microbios de la placa de los dientes. (Audio 15.65)

You need to brush your teeth after breakfast and lunch and before bed.
Debes cepillarte los dientes después del desayuno y el almuerzo y antes de acostarte. (Audio 15.66)

Let's brush the stained plaque bugs off your teeth!
Cepillemos a los microbios de la placa teñidos de tus dientes! (Audio 15.67)

Brush all your teeth using big circles with your toothbrush.
Cepilla todos tus dientes haciendo círculos grandes con tu cepillo de dientes. (Audio 15.68)

CARIES
CARIES (AUDIO 15.69)

Putting sugared drinks in a baby bottle causes tooth decay.
El poner bebidas azucaradas en el biberón causa caries dental.
(Audio 15.70)

Sealants can protect the chewing surfaces of permanent teeth from decay.
Los selladores pueden proteger las superficies de mascar de los dientes permanentes de las caries. (Audio 15.71)

Never put a child to bed with a bottle containing any liquid except water.
Nunca acueste a un(a) niño(a) a dormir con un biberón que contenga cualquier líquido excepto agua. (Audio 15.72) (Fig 15.1)

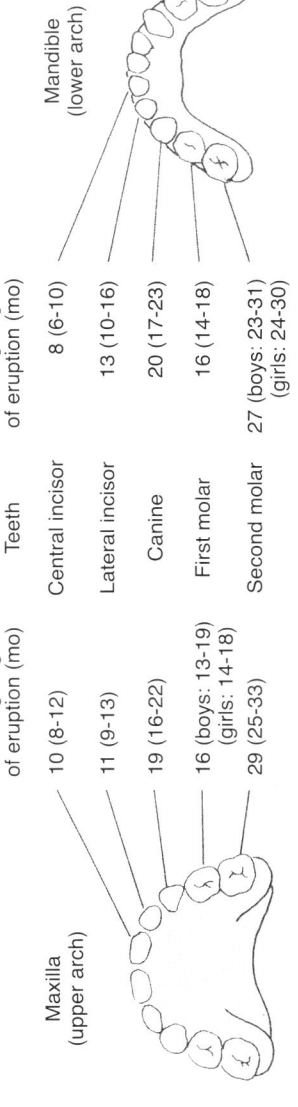

Fig. 15.1 Eruption sequence. *(From Wong's Nursing Care of Infants and Children, Eleventh Edition, Elsevier, 2018.)*

Chapter 16
Orthodontics

Capítulo 16
Ortodoncia (Audio 16.1)

ORTHODONTIC EXAMINATION
EXAMEN ORTODÓNTICO (AUDIO 16.2)

We will refer you to an orthodontist for _____. (See Box 16.1)
Lo(a) vamos a referir a un(a) ortodoncista para _____. (Vea el Cuadro 16.1) (Audio 16.3)

Would you like to improve your (smile/bite)?
¿Le gustaría mejorar su (sonrisa/mordedura)? (Audio 16.4)

Would you like to have better-looking teeth?
¿Le gustaría mejorar la apariencia de sus dientes? (Audio 16.5)

Do you think your teeth are (crooked/well aligned)?
¿Piensa que sus dientes están (torcidos/bien alineados)? (Audio 16.6)

Box 16.1
Reasons to refer a patient to an orthodontist
(Audio 16.52)

- A second opinion (Audio 16.53)
- An evaluation (Audio 16.54)
- Braces (Audio 16.55)
- Treatment (Audio 16.56)
- Uprighting (a molar/molars) (Audio 16.57)

Cuadro 16.1
Razones para referir a un(a) paciente a un(a) ortodoncista
(Audio 16.52)

- Una segunda opinión (Audio 16.53)
- Una evaluación (Audio 16.54)
- Frenillos/frenos/brackets (Audio 16.55)
- Tratamiento (Audio 16.56)
- Enderezar (un molar/molares) (Audio 16.57)

(Do you/Does your child) have any problems with the temporomandibular joint?
¿(Usted/Su niño(a)) tiene algún problema con la coyuntura temporomandibular? (Audio 16.7)

I will need to take impressions for study models.
Necesitaré tomar impresiones para modelos de estudio. (Audio 16.8)

The impression will need to stay in your mouth for _____ minutes until it is set.
La impresión debe permanecer en su boca por _____ minutos hasta que esté lista. (Audio 16.9)

I will need to take radiographs of your mouth and head.
Necesitaré tomar radiografías de su boca y cabeza. (Audio 16.10)

DISCUSSION OF FINDINGS
DISCUSIÓN DE LOS RESULTADOS (AUDIO 16.11)

(You/Your child) have/has _____. (See Box 16.2)
(Usted/Su niño(a)) tiene _____. (Vea el Cuadro 16.2) (Audio 16.12)

ORTHODONTIC TREATMENT PLANNING
PLANIFICACIÓN DEL TRATAMIENTO ORTODÓNTICO (AUDIO 16.13)

(You/Your child) will need to have (braces/teeth straightened).
(Usted/Su niño(a)) necesitará tener (frenillos/frenos/brackets/los dientes enderezados). (Audio 16.14)

Adults can wear braces too.
Los adultos también pueden usar (frenillos/frenos/brackets). (Audio 16.15)

(You/Your child) will need to wear braces for _____ (months/years).
(Usted/Su niño(a)) necesitará usar (frenillos/frenos/brackets) por _____ (meses/años). (Audio 16.16)

Box 16.2
Common orthodontic problems (Audio 16.58)

- Crossbite (Audio 16.59)
- Crowded teeth (Audio 16.60)
- Extra teeth (Audio 16.61)
- Missing teeth (Audio 16.62)
- Jaws that are out of alignment (Audio 16.63)
- Overbite (Audio 16.64)
- Overjet (Audio 16.65)

- Incorrect bite (Audio 16.66)

- Underbite (Audio 16.67)
- Tongue thrust (Audio 16.68)

- Spaces between the teeth (Audio 16.69)

Cuadro 16.2
Problemas ortodónticos comunes (Audio 16.58)

- Mordida cruzada (Audio 16.59)
- Dientes apiñados (Audio 16.60)
- Dientes adicionales (Audio 16.61)
- Dientes que faltan (Audio 16.62)
- (Mandíbulas/quijadas) desalineadas (Audio 16.63)
- Sobremordida (Audio 16.64)
- Sobremordida horizontal/ resalte (Audio 16.65)
- Mordida incorrecta (Audio 16.66)
- Submordida (Audio 16.67)
- Empuje de la lengua (Audio 16.68)
- Espacios entre los dientes (Audio 16.69)

(You/Your child) will need to wear headgear for _____ (weeks/months/hours per day).
(Usted/Su niño(a)) necesitará usar un aparato para la cabeza por _____ (semanas/meses/horas al día). (Audio 16.17)

(You need/Your child needs) to have a (space maintainer/ palatal expander/retainer).
(Usted/Su niño(a)) necesita un (mantenedor de espacio/expansor palatino/retenedor). (Audio 16.18)

(You need/Your child needs) to wear a (mouthguard/sports guard) to protect (your/his/her) teeth while playing sports.
(Usted/Su niño(a)) necesita usar (un protector/una guarda bucal/ una guarda deportiva) para proteger sus dientes mientras juega deportes. (Audio 16.19)

While (you are/your child is) in orthodontic treatment, thorough plaque removal is critical.
Mientras (usted/su niño(a)) está bajo tratamiento ortodóntico, es esencial remover la placa por completo. (Audio 16.20)

Avoiding certain (sticky/hard) foods is important while wearing braces.
El evitar alimentos (pegajosos/duros) es importante mientras usa (frenillos/frenos/brackets). (Audio 16.21)

ORTHODONTIC TREATMENT
TRATAMIENTO ORTODÓNTICO (AUDIO 16.22)

This is a picture of the braces that we will be putting on (your/your child's) teeth.
Ésta es una ilustración de los frenillos que le colocaremos a (usted/su niño(a)). (Audio 16.23)

Let me show you how we will attach the (brackets/bands) to (your/your child's) teeth. This will not hurt.
Permítame mostrarle cómo colocaremos (los brackets/las bandas) a (sus dientes/los dientes de su niño(a)). Esto no dolerá. (Audio 16.24)

Your teeth will feel different and will be sensitive for one to two days after we adjust your appliances.
Sus dientes se sentirán diferentes y estarán sensibles por uno a dos días después de que ajustemos los aparatos. (Audio 16.25)

You need to be careful with your appliances.
Usted necesita tener cuidado con sus aparatos. (Audio 16.26)

If a (bracket/band) comes loose, or if a wire gets bent, let us know right away.
Si (un bracket/una banda) se afloja, o si un alambre se tuerce, háganos saber inmediatamente. (Audio 16.27)

Let me show you how to attach an elastic band.
Permítame enseñarle cómo colocar una (banda/liga elástica). (Audio 16.28)

**To prevent tooth decay, you must brush your teeth _____
times every day as long as you have braces**.
Para prevenir caries, debe cepillarse los dientes _____ veces todos
los días mientras tenga (frenillos/frenos/brackets). (Audio 16.29)

Here is how you clean around the braces.
Así es cómo se limpia alrededor de los (frenillos/frenos/brackets).
(Audio 16.30)

**You need to rinse with this special mouthwash _____ times
every day**.
Usted necesita enjuagarse con este enjuague especial _____ veces al
día. (Audio 16.31)

ORAL SELF-CARE FOR ORTHODONTIC PATIENTS
CUIDADO ORAL PROPIO PARA PACIENTES
ORTODÓNTICOS (AUDIO 16.32)

**This is the most important time in your life for putting
extra effort into the care of your teeth**.
Éste es el momento más importante en su vida para poner esfuerzo
adicional en el cuidado de sus dientes. (Audio 16.33)

**At this point in your child's life, it is very important that he/
she take care to remove all of the plaque in his/her mouth**.
En este punto en la vida de su niño(a), es muy importante que él/ella
se concentre en remover toda la placa de su boca. (Audio 16.34)

**This is a good time to look at your child's teeth every day.
If the teeth don't look clean, send your child back to the
bathroom to brush again until they do look clean**.
Éste es un buen momento para que examine los dientes de su
niño(a) todos los días. Si los dientes no se ven limpios, envíe a su
niño(a) al baño nuevamente para que se los cepille de nuevo, hasta
que se vean limpios. (Audio 16.35)

**This is a time when a child has many interests, and personal
hygiene is not always one of them**.
Éste es un momento en que un(a) niño(a) tiene muchos intereses, y
la higiene personal no es siempre uno de ellos. (Audio 16.36)

Without extra care, serious problems can occur. It is not an easy task to keep teeth clean when braces are in place.

Sin un cuidado especial, pueden ocurrir problemas graves. No es fácil mantener limpios los dientes cuando hay (frenillos/frenos/ brackets). (Audio 16.37)

The (brackets/appliances) attached to the teeth trap food that will harm (your/your child's) teeth. This trapped food will become plaque, which will dissolve, decay, and rot your teeth. Plaque is a cause of mouth odor.

Los (brackets/aparatos) colocados en los dientes atrapan comida, la que dañarán (sus dientes/los dientes de su niño(a)). Esta comida atrapada se convertirá en placa, que disolverá, deteriorará, y pudrirá sus dientes. La placa es una causa del mal aliento. (Audio 16.38)

If you do not care for (your/your child's), teeth it can be expensive to fix them.

Si usted no cuida (sus dientes/los dientes de su niño(a)), puede ser muy caro arreglarlos. (Audio 16.39)

The sugars in food are especially harmful at this time. Avoid sugary liquids, such as soda, and even juice and milk, unless you brush or rinse right after.

Los azúcares en la comida son especialmente dañinos en este momento. Evite los líquidos con azúcar, tales como la soda e incluso el jugo y la leche; a menos que usted se cepille o se enjuague inmediatamente después de tomarlos. (Audio 16.40)

Avoid sticky candy and gum of all types.

Evite los dulces pegajosos y el chicle (goma de mascar) de todo tipo. (Audio 16.41)

Avoid other hard or crunchy foods, such as popcorn, heavy chips, or nuts.

Evite otras comidas duras o crujientes, tales como las palomitas de maíz, papitas (patatas fritas), o nueces. (Audio 16.42)

Never go to bed without cleaning your teeth well. Bedtime is the most important time for removing all plaque.

Nunca se acueste sin limpiarse bien los dientes. La hora de acostarse es la hora más importante para remover toda la placa. (Audio 16.43)

We would like you to use this special brush to reach all parts of the tooth. We would like you to use this brush like so.

Nos gustaría que use este cepillo especial para alcanzar todas las partes del diente. Nos gustaría que usara el cepillo de esta manera. (Audio 16.44)

We would like you to try to floss around all of your teeth. We have a floss threader that you will use to get through the wires.

Nos gustaría que trate de usar el hilo dental alrededor de todos sus dientes. Tenemos un enhebrador de hilo dental que usted usará para pasar a través de los alambres. (Audio 16.45)

We may recommend that you use a fluoride rinse. The rinse we would like you to use is _____;. You can purchase this in many types of stores without a prescription.

Es posible que le recomendemos que use un enjuague de fluoruro. El enjuague que quisiéramos que use es _____. Usted puede comprarlo en muchos tipos de tienda sin receta. (Audio 16.46)

We may recommend that you use a special, high-concentration fluoride toothpaste. This toothpaste is called _____ and it is available with a prescription. We will make this (toothpaste/fluoride rinse) available to you at a cost of _____ dollars.

Es posible que le recomendemos que use una pasta de dientes especial con una alta concentración de fluoruro. Esta pasta de dientes se llama _____, y está disponible con receta. Le podremos dar (esta pasta de dientes/este enjuague de fluoruro) a un costo de _____ dólares. (Audio 16.47)

After you use these fluoride products, do not eat, rinse, or drink for at least 30 minutes. A good time for the extra fluoride is immediately before you go to bed.

Después de usar estos productos de fluoruro, no coma, se enjuague, o beba durante al menos 30 minutos. Una buena hora para el fluoruro es inmediatamente antes de acostarse. (Audio 16.48)

With braces, it is somewhat harder to brush and floss, but you will need to do it.

Con (frenillos/frenos/brackets) es un poco más difícil cepillarse y usar hilo dental, pero debe hacerlo. (Audio 16.49)

Braces are hard to brush, but not brushing around braces can lead to (caries/tooth decay) or (gum disease/ periodontal disease).

Los (frenillos/frenos/brackets) son difíciles de cepillar, pero el no cepillar alrededor de los (frenillos/frenos/brackets) puede causar (caries/descomposición dental) o (enfermedad de las encías/ enfermedad periodontal). (Audio 16.50)

Brush your retainer twice daily to remove the plaque that forms on it.

Cepille su retenedor dos veces al día para remover la placa que se forma en él. (Audio 16.51)

Capítulo 17
Patología Oral(Bucal)/Medicina Oral(Bucal) (Audio 17.1)

MEDICAL-DENTAL CONNECTION AND CANCER TREATMENT
CONEXIÓN MÉDICO-DENTAL Y EL TRATAMIENTO PARA EL CÁNCER (AUDIO 17.2)

We will work with your (medical doctor/cancer specialist).
Trabajaremos con su (doctor(a)/especialista en cáncer). (Audio 17.3)

One's mouth should be healthy before one starts cancer treatment.
Su boca debe estar sana antes de comenzar tratamiento para el cáncer. (Audio 17.4)

The dentist will need to extract that tooth before cancer treatment starts.
El/La dentista necesitará extraer ese diente antes de comenzar con el tratamiento para el cáncer. (Audio 17.5)

Your teeth will need to be cleaned prior to cancer treatment.
Antes de comenzar el tratamiento para el cáncer debemos limpiarle los dientes. (Audio 17.6)

Cancer treatment can lead to increased _____. (See Box 17.1)
El tratamiento para el cáncer puede resultar en un aumento de _____. (Vea el Cuadro 17.1) (Audio 17.7)

Since you had cancer treatment, have you been having any problems with your mouth?
Desde que recibió tratamiento para el cáncer,¿ha tenido algún problema en la boca? (Audio 17.8)

Box 17.1
Possible side effects of cancer treatment (Audio 17.63)

- Bone infection (Audio 17.64)
- Caries/cavities (Audio 17.65)
- Dry mouth (Audio 17.66)
- Mouth sores (mucositis) (Audio 17.67)
- Tooth decay (Audio 17.68)

Cuadro 17.1
Los efectos secundarios posibles del tratamiento para el cáncer (Audio 17.63)

- Infección del hueso (Audio 17.64)
- Caries/cavidades (Audio 17.65)
- Boca reseca (Audio 17.66)
- Llagas en la boca (mucositis) (Audio 17.67)
- Descomposición de los dientes (Audio 17.68)

MEDICAL-DENTAL CONNECTION AND XEROSTOMIA (DRY MOUTH)
CONEXIÓN MÉDICO-DENTAL Y LA XEROSTOMÍA (BOCA RESECA) (AUDIO 17.9)

Medicine can cause dry mouth.
El medicamento puede causar boca reseca. (Audio 17.10)

Menopause can be a cause of dry mouth.
La menopausia puede ser una causa de la boca reseca. (Audio 17.11)

Mouth breathing can cause dry mouth.
El respirar por la boca puede causar boca reseca. (Audio 17.12)

Dry mouth can lead to increased _____. (See Box 17.2)
La boca reseca puede resultar en un aumento de _____. (Vea el Cuadro 17.2) (Audio 17.13)

Taking frequent sips of water during the day can alleviate the symptoms of dry mouth.
El beber pequeños tragos de agua frecuentemente durante el día puede aliviar los síntomas de la boca reseca. (Audio 17.14)

Box 17.2
Possible results of a dry mouth problem (Audio 17.69)

- Caries/cavities (Audio 17.70)

- Tooth decay (Audio 17.71)

- Gum/periodontal disease (Audio 17.72)

Cuadro 17.2
Resultados posibles del problema de boca reseca (Audio 17.69)

- Caries/cavidades (Audio 17.70)
- Descomposición de los dientes (Audio 17.71)
- Enfermedad de las encías/periodontal (Audio 17.72)

Drinking more water can help your dry mouth.
El beber más agua puede ayudar con la boca reseca. (Audio 17.15)

Mouthwashes with alcohol can cause soreness if your mouth is already dry.
Los enjuagues con alcohol pueden causar dolor si su boca ya está reseca. (Audio 17.16)

Do not suck on (sugared/sour) candy for your dry mouth.
No chupe dulces (azucarados/amargos) para la boca reseca. (Audio 17.17)

Many products are available for the relief of dry mouth.
Hay muchos productos disponibles para aliviar la boca reseca. (Audio 17.18)

Our (office/clinic) recommends these products for dry mouth.
Nuestra (oficina/clínica) recomienda estos productos para la boca reseca. (Audio 17.19)

Here's a sample product to treat your dry mouth.
Aquí tiene un producto de muestra para tratar su boca seca. (Audio 17.20)

MEDICAL-DENTAL CONNECTION AND DIABETES
CONEXIÓN MÉDICO-DENTAL Y LA DIABETES (AUDIO 17.21)

Diabetes delays normal healing after infection.
La diabetes retrasa la curación normal después de una infección. (Audio 17.22)

Diabetes can cause dry mouth.
La diabetes puede causar boca reseca. (Audio 17.23)

Diabetes increases the risk of gum disease.
La diabetes aumenta el riesgo de enfermedad de las encías. (Audio 17.24)

Regulating your blood sugar can reduce your risk of (gum/ periodontal) disease.
Regular el nivel de azúcar en la sangre puede reducir su riesgo de enfermedad (de las encías/periodontal). (Audio 17.25)

Controlling gum disease in your mouth can help you control your diabetes.
El controlar la enfermedad de las encías en su boca puede ayudarle a controlar su diabetes. (Audio 17.26)

Taking your diabetes medicine can keep your gums healthy.
El tomar sus medicamentos para la diabetes puede mantener sus encías saludables. (Audio 17.27)

MEDICAL-DENTAL CONNECTION AND SYSTEMIC DISEASE
CONEXIÓN MÉDICO-DENTAL Y LA ENFERMEDAD SISTÉMICA (AUDIO 17.28)

(Gum/Periodontal) disease increases the risk of (heart disease/stroke).
La enfermedad (de las encías/periodontal) aumenta el riesgo de (enfermedad del corazón/apoplejía). (Audio 17.29)

The bacteria associated with (gum/periodontal) disease are also associated with the development of dementia.
Las bacterias asociadas con la enfermedad (de las encías/periodontal) también están asociadas con el desarrollo de demencia. (Audio 17.30)

Medicine for the heart can cause increased bleeding during dental treatment.
La medicina para el corazón puede causar un aumento en el sangrado durante el tratamiento dental. (Audio 17.31)

Medicine for the heart can cause gum growth.
Los medicamentos para el corazón pueden provocar el crecimiento de las encías. (Audio 17.32)

Stomach problems can cause excess acid in your mouth.
Los problemas estomacales pueden causar exceso de ácido en la boca. (Audio 17.33)

Excess stomach acid in your mouth can cause (tooth decay/throat cancer).
El exceso de ácido del estómago en la boca puede causar (caries de los dientes/cáncer de la garganta). (Audio 17.34)

You need to get your acid reflux under control in order to protect your oral and systemic health.
Usted necesita tener su reflujo de ácido bajo control para proteger su salud oral y sistémica. (Audio 17.35)

BACTERIAL ENDOCARDITIS
ENDOCARDITIS BACTERIANA (AUDIO 17.36)

There are health conditions that can lead to a sluggish valve in your heart. If bacteria are introduced into your bloodstream, there is a chance that these bacteria will lodge in that sluggish valve and cause an inflammation of the lining of your heart. For that reason, if you have been diagnosed with any of the following conditions, you will need to be premedicated before some or all types of dental treatment.

Hay condiciones de salud que pueden causar que una válvula en su corazón trabaje más lentamente. Si se introducen bacterias en el torrente sanguíneo, existe la posibilidad de que estas bacterias se alojen en la válvula lenta y causen una inflamación en el revestimiento interno del corazón. Por esto, si le ha diagnosticado cualquiera de las siguientes condiciones, usted necesitará tomar una premedicación antes de algunos o todos los tipos de tratamiento dental. (Audio 17.37)

You have a condition in your heart that can lead to serious illness unless you take this (antibiotic/medication) before we treat you. Not taking these pills can cause serious illness, hospitalization, or even death.
Usted tiene una condición en su corazón que puede causar una enfermedad seria si no toma este (antibiótico/medicamento) antes de que le tratemos. El no tomar estas pastillas puede causar una enfermedad seria, hospitalización o hasta la muerte. (Audio 17.38)

We can give you a brochure explaining the importance of this medication.
Le podemos dar un folleto que explica la importancia de este medicamento. (Audio 17.39)

In order to prevent a condition called bacterial endocarditis, we follow the guidelines for premedication established by the American Heart Association.
Para prevenir la condición llamada endocarditis bacteriana, seguimos las guías para la premedicación establecidas por la Asociación Americana del Corazón. (Audio 17.40)

The condition that you have requiring this premedication is _____. (See Box 17.3)
La condición que usted tiene que requiere de esta premedicación es _____. (Vea el Cuadro 17.3) (Audio 17.41)

An item on your medical history indicates that we need more information about your _____.
Una entrada en su historial médico indica que necesitamos más información sobre su _____. (Audio 17.42)

We will need to call your physician to discuss premedication for the following condition: _____.
Necesitaremos llamar a su médico(a) para discutir la premedicación para la siguiente condición: _____. (Audio 17.43)

Box 17.3
Conditions requiring premedication before some or all dental treatment (Audio 17.73)

- Mitral valve prolapse (Audio 17.74)
- A replacement heart valve (Audio 17.75)
- Replacement joint, hip, or knee (Audio 17.76)
- Rheumatic heart disease (Audio 17.77)
- A history of subacute bacterial endocarditis (Audio 17.78)
- Intravascular access device (for chemotherapy, hemodialysis, or hyperalimentation) (Audio 17.79)
- Cerebrospinal fluid shunt (Audio 17.80)
- Hypertrophic cardiomyopathy (Audio 17.81)
- Complex cyanotic congenital heart disease (Audio 17.82)

Cuadro 17.3
Condiciones que requieren premedicación antes de algún o todo tratamiento dental (Audio 17.73)

- El prolapso de la válvula mitral (Audio 17.74)
- El reemplazo de una válvula del corazón (Audio 17.75)
- El reemplazo de una articulación, cadera, o rodilla (Audio 17.76)
- La enfermedad reumática del corazón (Audio 17.77)
- Un historial de endocarditis bacteriana subagudo (Audio 17.78)
- El dispositivo de acceso intravascular (por la quimoterapia, hemodiálisis, hiperalimentación) (Audio 17.79)
- El desvio del fluido cerebroespinal (Audio 17.80)
- La miocardiopatía hipertrófica (Audio 17.81)
- La cardiopatia congénita cianótica compleja (Audio 17.82)

We will keep the prescription information in your record so that we can help you by giving you a refill prescription.
Mantendremos la información de la receta en su historial para que le podamos ayudar dándole una receta de relleno. (Audio 17.44)

We will call in this prescription to your pharmacy.
Llamaremos para enviar esta receta a su farmacia. (Audio 17.45)

Do you have the phone number of your (pharmacy/ physician)?
¿Tiene el número de teléfono de su (farmacia/médico(a))? (Audio 17.46)

Do you know the name and location of your (pharmacy/ physician)?
¿Conoce el nombre y ubicación de su (farmacia/médico(a))? (Audio 17.47)

We will ask you to premedicate with this antibiotic called _____.
Le pediremos que tome esta premedicación del antibiótico llamado _____. (Audio 17.48)

You must take it _____ hours before treatment. Take _____ pills.
Usted lo debe tomar _____ horas antes del tratamiento. Tome _____ pastillas. (Audio 17.49)

We will not be able to treat you today without the premedication.
No le podremos tratar hoy sin la premedicación. (Audio 17.50)

We are happy to answer any questions that you might have.
Con gusto contestaremos cualquier pregunta que tenga. (Audio 17.51)

MEDICAL-DENTAL CONNECTION AND WOMEN'S ORAL HEALTH
CONEXIÓN MÉDICO-DENTAL Y LA SALUD ORAL DE LAS MUJERES (AUDIO 17.52)

_____ can affect the gums. (See Box 17.4)
_____ puede(n) afectar las encías. (Vea el Cuadro 17.4) (Audio 17.53)

Calcium is important for jaw health.
El calcio es importante para la salud de la mandíbula. (Audio 17.54)

Changes in a woman's hormones can cause an overreaction to plaque.
Los cambios en las hormonas de la mujer pueden causar una reacción excesiva a la placa. (Audio 17.55)

Box 17.4
Female health concerns that can affect the gums (Audio 17.83)

- Birth control pills (Audio 17.84)
- Estrogen (Audio 17.85)
- Hormone replacement (Audio 17.86)
- Hormone replacement therapy (Audio 17.87)
- Hormones (Audio 17.88)
- Menopause (Audio 17.89)
- Menses (Audio 17.90)
- Periods (Audio 17.91)
- Pregnancy (Audio 17.92)
- Progesterone (Audio 17.93)
- Puberty (Audio 17.94)
- Steroids (Audio 17.95)

Cuadro 17.4
Problemas de la salud femenina que pueden afectar las encías (Audio 17.83)

- Las pastillas anticonceptivas (Audio 17.84)
- El estrógeno (Audio 17.85)
- El reemplazo hormonal (Audio 17.86)
- La terapia para el reemplazo hormonal (Audio 17.87)
- Las hormonas (Audio 17.88)
- La menopausia (Audio 17.89)
- La menstruación (Audio 17.90)
- Los períodos (Audio 17.91)
- El embarazo (Audio 17.92)
- La progesterona (Audio 17.93)
- La pubertad (Audio 17.94)
- Los esteroides (Audio 17.95)

Changes in a woman's hormones can cause the gums to be red, to be sore, or to bleed.
Los cambios en las hormonas de la mujer pueden causar que las encías se pongan rojas y adoloridas, o que sangren. (Audio 17.56)

(Gum/Periodontal) disease can lead to (low-birth-weight/ premature) babies.
La enfermedad (de las encías/periodontal) puede causar que los bebés nazcan (con un peso natal bajo/prematuros). (Audio 17.57)

Teeth are lost due not to pregnancy but to other factors.
Los dientes no se pierden a causa del embarazo, sino a causa de otros factores. (Audio 17.58)

Your health during pregnancy can affect your baby's teeth.
Su salud durante el embarazo puede afectar los dientes de su bebé. (Audio 17.59)

Due to your pregnancy, we need to check with your medical doctor.
Debido a su embarazo, necesitamos hablar con su doctor(a). (Audio 17.60)

Due to the medicine, you need to wait _____ hours before nursing.
Debido a la medicina, usted debe esperar _____ horas antes de dar pecho. (Audio 17.61)

We recommend that you pump your breast milk and dispose of it for up to _____ hours after taking the medicine.
Le recomendamos que extraiga su leche materna y la deseche hasta por _____ horas después de tomar la medicina. (Audio 17.62)

Chapter 18
Oral Radiology

Capítulo 18
Radiología Oral (Audio 18.1)

Many diseases of the teeth can't be seen when your dentist (looks at/examines) your mouth.
Muchas enfermedades de los dientes no pueden verse cuando su dentista (observa/examina) su boca. (Audio 18.2)

Radiographs can detect damage not visible during a regular exam.
Las radiografías pueden detectar el daño no visible durante un examen regular. (Audio 18.3)

We need to take some intraoral radiographs to see if there are any (cavities/bone loss).
Necesitamos tomar algunas radiografías intraorales para ver si hay (caries/pérdida de hueso). (Audio 18.4)

Radiographs also help us record your dental health.
Las radiografías también pueden ayudarnos a registrar su salud dental. (Audio 18.5)

When did you last have radiographs taken?
¿Cuándo fue la última vez que le tomaron radiografías? (Audio 18.6)

What types of radiographs were taken? What part was included?
¿Qué tipos de radiografías le tomaron? ¿Qué parte fue incluida? (Audio 18.7)

Can you have your radiographs sent to us?
¿Puede hacer que nos envíen sus radiografías? (Audio 18.8)

We will need your permission to have radiographs (sent/taken).
Necesitaremos su permiso para que las radiografías sean (enviadas/tomadas). (Audio 18.9)

We need to take a complete series of radiographs (about ___ images).
Necesitamos tomar una serie completa de radiografías (alrededor de _____ imágenes). (Audio 18.10)

A complete series of radiographs shows the teeth and jawbone.
Una serie completa de radiografías muestra los dientes y el hueso de la mandíbula. (Audio 18.11)

We need to take bitewings (about ___ images).
Necesitamos tomar radiografías interproximales (alrededor de _____ imágenes). (Audio 18.12)

Bitewings can show tooth decay between the teeth.
Las radiografías interproximales pueden mostrar caries entre los dientes. (Audio 18.13)

We need to take radiographs of the root of the tooth.
Necesitamos tomar radiografías de la raíz del diente. (Audio 18.14)

We need to take a (pan/panoramic) radiograph.
Necesitamos tomar una radiografía panorámica. (Audio 18.15)

We need to take a radiograph of your entire mouth, teeth, and bone structure.
Necesitamos tomar una radiografía de toda la boca, los dientes y huesos. (Audio 18.16)

The panoramic radiograph shows (jawbones/third molars/ wisdom teeth).
La radiografía panorámica muestra (los huesos de la mandíbula/ los terceros molares/las muelas cordales/las muelas de juicio). (Audio 18.17)

The panoramic radiograph does not provide a detailed view of your teeth and jaws.
La radiografía panorámica no proporciona una vista detallada de sus dientes y su mandíbula. (Audio 18.18)

The dentist can't treat you properly if you refuse to take the radiograph.
El/La dentista no puede tratarle apropiadamente si usted se niega a tomarse las radiografías. (Audio 18.19)

Without radiographs, we cannot do a proper and complete dental exam.
Sin radiografías no podemos hacer un examen dental adecuado y completo. (Audio 18.20)

After the appropriate radiographs, I can develop a treatment plan.
Después de tener las radiografías apropiadas, yo podré desarrollar un plan de tratamiento. (Audio 18.21)

RADIOGRAPHIC PROCEDURES
PROCEDIMIENTOS RADIOGRÁFICOS (AUDIO 18.22)

Please remove your ___. (See Box 18.1)
Por favor quítese su(s) _____. (Vea el Cuadro 18.1) (Audio 18.23)

I will place the lead apron on you as a protection.
Le colocaré el delantal de plomo como protección. (Audio 18.24)

Box 18.1 Common items that patients must remove during radiographic procedures (Audio 18.62)	**Cuadro 18.1 Artículos comunes que los pacientes deben quitarse durante los procedimientos radiográficos (Audio 18.62)**

- Appliance (Audio 18.63)
- Cap/hat (Audio 18.64)
- Denture (Audio 18.65)

- Earring (Audio 18.66)

- Glasses (Audio 18.67)

- Lipstick (Audio 18.68)
- Necklace (Audio 18.69)
- Retainer (Audio 18.70)

- Aparato (Audio 18.63)
- Gorro/gorra (Audio 18.64)
- Dentadura/caja postiza/placa (Audio 18.65)
- Arete/pendiente/aros (Audio 18.66)
- Gafas/lentes/anteojos (Audio 18.67)
- Lápiz labial (Audio 18.68)
- Collar/cadena (Audio 18.69)
- Retenedor (Audio 18.70)

A lead apron is no longer recommended for radiographs.
Ya no se recomienda el uso de un delantal de plomo para las
radiografías. (Audio 18.25)

**No one except the patient can be in the room during the
x-ray examination**.
Nadie excepto el paciente puede estar en el cuarto durante el
examen radiográfico. (Audio 18.26)

**For my protection, I will be leaving the room during the
x-ray examination**.
Para mi protección, saldré del cuarto durante el examen
radiográfico. (Audio 18.27)

Do you gag when getting dental radiographs?
¿Le dan náuseas cuando le hacen radiografías dentales? (Audio 18.28)

**We will use (nitrous oxide/topical spray) to help keep you
from gagging**.
Usaremos (óxido nitroso/anestésico tópico) para prevenirle las
náuseas. (Audio 18.29)

I need to place the x-ray sensor here.
Necesito colocar el sensor de radiografías aquí. (Audio 18.30)

**It may be uncomfortable, but it will be only for a short
time**.
Puede ser incómodo, pero será sólo por un momento. (Audio 18.31)

**Bite down slowly on the sensor (guide/holder/packet) and
hold your bite**.
Muerda lentamente en el sensor (guía/esta agarradera/este paquete)
y mantenga la mordida. (Audio 18.32)

Put your chin here and hold it.
Coloque la barbilla aquí y mantela. (Audio 18.33)

(Lower/Raise) your chin.
(Suba/Baje) la barbilla. (Audio 18.34)

Hold still for the radiographs.
Manténgase quieto(a) para las radiografías. (Audio 18.35)

Movement can make the radiographs useless.
El movimiento puede inutilizar las radiografías. (Audio 18.36)

Breathe through your nose while we take the radiographs.
Respire por la nariz mientras le tomamos las radiografías.
(Audio 18.37)

The machine will rotate around you while it takes the radiographs.
La máquina rotará alrededor de usted mientras toma las radiografías.
(Audio 18.38)

The machine will rotate for ___ seconds.
La máquina rotará por _____ segundos. (Audio 18.39)

Place your tongue on the roof of your mouth while the machine rotates around you.
Coloque la lengua en el (cielo/techo) de su boca mientras la máquina gira alrededor de usted. (Audio 18.40)

Put your tongue on the roof of your mouth.
Ponga su lengua contra el (paladar/techo de su boca). (Audio 18.41)

The machine will not touch you while taking radiographs.
La máquina no le tocará mientras está tomando las radiografías.
(Audio 18.42)

You will not feel the x-ray as I take the radiograph.
Usted no sentirá los rayos-x mientras tomo la radiografía. (Audio 18.43)

Are you comfortable with the sensor?
¿Está cómodo(a) con el sensor? (Audio 18.44)

Let me know if you are not comfortable while I am taking the radiograph.
Hágame saber si no está cómodo(a) mientras tomo la radiografía.
(Audio 18.45)

I will be gentle when taking the radiograph.
Seré cuidadoso(a) mientras tomo la radiografía. (Audio 18.46)

We had a (developing/positioning) error and need to retake the radiograph.
Tuvimos un error de (revelado/posición) y necesitamos volver a tomar la radiografía. (Audio 18.47)

We need to retake the radiograph.
Necesitamos volver a tomar la radiografía. (Audio 18.48)

We will be taking periodic radiographs of you every _____ (years/months).
Le tomaremos radiografías periódicamente cada _____ (años/meses). (Audio 18.49)

Due to your high risk for (caries/periodontal disease), we will need to take radiographs more often.
Debido a su alto riesgo de (caries/enfermedad periodontal), necesitaremos tomar radiografías con más frecuencia. (Audio 18.50)

We will mount your radiograph.
Montaremos su radiografía. (Audio 18.51)

We use digital radiographs, which are the latest technology.
Usaremos radiografías digitales, que son la última tecnología. (Audio 18.52)

You will receive less radiation with digital radiographs.
Recibirá menos radiación con las radiografías digitales. (Audio 18.53)

Our computer will store your digital radiographs.
Nuestra computadora guardará sus radiografías digitales. (Audio 18.54)

Let's look at your radiographs.
Miremos sus radiografías. (Audio 18.55)

When taking radiographs, we take every precaution for your safety.
Cuando tomamos radiografías, tomamos todas las precauciones para su seguridad. (Audio 18.56)

We use the latest technology and most appropriately sized sensors in order to reduce the number of radiographs needed.
Utilizamos lo más nuevo en tecnología y sensores de tamaño más adecuado para reducir el número de radiografías necesarias. (Audio 18.57)

We follow the manufacturer's recommendations for taking and processing the radiographs.
Nosotros seguimos las recomendaciones del fabricante para tomar y procesar las radiografías. (Audio 18.58)

DISCUSSION OF RADIOGRAPHIC FINDINGS
DISCUSIÓN DE LOS RESULTADOS
RADIOGRÁFICOS (AUDIO 18.59)

A radiograph may show ___. (See Box 18.2)
Una radiografía puede mostrar _____. (Vea el Cuadro 18.2)
(Audio 18.60)

Look at this/these ___ on the radiograph. (See Box 18.2)
Observe (este/esta/estos) _____ en la radiografía. (Vea el
Cuadro 18.2) (Audio 18.61)

Box 18.2 **Common radiographic** **findings (Audio 18.71)**	**Cuadro 18.2** **Hallazgos radiográficos** **comunes (Audio 18.71)**

• Abscess (Audio 18.72)
• Horizontal bone loss
  (Audio 18.73)
• Vertical bone loss
  (Audio 18.74)
• Bone density (Audio 18.75)
 	
• Cyst (Audio 18.76)
• Dark area (radiolucency)
  (radiolucent)
  (Audio 18.77)
• Developmental problem
  (Audio 18.78)
• Extra teeth (supernumerary)
  (Audio 18.79)
 	
• Filling (restoration)
  (Audio 18.80)
• Gum disease (periodontal
  disease) (Audio 18.81)
	• Absceso (Audio 18.72)
	• Pérdida de hueso horizontal
	  (Audio 18.73)
	• Pérdida de hueso vertical
	  (Audio 18.74)
	• Densidad de hueso
	  (Audio 18.75)
	• Quiste (Audio 18.76)
	• Área oscura (radiolucidez)
	  (radiotransparente)
	  (Audio 18.77)
	• Problemas de desarrollo
	  (Audio 18.78)
	• Dientes adicionales
	  (supernumeraries)
	  (Audio 18.79)
	• Empaste/relleno/calza
	  (restauración) (Audio 18.80)
	• Enfermedad de las encías
	  (enfermedad periodontal)
	  (Audio 18.81)

(Continued)

Box 18.2
Common radiographic findings—cont'd

- Infection in the bone (Audio 18.82)
- Implant (Audio 18.83)
- Impacted tooth (Audio 18.84)
- Tooth decay around filling (caries around filling) (Audio 18.85)

- Tooth decay between the teeth (caries between the teeth) (Audio 18.86)
- Tumor (cancer) (Audio 18.87)
- Unerupted tooth (Audio 18.88)
- Widening of the periodontal ligament (Audio 18.89)

- White area (radiopacity) (radiopaque) (Audio 18.90)
- Wisdom teeth (third molars) (Audio 18.91)

Cuadro 18.2
Hallazgos radiográficos comunes—continuación

- Infección del hueso (Audio 18.82)
- Implante (Audio 18.83)
- Diente impactado (Audio 18.84)
- Caries dental alrededor de el empaste/relleno/calza (caries alrededor del empaste) (Audio 18.85)
- Caries dental entre los dientes (caries entre los dientes) (Audio 18.86)
- Tumor (cáncer) (Audio 18.87)
- Diente retenido (Audio 18.88)
- Ensanchamiento del ligamento periodontal (Audio 18.89)
- Área blanca (radioopacidad) (radioopaco) (Audio 18.90)
- Muelas cordales/muelas del juicio (terceros molares) (Audio 18.91)

Chapter 19
Consultation and Referral

Capítulo 19
Consulta y Referencia (Audio 19.1)

We will need to consult a(n) _____ before we proceed with dental treatment. (See Box 19.1)

Necesitaremos consultar con un(a) _____ antes de proceder con el tratamiento dental. (Vea el Cuadro 19.1) (Audio 19.2)

Due to your health, we will need to refer you to a(n) _____, who will be better able to treat you. (See Box 19.1)

Debido a su salud, necesitaremos enviarle a un(a) _____, quien será más capacitado(a) para tratarle. (Vea el Cuadro 19.1) (Audio 19.3)

Box 19.1
Types of specialists
(Audio 19.10)

- Braces specialist (orthodontist) (Audio 19.11)
- Dental specialist (Audio 19.12)
- General dentist (Audio 19.13)
- Denture specialist (prosthodontist) (Audio 19.14)
- Dermatologist (Audio 19.15)
- Gum specialist (periodontist) (Audio 19.16)
- Medical doctor (Audio 19.17)
- Oral surgeon (Audio 19.18)
- Root canal specialist (endodontist) (Audio 19.19)

Cuadro 19.1
Tipos de especialistas
(Audio 19.10)

- Especialista en frenillos (ortodoncista) (Audio 19.11)
- Especialista dental (Audio 19.12)
- Dentista general (Audio 19.13)
- Especialista en dentaduras (prostodoncista) (Audio 19.14)
- Dermatólogo(a) (Audio 19.15)
- Especialista en encías (periodoncista) (Audio 19.16)
- Doctor(a)/médico(a) (Audio 19.17)
- Cirujano(a) oral (Audio 19.18)
- Especialista en tratamientos de (endodoncia/conducto) (endodoncista) (Audio 19.19)

Have you ever been asked to visit a(n) _____? (See Box 19.1)
¿Alguna vez le han pedido que visite a un(a) _____? (Vea el Cuadro 19.1) (Audio 19.4)

Have you ever visited a(n) _____? (See Box 19.1)
¿Alguna vez ha visitado a un(a) _____? (Vea el Cuadro 19.1) (Audio 19.5)

Does your _____ know about this? (See Box 19.1)
¿Su _____ sabe acerca de esto? (Vea el Cuadro 19.1) (Audio 19.6)

We will need to refer you to a(n) _____. (See Box 19.1)
Necesitaremos enviarlo(a) a un(a) _____. (Vea el Cuadro 19.1) (Audio 19.7)

You need to sign this permission form so we can obtain information from the _____. (See Box 19.1)
Usted necesita firmar este formulario de permiso para que podamos obtener información del/de la _____. (Vea el Cuadro 19.1) (Audio 19.8)

You need to see your medical doctor about your high blood pressure (now/in) _____ (days/in) _____ weeks.
Necesita ver a su doctor(a) por su alta presión arterial (ahora/en) _____ (días/en) _____ semanas. (Audio 19.9)

PART III
Medical Terminology

PARTE III
Terminología Médica
(Audio 20.1)

Chapter 20
Review of Medical History

Capítulo 20
Revisión del Historial Médico (Audio 20.2)

TAKING A PATIENT HISTORY
REGISTRANDO EL HISTORIAL DEL PACIENTE
(AUDIO 20.3)

Dental History
Historial Dental (Audio 20.4)

Before we can treat you we need to have some information about your dental health. I will ask you a few questions that are on this questionnaire, and I can then complete the form for you.
Antes de que podamos tratarle, necesitamos tener cierta información sobre su salud dental. Le haré algunas preguntas de este cuestionario, y luego completaré el formulario por usted. (Audio 20.5)

Are you in any discomfort at this time? If yes, where is the discomfort?
¿Tiene algúna molestia en este momento? Si es así, ¿dónde tiene el malestar? (Audio 20.6)

What type of discomfort is it? Is it a sharp pain?
¿Qué tipo de malestar es? ¿Es un dolor agudo? (Audio 20.7)

Is this tooth sensitive to heat? Cold? When you bite?
¿Es este diente sensible a lo caliente? ¿Al frío? ¿Cuando muerdes? (Audio 20.8)

Has there been any (inflammation/swelling) in this area? Is it bleeding?
¿Ha habido alguna (inflamación/hinchazón) en esta área? ¿Le sangra? (Audio 20.9)

How long has it been bothering you? What relieves the discomfort?
¿Hace cuánto tiempo que le molesta? ¿Qué alivia el malestar? (Audio 20.10)

How long since you have been to a dentist?
¿Hace cuánto tiempo que no visitaba a un(a) dentista/odontolgo(a)?
(Audio 20.11)

What procedures were performed at that dental visit?
¿Qué procedimientos se realizaron en esa visita al dentista?
(Audio 20.12)

Did you have radiographs taken?
¿Le tomaron radiografías? (Audio 20.13)

How often did you visit a dentist before then?
¿Con qué frecuencia visitó a un dentista antes de ese entonces?
(Audio 20.14)

Have you lost any teeth? Why?
¿Ha perdido algún diente? ¿Por qué? (Audio 20.15)

Have the teeth that you lost ever been replaced? With a removable partial denture? Bridge? Full denture?
¿Han sido reemplazados los dientes que perdió? ¿Con una
dentadura (prótesis) parcial removible? ¿Puente? ¿Dentadura
(prótesis) completa? ¿Placa? (Audio 20.16)

Are your teeth sensitive to _____? (See Box 20.1)
¿Son sus dientes sensibles al/a lo/a los _____? (Vea el Cuadro 20.1)
(Audio 20.17)

Box 20.1 **Things that teeth can be sensitive to (Audio 20.159)**	**Cuadro 20.1** **Cosas a las que los dientes pueden ser sensibles (Audio 20.159)**
• Air (Audio 20.160)	• Aire (Audio 20.160)
• Biting (Audio 20.161)	• Morder (Audio 20.161)
• Cold (Audio 20.162)	• Frío (Audio 20.162)
• Drinking (Audio 20.163)	• Beber (Audio 20.163)
• Hot (Audio 20.164)	• Caliente (Audio 20.164)
• Sour things (Audio 20.165)	• Amargo (Audio 20.165)
• Sweets (Audio 20.166)	• Dulces (Audio 20.166)

Have you had your teeth straightened? When?
¿Le han enderezado los dientes? ¿Cuándo? (Audio 20.18)

How often do you brush your teeth?
¿Con qué frecuencia se cepilla los dientes? (Audio 20.19)

How do you brush your teeth?
¿Cómo se cepilla los dientes? (Audio 20.20)

How long do you use your toothbrush before replacing it?
¿Por cuánto tiempo usa su cepillo de dientes antes de reemplazarlo?
(Audio 20.21)

Do you use a between-the-teeth stimulator?
¿Usa un estimulador interdental? (Audio 20.22)

Do you use dental floss?
¿Usa hilo dental? (Audio 20.23)

Do you have bleeding gums? When?
¿Le sangran las encías? ¿Cuándo? (Audio 20.24)

Do you eat between meals?
¿Come entre comidas? (Audio 20.25)

Do you brush your teeth after eating snacks?
¿Se cepilla los dientes después de haber comido bocadillos?
(Audio 20.26)

Does food wedge between your teeth? Where?
¿Se acumula comida entre sus dientes? ¿Dónde? (Audio 20.27)

Do you grind or clench your teeth? When?
¿Rechina o aprieta los dientes? ¿Cuándo? (Audio 20.28)

Have you ever had gum treatments?
¿Ha tenido en algún momento tratamiento para las encías?
(Audio 20.29)

Do you feel you have had bad breath at times?
¿Sientes que tienes mal aliento en ocasiones? (Audio 20.30)

Do you sometimes have an unpleasant taste in your mouth?
¿Tiene a veces un sabor desagradable en la boca? (Audio 20.31)

Do you have any pain around your ears? Do you hear popping, clicking, or snapping noises when you chew?
¿Tiene algún dolor alrededor de los oídos? ¿Escucha sonidos como estallidos, chasquidos, o crujidos al masticar? (Audio 20.32)

Are you aware of any swelling or lumps in your mouth?
¿Sabe de alguna hinchazón o absceso en su boca? (Audio 20.33)

Do you have or have you ever had any of the following habits? (See Box 20.2)
¿Tiene o ha tenido alguno de los siguientes hábitos? (Vea el Cuadro 20.2) (Audio 20.34)

TREATMENT GOALS
OBJETIVOS DEL TRATAMIENTO (AUDIO 20.35)

How do you feel about your teeth?
¿Cómo se siente sobre sus dientes? (Audio 20.36)

Do you like the way your teeth look?
¿Le gusta como se ven sus dientes? (Audio 20.37)

Do you want to keep the natural teeth you have?
¿Quiere mantener los dientes naturales que tiene? (Audio 20.38)

Do you want to avoid dental discomfort you may have experienced in the past?
¿Quiere evitar las molestias dentales que puede haber experimentado en el pasado? (Audio 20.39)

Do you want to avoid dentures?
¿Quiere evitar las dentaduras (postizas)? (Audio 20.40)

Do you want to have pleasant breath?
¿Quiere tener un aliento agradable? (Audio 20.41)

If you have children, do you want to learn how to help them keep their teeth for a lifetime without discomfort?
Si tiene niños, ¿quiere aprender cómo ayudarles a conservar sus dientes toda la vida sin molestias? (Audio 20.42)

Box 20.2
Oral habits
(Audio 20.167)

- Biting fingernails
  (Audio 20.168)
- Biting hairpins
  (Audio 20.169)

- Biting lips (Audio 20.170)
- Biting thread (Audio 20.171)
- Cheek or tongue chewing
  (Audio 20.172)
- Chewing on pencils/pens
  (Audio 20.173)
- Chewing on seeds/nuts/ice
  (Audio 20.174)
- Drinking tea/coffee
  (Audio 20.175)
- Excessive gum chewing
  (Audio 20.176)
- Excessive mouth breathing
  (Audio 20.177)
- Finger sucking
  (Audio 20.178)
- Grinding/clenching
  (Audio 20.179)
- Mint/hard candy use
  (Audio 20.180)
- Opening containers/
  plastic bags with teeth
  (Audio 20.181)
- Thumb sucking
  (Audio 20.182)
- Tobacco use (Audio 20.183)

Cuadro 20.2
Hábitos orales
(Audio 20.167)

- Morderse las uñas
  (Audio 20.168)
- Morder horquillas/
  pasador/incaibles para pelo
  (Audio 20.169)
- Morderse los labios
  (Audio 20.170)
- Morder hilo (Audio 20.171)
- Masticarse las mejillas o la
  lengua (Audio 20.172)
- Masticar lápices/bolígrafos
  (Audio 20.173)
- Masticar semillas/nueces/
  hielo (Audio 20.174)
- Beber té/café (Audio 20.175)
- Masticar chicle excesivamente
  (Audio 20.176)
- Respirar por la boca en
  exceso (Audio 20.177)
- Chuparse los dedos
  (Audio 20.178)
- Rechinar/apretar
  (Audio 20.179)
- Uso de mentas/dulces duras
  (Audio 20.180)
- Abrir envases/bolsas
  plásticas con los dientes
  (Audio 20.181)
- Chuparse el dedo gordo
  (Audio 20.182)
- Uso de tabaco (Audio 20.183)

MEDICAL HISTORY
HISTORIAL MÉDICO (AUDIO 20.43)

We need to have some information about your general health. I am going to help you fill out this form, and I need to ask you some questions.
Necesitamos tener cierta información sobre su salud general. Yo le voy a ayudar a llenar este formulario, y necesito hacerle algunas preguntas. (Audio 20.44)

What was the date of your last physical examination?
¿Cuál fue la fecha de su último examen físico? (Audio 20.45)

Who is your (physician/medical doctor)?
¿Quién es su (médico(a)/doctor(a))? (Audio 20.46)

What is your birth date? Age?
¿Cuál es su fecha de nacimiento? ¿Edad? (Audio 20.47)

Do you have or have you had any of the following?
¿Usted tiene o ha tenido alguno de los siguientes? (Audio 20.48)

Any heart problems? If yes, when? What type of problems? Heart murmur? Pacemaker?
¿ Algún problema cardíaco? Si sí, ¿cuándo? ¿Qué tipo de problema? ¿Soplo cardíaco? ¿Marcapasos? (Audio 20.49)

Have you ever had rheumatic fever?
¿Ha tenido alguna vez fiebre reumática? (Audio 20.50)

Do you have any prosthetic devices?
¿Tiene algún aparato prostético? (Audio 20.51)

Have you ever been advised to take a premedication prior to dental treatment?
¿Le han aconsejado alguna vez que tome premedicación antes del tratamiento dental? (Audio 20.52)

Have you ever had hepatitis B? Hepatitis C?
¿Ha tenido alguna vez hepatitis B? ¿Hepatitis C? (Audio 20.53)

Do you have high blood pressure? If yes, are you on any medication? If yes, what are you taking, when, and how often?
¿Tiene la presión arterial alta? Si es así, ¿toma medicamentos? Si es así, ¿qué está tomando, cuándo, y con qué frecuencia? (Audio 20.54)

Do you have low blood pressure? If yes, are you being treated by a doctor? If yes, are you on any medication? If yes, what medication? How much and how often do you take it?
¿Tiene la presión arterial baja? En caso afirmativo, ¿está siendo tratado por un médico? Si sí, ¿está usted tomando algún medicamento? Si sí, ¿qué medicamento? ¿Cuánto y con qué frecuencia lo tomas? (Audio 20.55)

Do you have any circulatory problems? If yes, what type of problem are you having?
¿Tiene algún problema circulatorio? Si es así, ¿qué tipo de problema tiene? (Audio 20.56)

Do you have any nervous problems? If yes, what type of problem are you having?
¿Tiene algún problema nervioso? Si es así, ¿qué tipo de problema tiene? (Audio 20.57)

Have you ever had radiation treatment? If yes, when was the treatment? For what was the radiation treatment done?
¿Alguna vez ha recibido tratamiento de radiación? En caso afirmativo, ¿cuándo fue el tratamiento? ¿Para qué le hicieron el tratamiento de radiación? (Audio 20.58)

Have you ever experienced excessive bleeding? If yes, when and where?
¿Alguna vez ha experimentado sangrado excesivo? Si si, ¿cuándo y dónde? (Audio 20.59)

Have you been diagnosed with AIDS? When were you diagnosed? Are you under any treatment?
¿Ha sido diagnosticado(a) con SIDA? ¿Cuándo fue diagnosticado(a)? ¿Está bajo(a) algún tratamiento? (Audio 20.60)

MEDICATIONS AND ALLERGIES
MEDICAMENTOS Y ALERGIAS (AUDIO 20.61)

Are you currently taking any medication(s)? If yes, what is it?
¿Está tomando medicamento(s) actualmente? Si es así, ¿qué medicamento? (Audio 20.62)

Do you have any allergies to anesthetic? If yes, what type of anesthetic?
¿Tiene alergia a algún anestésico? Si es así, ¿a qué tipo de anestésico? (Audio 20.63)

Do you have any allergies to medicine or drugs? If yes, which ones?
¿Tiene alergia a algún medicamento o droga? Si sí, ¿a cuáles? (Audio 20.64)

Do you have any other allergies? If yes, what are they?
¿Tiene otras alergias? Si es así, ¿cuáles son? (Audio 20.65)

VITAL SIGNS
SIGNOS VITALES (AUDIO 20.66)

I will be taking your _____ to record a baseline reading. (See Box 20.3)
Le tomaré _____ para registrar una lectura de referencia. (Vea el Cuadro 20.3) (Audio 20.67)

Today's baseline reading for your _____ was not in the normal range; what do you think made this happen? (See Box 20.3)
La lectura inicial de hoy de _____ no estaba en el rango normal; ¿por qué cree que ocurrió esto? (Vea el Cuadro 20.3) (Audio 20.68)

A baseline reading that is not in the normal range may indicate _____. (See Box 20.4)
Una lectura inicial que no está en el rango normal puede indicar _____. (Vea el Cuadro 20.4) (Audio 20.69)

Temperature
Temperatura (Audio 20.70)

We use a disposable sheath over the thermometer for your protection.
Utilizaremos una funda desechable sobre el termómetro para su protección. (Audio 20.71)

Box 20.3
Types of health assessment readings (Audio 20.184)

- Blood pressure (Audio 20.185)
- Pulse (Audio 20.186)
- Respiration (Audio 20.187)
- Temperature (Audio 20.188)

Cuadro 20.3
Tipos de lecturas de evaluaciones de salud (Audio 20.184)

- La presión arterial (Audio 20.185)
- El pulso (Audio 20.186)
- La respiración (Audio 20.187)
- La temperatura (Audio 20.188)

Box 20.4
Types of problems that can be detected by an abnormal baseline reading (Audio 20.189)

- Health problems (Audio 20.190)
- A need for you to see your medical doctor (Audio 20.191)
- That you are not taking your medicine (Audio 20.192)
- An undiagnosed condition (Audio 20.193)

Cuadro 20.4
Tipos de problemas que pueden ser detectados por una lectura base anormal (Audio 20.189)

- Problemas de salud (Audio 20.190)
- La necesidad de ver a su doctor(a)/médico(a) (Audio 20.191)
- Que no se está tomando sus medicamentos (Audio 20.192)
- Una condición no diagnosticada (Audio 20.193)

Open your mouth, and I will place the thermometer under your tongue.
Abra la boca y colocaré el termómetro debajo de su lengua. (Audio 20.72)

Hold the thermometer with your lips closed.
Sostenga el termómetro con los labios cerrados. (Audio 20.73)

Don't bite the thermometer.
No muerda el termómetro. (Audio 20.74)

I will be leaving the thermometer in your mouth for 3 minutes.
Dejaré el termómetro en su boca por 3 minutos. (Audio 20.75)

Open your mouth so I can remove the thermometer.
Abra la boca para que yo pueda sacar el termómetro. (Audio 20.76)

I am going to place the thermometer in your ear.
Voy a colocar el termómetro en su oído. (Audio 20.77)

Your temperature today is _____ °(C/F).
Su temperatura de hoy es _____ °(C/F). (Audio 20.78)

Your temperature is (high/raised/normal).
Su temperatura está (alta/elevada/normal). (Audio 20.79)

A raised temperature can be a sign of infection.
Una temperatura elevada puede ser una señal de infección.
(Audio 20.80)

Pulse
Pulso (Audio 20.81)

To get a pulse, I need to hold your wrist with the palm down.
Para obtener un pulso, necesitaré sostener su muñeca con la palma hacia abajo. (Audio 20.82)

With my fingers, I will be applying slight, temporary pressure to your wrist in order to take your pulse.
Le aplicaré una presión leve y temporal en la muñeca con los dedos para tomarle el pulso. (Audio 20.83)

Your pulse today is _____ beats per minute.
Su pulso de hoy es _____ latidos por minuto. (Audio 20.84)

Your pulse today feels _____. (See Box 20.5)
Su pulso de hoy se siente _____. (Vea el Cuadro 20.5)
(Audio 20.85)

Respiration
Respiración (Audio 20.86)

Your respiration rate is _____ breaths per minute.
Su ritmo de respiración es _____ respiraciones por minuto.
(Audio 20.87)

**Box 20.5
Descriptions of pulse
and respiration
readings
(Audio 20.194)**

- Bounding (Audio 20.195)
- Fast (Audio 20.196)
- Faster (Audio 20.197)
- Irregular (Audio 20.198)
- Regular (Audio 20.199)
- Normal (Audio 20.200)
- Slow (Audio 20.201)
- Slower (Audio 20.202)
- Thready (Audio 20.203)
- Weak (Audio 20.204)

**Cuadro 20.5
Descripciones de
las lecturas de
pulso y respiración
(Audio 20.194)**

- Saltón (Audio 20.195)
- Rápido (Audio 20.196)
- Más rápido (Audio 20.197)
- Irregular (Audio 20.198)
- Regular (Audio 20.199)
- Normal (Audio 20.200)
- Lento (Audio 20.201)
- Más lento (Audio 20.202)
- Filiforme (Audio 20.203)
- Débil (Audio 20.204)

**Your respiration today was _____. Your respiration today
shows _____. (See Boxes 20.5 and 20.6)**
Su respiración hoy estaba _____. Su respiración hoy demuestra
_____. (Vea los Cuadros 20.5 y 20.6) (Audio 20.88)

Blood Pressure
Presión Arterial (Audio 20.89)

**To take your blood pressure, I will need your (left/right)
arm supported and the palm turned up**.
Para tomarle la presión arterial, necesitaré que apoye el brazo
(izquierdo/derecho) y que ponga la palma hacia arriba. (Audio 20.90)

**You need to expose your (left/right) arm fully before I can
take your blood pressure**.
Debe exponer completamente su brazo (izquierdo/derecho) antes
de que pueda tomarle la presión arterial. (Audio 20.91)

**(Push up/Roll up) your (left/right) shirt sleeve so I can take
your blood pressure**.
(Súbase/Enróllese) la manga (izquierda/derecha) para que pueda
tomarle la presión arterial. (Audio 20.92)

Box 20.6
Terms used to describe breathing (Audio 20.205)

- Dyspnea (Audio 20.206)
- Tachypnea (Audio 20.207)
- Hyperventilation (Audio 20.208)

Cuadro 20.6
Términos usados para describir la respiración (Audio 20.205)

- Disnea (Audio 20.206)
- Taquipnea (Audio 20.207)
- Hiperventilación (Audio 20.208)

Take off your jacket so I can take your blood pressure.
Quítese la chaqueta para que pueda tomarle la presión arterial. (Audio 20.93)

I will place this cuff over your arm in order to take your blood pressure.
Le colocaré este brazalete alrededor del brazo para tomarle la presión arterial. (Audio 20.94)

I will pump up this cuff so I can take your blood pressure.
Inflaré esta brazalete para tomarle la presión arterial. (Audio 20.95)

You will feel slight, temporary pressure on your arm while I take your blood pressure.
Sentirá una presión leve y temporal en su brazo mientras le tomo la presión arterial. (Audio 20.96)

I will put this meter on the inside of your elbow in order to take your blood pressure.
Le colocaré este metro sobre la parte interior del codo para tomarle la presión arterial. (Audio 20.97)

Do you have higher blood pressure in a doctor's office?
¿Tiene la presión arterial más alta en la oficina del médico? (Audio 20.98)

Do you get a "white coat" reading?
¿Usted obtiene una lectura de "bata blanca"? (Audio 20.99)

We will need to use another cuff to get a more accurate reading.
Necesitaremos usar otra brazalete de presion para obtener una lectura más precisa. (Audio 20.100)

I will place this blood pressure device over your wrist to take your reading automatically.
Le colocaré este aparato de presión arterial sobre la muñeca para obtener una lectura automáticamente. (Audio 20.101)

Your blood pressure reading is _____ over _____.
Su lectura de presión arterial es _____ sobre _____. (Audio 20.102)

The top figure is called the systolic, and it represents the heart at work.
La figura de arriba se llama sistólica, y representa al corazón trabajando. (Audio 20.103)

The lower figure is called the diastolic, and it represents the heart at rest.
La figura de abajo se llama diastólica, y representa al corazón en descanso. (Audio 20.104)

Your blood pressure today is _____.
Su presión arterial hoy es _____. (Audio 20.105)

You have a _____ blood pressure. (See Box 20.7)
Usted tiene una presión arterial _____. (Vea el Cuadro 20.7) (Audio 20.106)

Box 20.7 Descriptions of blood pressure readings (Audio 20.209)

- High (Audio 20.210)
- Higher (Audio 20.211)
- Increased (Audio 20.212)
- Low (Audio 20.213)
- Lower (Audio 20.214)
- Normal (Audio 20.215)
- Raised (Audio 20.216)

Cuadro 20.7 Descripciones de las lecturas de presión arterial (Audio 20.209)

- Alta (Audio 20.210)
- Más alta (Audio 20.211)
- Aumentada (Audio 20.212)
- Baja (Audio 20.213)
- Más baja (Audio 20.214)
- Normal (Audio 20.215)
- Elevada (Audio 20.216)

A high blood pressure reading may mean that you have hypertension.
Una lectura de presión arterial alta puede indicar que usted tiene hipertensión/presion alta. (Audio 20.107)

As a precaution, we will need to take your blood pressure (before/during/after) dental treatment.
Como precaución, necesitaremos tomarle la presión arterial (antes/durante/después) del tratamiento dental. (Audio 20.108)

Rest, and we will take your blood pressure again.
Descanse y le tomaremos la presión arterial nuevamente. (Audio 20.109)

EXTRAORAL ASSESSMENT
EVALUACIÓN EXTRAORAL (AUDIO 20.110)

I will be (examining/palpating) your _____ to get some information about your health. (See Box 20.8)
(Examinaré/Palparé) su _____ para obtener información sobre su salud. (Vea el Cuadro 20.8) (Audio 20.111)

For your protection I will be wearing gloves while I (examine/palpate) your _____. (See Box 20.8)
Para su protección, usaré guantes mientras le (examino/palpo) su _____. (Vea el Cuadro 20.8) (Audio 20.112)

With my fingers, I will be putting slight, temporary pressure on your face and neck in order to examine you.
Le pondré una presión leve y temporal con los dedos sobre su cara y cuello para examinarle. (Audio 20.113)

Remove your (hat/hearing aid/headphones/lipstick).
Quítese el (sombrero/audífono/audifonos/lápiz de labio/ lápiz labial). (Audio 20.114)

Loosen your tie.
Suéltese la corbata. (Audio 20.115)

Sit upright.
Siéntese derecho(a). (Audio 20.116)

Don't lean back.
No se recueste. (Audio 20.117)

Face me.
Míreme. (Audio 20.118)

Are you comfortable while I check your _____? (See Box 20.8)
¿Está cómodo(a) mientras le examino su _____? (Vea el
Cuadro 20.8) (Audio 20.119)

Box 20.8 Extraoral structures (Audio 20.217)

- Cheek (Audio 20.218)
- Chin (Audio 20.219)
- Ear (Audio 20.220)
- Eye (Audio 20.221)
- Face (Audio 20.222)
- Forehead (Audio 20.223)
- Jaw (Audio 20.224)
- Joint (temporomandibular) (Audio 20.225)

- Lip (Audio 20.226)
- Lymph node (Audio 20.227)
- Mouth (Audio 20.228)
- Muscle (Audio 20.229)
- Neck (Audio 20.230)
- Nose (Audio 20.231)
- Salivary gland (Audio 20.232)
- Scalp (Audio 20.233)
- Sinus (Audio 20.234)
- Thyroid (Audio 20.235)
- Tongue (Audio 20.236)

Cuadro 20.8 Estructuras extraorales (Audio 20.217)

- Cachete/mejilla (Audio 20.218)
- Barbilla/menton (Audio 20.219)
- Oído (Audio 20.220)
- Ojo (Audio 20.221)
- Cara (Audio 20.222)
- Frente (Audio 20.223)
- Mandíbula/quijada (Audio 20.224)
- Articulación (temporomandibular) (Audio 20.225)

- Labio (Audio 20.226)
- Nódulo linfático/ganglio linfático (Audio 20.227)
- Boca (Audio 20.228)
- Músculo (Audio 20.229)
- Cuello (Audio 20.230)
- Nariz (Audio 20.231)
- Glándula salival (Audio 20.232)
- Cuero cabelludo (Audio 20.233)
- Seno (Audio 20.234)
- Tiroides (Audio 20.235)
- Lengua (Audio 20.236)

Let me know if you feel uncomfortable while I check your _____. (See Box 20.8)
Hágame saber si se siente incómodo(a) mientras le examino su _____. (Vea el Cuadro 20.8) (Audio 20.120)

I will be gentle when (examining/palpating) your _____. (See Box 20.8)
Seré cuidadoso(a) al (examinar/palpar) su _____. (Vea el Cuadro 20.8) (Audio 20.121)

Do you feel any pain when I press here?
¿Siente algún dolor cuando presiono aquí? (Audio 20.122)

Do you feel pain when you do that?
¿Siente algún dolor cuando hace esto? (Audio 20.123)

Did you notice this?
¿Usted notó esto? (Audio 20.124)

Does this bother you?
¿Esto le molesta? (Audio 20.125)

How long have you had this? (See Box 20.9)
¿Por cuánto tiempo ha tenido esto? (Vea el Cuadro 20.9) (Audio 20.126)

Has this shown _____? (See Box 20.9)
¿Esto le ha mostrado _____? (Vea el Cuadro 20.9) (Audio 20.127)

Have you had (lip/skin/oral) cancer?
¿Ha tenido cáncer (del labio/de la piel/de la boca)? (Audio 20.128)

Has this lymph node become enlarged before?
¿Este nódulo linfático se ha agrandado antes? (Audio 20.129)

Have you had trauma to your _____? (See Box 20.8)
¿Ha tenido algún trauma en su _____? (Vea el Cuadro 20.8) (Audio 20.130)

Have you had treatment for this?
¿Ha tenido tratamiento para esto? (Audio 20.131)

Bend your head (forward/backward).
Incline la cabeza hacia (adelante/atrás). (Audio 20.132)

**Box 20.9
Common symptoms
and conditions
(Audio 20.237)**

- Abscess formation
  (Audio 20.238)
- Ache (Audio 20.239)

- Bleeding (Audio 20.240)
- Burning (Audio 20.241)
- Change in color
  (Audio 20.242)
- Enlargement
  (Audio 20.243)
- Growth (Audio 20.244)
- Healing (Audio 20.245)
- Infection (Audio 20.246)
- Inflammation
  (Audio 20.247)
- Itching (Audio 20.248)
- Numbness (paresthesia)
  (Audio 20.249)

- Pain (Audio 20.250)
- Sensitivity (Audio 20.251)

- Swelling (Audio 20.252)

- Soreness (Audio 20.253)
- Tingling (Audio 20.254)
- Ulceration (Audio 20.255)

**Cuadro 20.9
Síntomas y condiciones
comunes
(Audio 20.237)**

- Una formación de absceso
  (Audio 20.238)
- Un dolor constante
  (Audio 20.239)
- Un sangrado (Audio 20.240)
- Una quemazón (Audio 20.241)
- Un cambio en color
  (Audio 20.242)
- Un agrandamiento
  (Audio 20.243)
- Un crecimiento (Audio 20.244)
- Una curación (Audio 20.245)
- Una infección (Audio 20.246)
- Una inflamación
  (Audio 20.247)
- Un picor (Audio 20.248)
- Un adormecimiento/
  entumecimiento (parestesia)
  (Audio 20.249)
- Un dolor (Audio 20.250)
- Una sensibilidad
  (Audio 20.251)
- Una hinchazón
  (Audio 20.252)
- Un dolor (Audio 20.253)
- Un hormigueo (Audio 20.254)
- Una ulceración (Audio 20.255)

Turn your head to the (right/left).
Volte la cabeza hacia la (derecha/izquierda). (Audio 20.133)

I will be checking your (hairline/outer ear).
Le examinaré su (línea capilar/linea de cabello/oreja). (Audio 20.134)

I will be placing my fingers in your outer ears and pressing forward so that I can check your joint.
Colocaré mis dedos en sus orejas y presionaré hacia adelante para examinar su articulación. (Audio 20.135)

(Open/Close) your (mouth/eyes).
(Abra/Cierre) la (boca/los ojos). (Audio 20.136)

Move your lower jaw to the (right/left).
Mueva la (quijada/mandibula) hacia la (derecha/izquierda).
(Audio 20.137)

Move your lower jaw (forward/backward).
Mueva la (quijada/mandibula) adelante/atrás. (Audio 20.138)

Put your teeth together and bite down hard.
Junte los dientes y muerda fuerte. (Audio 20.139)

Do you hear (anything/a noise) when you (open/close) your mouth?
¿Escucha (algo/un ruido) cuando (abre/cierra) la boca?
(Audio 20.140)

Do you have joint problems? On which side? How often?
¿Tiene problemas en las articulaciones? ¿En qué lado? ¿Con qué frecuencia? (Audio 20.141)

Do you have jaw pain in the morning?
¿Tiene dolor en la quijada por la mañana? (Audio 20.142)

I will need to check your lower neck area but not any lower than that.
Necesitaré examinarle la parte baja del cuello, pero no más abajo que eso. (Audio 20.143)

Raise your shoulders.
Levante los hombros. (Audio 20.144)

I will place my fingers on your neck while you swallow.
Le colocaré los dedos sobre el cuello mientras usted traga.
(Audio 20.145)

Drink some water from this glass. Swallow again.
Bebe un poco de agua de este vaso. Trague otra vez. (Audio 20.146)

DISCUSSION OF EXTRAORAL FINDINGS
DISCUSIÓN DE LOS RESULTADOS EXTRAORALES
(AUDIO 20.147)

You show _____. (See Box 20.10)
Usted muestra _____. (Vea el Cuadro 20.10) (Audio 20.148)

This lesion shows _____. (See Box 20.10)
Esta lesión muestra _____. (Vea el Cuadro 20.10) (Audio 20.149)

You have _____. (See Box 20.10)
Usted tiene _____. (Vea el Cuadro 20.10) (Audio 20.150)

OVERALL HEALTH DISCUSSION
DISCUSIÓN DE LA SALUD EN GENERAL
(AUDIO 20.151)

You have a (low/moderate/high) risk of medical complications.
Usted tiene un riesgo (bajo/moderado/alto) de complicaciones
médicas. (Audio 20.152)

**Due to your health concerns, we will need to see you
immediately for emergency dental care**.
Debido a sus condiciones de salud, necesitaremos verle
inmediatamente para atención dental de emergencia. (Audio 20.153)

**Due to your health, we will take precautions in our (office/
clinic) to reduce the risk of complications**.
Debido a su salud, tomaremos precauciones en nuestra (oficina/
clínica) para reducir el riesgo de complicaciones. (Audio 20.154)

**We have determined that your health needs to (improve/
get better) before you undergo dental treatment**.
Hemos determinado que su salud necesita mejorar antes de que
podamos realizarle su tratamiento dental. (Audio 20.155)

Your blood pressure is too high for us to treat you today.
Su presión arterial está demasiado alta para que podamos tratarlo(a)
hoy. (Audio 20.156)

You need to see your physician.
Usted necesita ver a su médico(a). (Audio 20.157)

Box 20.10
Common extraoral findings (Audio 20.256)

- Acne (Audio 20.257)
- Birthmark (Audio 20.258)

- Bleeding (hemorrhage) (Audio 20.259)
- Blister (vesicle) (Audio 20.260)
- Bruise (hematoma) (Audio 20.261)
- Cold sore (Audio 20.262)

- Dryness (Audio 20.263)
- Freckle (Audio 20.264)
- Lesion (Audio 20.265)
- Mole (nevus) (Audio 20.266)
- Patch (macule/papule) (Audio 20.267)
- Petechiae (Audio 20.268)
- Redness/red (Audio 20.269)

- Ruddy (Audio 20.270)
- Scar (Audio 20.271)
- Spider vein (Audio 20.272)

- Swelling (Audio 20.273)
- Tumor (cancer) (Audio 20.274)
- Ulcer (Audio 20.275)

Cuadro 20.10
Hallazgos extraorales comunes (Audio 20.256)

- Un acné (Audio 20.257)
- Una marca de nacimiento (Audio 20.258)
- Un sangrado (hemorragia) (Audio 20.259)
- Una ampolla (vesícula) (Audio 20.260)
- Un(a) moretón (hematoma) (Audio 20.261)
- Un herpes labial (Audio 20.262)
- Una sequedad (Audio 20.263)
- Una peca (Audio 20.264)
- Una lesión (Audio 20.265)
- Un lunar (nevo) (Audio 20.266)
- Un parche (mácula/pápula) (Audio 20.267)
- Una petequia (Audio 20.268)
- Un enrojecimiento/rojo (Audio 20.269)
- Un rojizo (Audio 20.270)
- Una cicatriz (Audio 20.271)
- Una vena de araña (Audio 20.272)
- Una hinchazón (Audio 20.273)
- Un tumor (cáncer) (Audio 20.274)
- Una úlcera (Audio 20.275)

You need to be premedicated with an antibiotic before we can treat you.

Usted necesita ser premedicado(a) con un antibiótico antes de que podamos tratarle. (Audio 20.158)

Chapter 21
Medications and Pharmacy

Capítulo 21
Medicamentos y Farmacia (Audio 21.1)

MEDICATIONS AND ALLERGIES
MEDICAMENTOS Y ALERGIAS (AUDIO 21.2)

Are you currently taking any medication(s)? If yes, what is it?
¿Está tomando algún(os) medicamento(s)? Si es así, ¿qué
medicamento? (Audio 21.3)

**Do you have any allergies to anesthetic? If yes, what type of
anesthetic?**
¿Tiene alergias a algún anestésico? Si es así, ¿a qué tipo de
anestésico? (Audio 21.4)

**Do you have any allergies to medicine or drugs? If yes,
which ones?**
¿Tiene alergias a algún medicamento o drogas? Si es así, ¿a cuáles?
(Audio 21.5)

Do you have any other allergies? If yes, what are they?
¿Tiene otras alergias? Si es así, ¿cuáles son? (Audio 21.6)

Have you taken any aspirin in the past 3 days?
¿Ha tomado aspirina en los últimos 3 días? (Audio 21.7)

Are you currently taking Coumadin (blood thinners)?
¿Está tomando Coumadin (anticoagulants) actualmente? (Audio 21.8)

**I am going to give you a prescription for a fluoride
toothpaste. I would like you to use it twice daily for
2 minutes each time. Do not rinse, drink, or eat for
30 minutes afterwards**.
Voy a darle una receta para una pasta dental con fluoruro. Me
gustaría que la usara dos veces al día durante 2 minutos cada vez.
No se enjuague, beba o coma por 30 minutos después. (Audio 21.9)

Please rinse with this mouthwash for 30 seconds twice daily.
Por favor enjuáguese con este enjuague bucal durante 30 segundos
dos veces al día. (Audio 21.10)

INFECTIONS
INFECCIONES (AUDIO 21.11)

Have you had a fever?
¿Ha tenido fiebre? (Audio 21.12)

What was your temperature?
¿Cuál fue su temperatura? (Audio 21.13)

Have you noticed any swelling? Where?
¿Ha tenido alguna hinchazón? ¿Dónde? (Audio 21.14)

Have you had a sore throat?
¿Ha tenido dolor de garganta? (Audio 21.15)

Have you noticed any redness?
¿Ha notado algún enrojecimiento? (Audio 21.16)

Do you frequently get cold sores?
¿Tiene (herpes labial/fuegos) con frecuencia? (Audio 21.17)

Was there a blister?
¿Hubo una ampolla allí? (Audio 21.18)

I would like you to take this medicine as directed.
Me gustaría que tomara este medicamento según las indicaciones.
(Audio 21.19)

Have you ever taken _____**? (See Box 21.1)**
¿Alguna vez ha tomado _____? (Vea el Cuadro 21.1)
(Audio 21.20)

This is an antibiotic. Please take the medicine until it is all gone.
Este es un antibiótico. Por favor tome el medicamento hasta que se acabe. (Audio 21.21)

This is an antiviral medication.
Este es un medicamento antiviral. (Audio 21.22)

This is an antifungal medication.
Este es un medicamento (antifúngico/antimicótico). (Audio 21.23)

Box 21.1
Antimicrobials
(Audio 21.28)

- Acyclovir (Zovirax) (Audio 21.29)
- Amoxicillin (Audio 21.30)
- Ampicillin (Audio 21.31)
- Azithromycin (Zithromax) (Audio 21.32)
- Clindamycin (Audio 21.33)
- Erythromycin (Audio 21.34)
- Fluconazole (Diflucan) (Audio 21.35)
- Metronidazole (Audio 21.36)
- Nystatin (Audio 21.37)
- Penicillin (Audio 21.38)
- Valacyclovir (Valtrex) (Audio 21.39)

Cuadro 21.1
Antimicrobianos
(Audio 21.28)

- Aciclovir (Zovirax) (Audio 21.29)
- Amoxicilina (Audio 21.30)
- Ampicilina (Audio 21.31)
- Azitromicina (Zithromax) (Audio 21.32)
- Clindamicina (Audio 21.33)
- Eritromicina (Audio 21.34)
- Fluconazol (Diflucan) (Audio 21.35)
- Metronidazol (Audio 21.36)
- Nistatina (Audio 21.37)
- Penicilina (Audio 21.38)
- Valaciclovir (Valtrex) (Audio 21.39)

PAIN
DOLOR (AUDIO 21.24)

On a scale of 1 to 10, where 10 is the worst pain and 1 is the least, how would you rate your pain right now?
En una escala del 1 al 10, donde 10 es el peor dolor y 1 es un dolor menor, ¿cómo calificaría usted su dolor en este momento? (Audio 21.25)

I am going to give you a prescription for _____ to relieve your pain. (See Box 21.2)
Voy a darle una receta para _____ para aliviar su dolor. (Vea el Cuadro 21.2) (Audio 21.26)

Only take the pain medicine if you have pain.
Sólo tome el medicamento si tiene dolor. (Audio 21.27)

Box 21.2
Pain medicine
(Audio 21.40)

- Acetaminophen (Tylenol)
  (Audio 21.41)
- Excedrin (Audio 21.42)
- Hydrocodone (Audio 21.43)
- Ibuprofen (Motrin)
  (Audio 21.44)
- Lidocaine (Audio 21.45)
- Local anesthetic
  (Audio 21.46)
- Narcotic (Audio 21.47)
- Oxycodone (Audio 21.48)
- Tylenol with codeine
  (Audio 21.49)
- Vicodin/Lortab
  (Audio 21.50)

Cuadro 21.2
Medicamentos para el
dolor (Audio 21.40)

- Acetaminofeno/paracetamol
  (Tylenol) (Audio 21.41)
- Excedrin (Audio 21.42)
- Hidrocodona (Audio 21.43)
- Ibuprofeno (Motrin)
  (Audio 21.44)
- Lidocaína (Audio 21.45)
- Anestesia local
  (Audio 21.46)
- Narcótico (Audio 21.47)
- Oxicodona (Audio 21.48)
- Tylenol con codeína
  (Audio 21.49)
- Vicodin/Lortab
  (Audio 21.50)

Chapter 22
Diet and Nutrition

Capítulo 22
Dieta y Nutrición (Audio 22.1)

DENTAL DISEASE AND DIET
LA ENFERMEDAD DENTAL Y LA DIETA
(AUDIO 22.2)

The sugars are the cause of acid production by the plaque. They are nowt the cause of plaque.
Los alimentos azucarados pueden causar que la placa produzca ácidos. (Audio 22.3)

It is not how many pieces of candy you eat that matters. It is how sticky the candy is and how long you chew it.
No es cuántos pedazos de dulce coma lo que importa. Es cuán pegajoso el dulce es y por cuánto tiempo lo mastica. (Audio 22.4)

Starches, such as bread, crackers, and cereal, also cause acids to form in plaque. Foods eaten as part of a meal cause less damage.
Los almidones, tales como el pan, las galletas y el cereal, también causan la formación de ácidos en la placa. Los alimentos que se comen como parte de una comida causan menos daño. (Audio 22.5)

(Saliva/Brushing/Rinsing) helps wash foods from the teeth and helps reduce acids.
(La saliva/El cepillar/El enjuagar) ayuda a lavar la comida de los dientes y ayuda a reducir los ácidos. (Audio 22.6)

One way to prevent (caries/decay/gum disease/periodontal disease) is to eat a healthy diet and limit your consumption of snacks.
Una manera de prevenir (las caries/la descomposición/la enfermedad de las encías/la enfermedad periodontal) es comiendo una dieta saludable y limitando el consumo de (bocadillos/botanas). (Audio 22.7)

If you need a snack, choose raw vegetables or fresh fruit.
Si necesita un bocadillo, escoja vegetales crudos o frutas frescas. (Audio 22.8)

When you snack often, acid can attack your teeth all day long.
Cuando come bocadillos frecuentemente, los ácidos pueden atacar sus dientes todo el día. (Audio 22.9)

Rinse well with water after any snack.
Enjuáguese bien con agua después de cualquier bocadillo. (Audio 22.10)

After many acid attacks from plaque, your teeth decay.
Después de muchos ataques de ácidos de la placa, sus dientes se deterioran. (Audio 22.11)

Soda, especially diet soda, has acids that decay your teeth.
La (soda/refrescos), especialmente la soda de dieta, tienen ácidos que deterioran los dientes. (Audio 22.12)

Hidden sugar that can cause tooth decay is also found in _____. (See Box 22.1)
El azúcar occulta que puede causar caries dental también se encuentra en _____. (Vea el Cuadro 22.1) (Audio 22.13)

To help prevent tooth decay, we will be taking a dietary history.
Para ayudar a prevenir la caries dental, realizaremos un historial dietético. (Audio 22.14)

Let's discuss sugar substitutes.
Hablemos sobre los sustitutos del azúcar. (Audio 22.15)

CHILDREN AND DIET
LOS NIÑOS Y LA DIETA (AUDIO 22.16)

Never allow your child to fall asleep with a bottle containing milk, formula, or fruit juice.
Nunca permita que su niño(a) se duerma con un biberón que contenga leche, fórmula o jugo de fruta. (Audio 22.17)

Avoid filling your child's bottle with sugar water or soda.
Evite llenar el biberón de su niño(a) con agua azucarada o soda. (Audio 22.18)

Box 22.1
Sources of hidden sugar (Audio 22.24)

- Breath mints (Audio 22.25)

- Ketchup (Audio 22.26)
- Chewing tobacco (Audio 22.27)
- Cough drops (Audio 22.28)
- Fruit drinks (check the label) (Audio 22.29)

- Gum (Audio 22.30)

- Medicine (Audio 22.31)

- Soft drinks (soda) (Audio 22.32)
- Sugared coffee (Audio 22.33)

- Sugared tea (Audio 22.34)
- White bread (Audio 22.35)

Cuadro 22.1
Fuentes de azúcar escondido (Audio 22.24)

- Las mentas de aliento (Audio 22.25)
- El catsup (Audio 22.26)
- El tabaco de mascar (Audio 22.27)
- Las pastillas contra la tos (Audio 22.28)
- Las bebidas de frutas (verifique la etiqueta) (Audio 22.29)
- El chicle (goma de mascar) (Audio 22.30)
- Los medicamentos (Audio 22.31)
- Las gaseosas/los refrescos (soda) (Audio 22.32)
- El café endulzado (Audio 22.33)
- El té endulzado (Audio 22.34)
- El pan blanco (Audio 22.35)

If you must give your baby a bottle at bedtime, make sure it contains only water.
Si tiene que darle un biberóna a su bebé a la hora de dormir, asegúrese de que sólo contenga agua. (Audio 22.19)

Never dip the pacifier into sugar or honey.
Nunca sumerja el chupete en azúcar o miel. (Audio 22.20)

Have your child begin drinking from a cup by his/her first birthday.
Haga que su niño(a) comience a beber de un vaso antes de su primer cumpleaños. (Audio 22.21)

Eating a healthy, balanced diet helps keep our teeth and gums free of disease.

El consumir una dieta saludable y balanceada ayuda a mantener sus dientes y encías libres de enfermedades. (Audio 22.22)

Let's not feed the plaque bugs!

¡No alimentemos a los microbios de la placa! (Audio 22.23)

PART IV

Office Administration and General Communication

PARTE IV

Administración de la Oficina y Comunicación General
(Audio 23.1)

Chapter 23
Addressing the Patient with Courtesy

Capítulo 23
Dirigiéndose al Paciente con Cortesía (Audio 23.2)

GREETING THE PATIENT
SALUDO AL PACIENTE (AUDIO 23.3)

Good (morning/afternoon/evening).
Buenos(as) (días/tardes/noches). (Audio 23.4)

It is nice to meet you.
Es un gusto conocerle. (Audio 23.5)

Hello, _____. I am _____
Hola, _____. Yo soy _____. (Audio 23.6)

I am the _____ and I will be working with you today.
(See Box 23.1)
Yo soy el/la _____ y estaré trabajando con usted hoy. (Vea el
Cuadro 23.1) (Audio 23.7)

Welcome to our office.
Bienvenido(a) a nuestra oficina. (Audio 23.8)

I'm sorry you had to wait. We are very busy today.
Disculpe que haya tenido que esperar. Estamos muy ocupados hoy.
(Audio 23.9)

Box 23.1 Members of the dental team (Audio 23.73)	Cuadro 23.1 Miembros del equipo dental (Audio 23.73)
• Dentist (Audio 23.74)	• Dentista/odontologo(a) (Audio 23.74)
• Dental hygienist (Audio 23.75)	• Higienista dental (Audio 23.75)
• Dental assistant (Audio 23.76)	• Asistente dental (Audio 23.76)
• Office manager (Audio 23.77)	• Encargado(a) de la oficina (Audio 23.77)

How are you today?
¿Cómo se encuentra hoy? (Audio 23.10)

Have you been seen by Dr. _____ before?
¿Ha sido atendido por el Dr./la Dra. _____ antes? (Audio 23.11)

Is this your first visit to the office?
¿Es ésta su primera visita a la oficina? (Audio 23.12)

Come in, Mr./Mrs./Miss _____.
Entre, Sr./Sra./Srta. _____. (Audio 23.13)

Mr./Mrs./Miss _____, this is Dr. _____. Dr. _____, this is Mr./ Mrs./Miss _____.
Sr./Sra./Srta. _____, éste/a es el/la Dr(a). _____. Dr(a)._____, éste/a es el/la Sr./Sra./Srta. _____. (Audio 23.14)

Dr. _____ is going to be treating you today.
El Dr./La Dra. _____ le va a tratar hoy. (Audio 23.15)

Thank you for being such a (cooperative/good) patient today.
Gracias por ser un(a) paciente tan (cooperativo(a)/bueno(a)) hoy. (Audio 23.16)

You did great today.
Hiciste muy bien hoy. (Audio 23.17)

Do you have any questions about your treatment today?
¿Tiene preguntas sobre el tratamiento de hoy? (Audio 23.18)

It was a pleasure meeting you.
Fue un placer conocerle. (Audio 23.19)

I look forward to seeing you at your next appointment.
Estaré a la espera de verle en su próxima cita. (Audio 23.20)

UNDERSTANDING THE PATIENT
ENTENDIENDO AL PACIENTE (AUDIO 23.21)

Do you prefer to speak Spanish or English?
¿Prefiere hablar en español o en inglés? (Audio 23.22)

Please repeat what you told me.
Repita lo que me dijo, por favor. (Audio 23.23)

I didn't understand you completely. You told me that _____, correct?
No le entendí completamente. ¿Me dijo que _____, correcto? (Audio 23.24)

I still don't understand you.
Todavía no le entiendo. (Audio 23.25)

I didn't understand anything you said to me.
No entendí nada de lo que me dijo. (Audio 23.26)

My Spanish is limited, so please use (simple/everyday) words.
Mi español es limitado, así que por favor hábleme con palabras (sencillas/comunes). (Audio 23.27)

Please speak more slowly.
Hable más despacio, por favor. (Audio 23.28)

I'm not familiar with that word.
No conozco esa palabra. (Audio 23.29)

What is the meaning of that word?
¿Qué (significa/quiere decir) esa palabra? (Audio 23.30)

I cannot hear you. Please speak louder.
No puedo oírle. Hable más fuerte, por favor. (Audio 23.31)

I did not say that (to you).
No (le) dije eso. (Audio 23.32)

I need a (translator/interpreter)—wait a minute.
Necesito un (traductor/intérprete)—espere un minuto. (Audio 23.33)

Is this correct?
¿Es ésto correcto? (Audio 23.34)

POSITIONING THE PATIENT
ACOMODAR AL PACIENTE (AUDIO 23.35)

_____ (Name), please sit in the chair.
_____ (Nombre), por favor siéntese en la silla. (Audio 23.36)

May I take your _____? (See Box 23.2)
¿Puedo tomar su(s) _____? (Vea el Cuadro 23.2) (Audio 23.37)

**I will put your _____ here where (it/they) will be safe.
(See Box 23.2)**
Pondré su(s) _____ aquí, donde estará(n) seguro(s)/segura(s). (Vea el
Cuadro 23.2) (Audio 23.38)

I am going to (lower/raise) the chair.
Voy a (subir/bajar) la silla. (Audio 23.39)

**I am going to tilt the chair back so you will feel like you are
lying down.**
Voy a reclinar la silla, así que sentirá que se está acostando.
(Audio 23.40)

**In this position, it will be easier for us to examine your
mouth.**
En esta posición será más fácil para examinarle la boca.
(Audio 23.41)

I am going to tilt you forward now.
Voy a inclinarle hacia adelante ahora. (Audio 23.42)

You may get up now.
Se puede levantar ahora. (Audio 23.43)

Do you feel dizzy?
¿Se siente mareado(a)? (Audio 23.44)

**Box 23.2
Patient items that may
need to be removed
during treatment
(Audio 23.78)**

- Glasses (Audio 23.79)

- Purse (Audio 23.80)
- Cane (Audio 23.81)
- Walker (Audio 23.82)
- Crutches (Audio 23.83)

**Cuadro 23.2
Artículos del paciente que
quizás deben removerse
durante el tratamiento
(Audio 23.78)**

- Lentes/anteojos/gafas
  (Audio 23.79)
- Bolso(a) (Audio 23.80)
- Bastón (Audio 23.81)
- Andador (Audio 23.82)
- Muletas (Audio 23.83)

Are you comfortable?
¿Está cómodo(a)? (Audio 23.45)

Turn your head toward me so I can see the tooth better.
Volte la cabeza hacia mí para que pueda ver el diente mejor.
(Audio 23.46)

Turn your head toward the doctor.
Volte la cabeza hacia el/la doctor(a). (Audio 23.47)

(Rest/Tilt/Lift) your head.
(Descanse/Incline/Levante) la cabeza. (Audio 23.48)

Open your mouth. Open wider. Open more.
Abra la boca. Abra más grande. Abra más. (Audio 23.49)

Close your mouth.
Cierre la boca. (Audio 23.50)

Tilt your chin down.
Incline la barbilla hacia abajo. (Audio 23.51)

Rinse your mouth. Swish the water around in your mouth.
Enjuáguese la boca. Agite el agua en su boca. (Audio 23.52)

Hold very still.
Manténgase quieto(a). (Audio 23.53)

Hold still and don't move.
Manténgase quieto y no se mueva. (Audio 23.54)

You need to rinse out your mouth.
Necesita enjuagarse la boca. (Audio 23.55)

Here is some water in a cup.
Aquí tiene un poco de agua en una taza. (Audio 23.56)

Swish the water around in your mouth, and then place this saliva ejector in your mouth; the water will then be suctioned out.
Agite el agua en su boca, y luego coloque este eyector de saliva en su boca y el agua será succionada. (Audio 23.57)

Do not close on the saliva ejector.
No cierre en el eyector de saliva. (Audio 23.58)

The first thing that we will do is clean the area with this gauze.
Lo primero que haremos será limpiar el área con esta gaza.
(Audio 23.59)

I am going to use this suction tip in your mouth to remove the (water/saliva).
Voy a usar esta punta de succión en su boca para remover (el agua/la saliva). (Audio 23.60)

If you can turn toward me, I can remove the water more easily.
Si voltea hacia mí, puedo remover el agua más fácilmente. (Audio 23.61)

BIDDING FAREWELL
DESPEDIDA (AUDIO 23.62)

Thank you very much.
Muchas gracias. (Audio 23.63)

You're welcome. (It was nothing.)
De nada. (No fue nada.) (Audio 23.64)

Don't mention it. (You're welcome.)
No hay de qué. (De nada.) (Audio 23.65)

It was a pleasure serving you.
Fue un placer haberle atendido. (Audio 23.66)

You are very kind.
Usted es muy amable. (Audio 23.67)

Very nice meeting you.
Mucho gusto en conocerlo(a). (Audio 23.68)

Same to you.
Igualmente. (Audio 23.69)

See you later.
Hasta luego. (Audio 23.70)

Until next time. (See you soon.)
Hasta la próxima vez. (Hasta pronto.) (Audio 23.71)

Goodbye.
Adiós. (Audio 23.72)

Chapter 24
HIPAA and Informed Consent

Capítulo 24
HIPAA y Consentimiento Informado (Audio 24.1)

HIPAA AND THE HEALTH AND MEDICAL HISTORY FORMS
HIPAA Y LOS FORMULARIOS DEL HISTORIAL MÉDICO Y DE SALUD (AUDIO 24.2)

I have some paperwork that needs to be completed.
Tengo algunos papeles que debemos completar. (Audio 24.3)

We need to have you (complete/fill out) these forms.
Necesitamos que usted (complete/llene) estos formularios.
(Audio 24.4)

This is the health history form from your last visit. I would like to verify that it is still accurate.
Éste es el formulario del historial de salud de su última visita. Me gustaría verificar que sigue siendo correcto. (Audio 24.5)

Are you able to complete these forms? Do you need help from me?
¿Puede completar estos formularios? ¿Necesita de mi ayuda?
(Audio 24.6)

We need to have some personal history for our records.
Necesitamos tener cierto historial personal para nuestros (archivos/registros). (Audio 24.7)

Our office policy is consistent with the federal guidelines of the Health Insurance Portability and Accountability Act of 1996 (HIPAA).
Nuestra política de la oficina concuerda con las guías federales de la Ley de Portabilidad y Responsabilidad del Seguro Médico de 1996 (HIPAA por sus siglas en inglés). (Audio 24.8)

We will ensure the confidentiality of your health information.
Le aseguramos la confidencialidad de su información de salud.
(Audio 24.9)

Your health plan requires this information.
Su plan de salud requiere esta información. (Audio 24.10)

What is your name? First name? Middle name? Last name?
¿Cómo se llama? ¿Cuál es su nombre de pila? ¿Su segundo nombre?
¿Su apellido? (Audio 24.11)

How do you spell your name?
¿Cómo se deletrea su nombre? (Audio 24.12)

What is your address? City? State? Zip code?
¿Cuál es su dirección? ¿Ciudad? ¿Estado? ¿Código postal?
(Audio 24.13)

What is your phone number? What is the area code?
¿Cuál es su número de teléfono? ¿Cuál es el código de área?
(Audio 24.14)

What is your birth date?
¿Cuál es su fecha de nacimiento? (Audio 24.15)

Who is responsible for this account?
¿Quién es responsable por esta cuenta? (Audio 24.16)

[If this is a child] What is the child's nickname?
[Si éste es un(a) niño(a)] ¿Cuál es el apodo (del niño/de la niña)?
(Audio 24.17)

**Are you the parent or responsible guardian for this
(patient/child)?**
¿Es usted el padre o guardián responsable de este(a) (paciente/
niño(a))? (Audio 24.18)

Are you covered by insurance?
¿Está usted cubierto(a) por un seguro? (Audio 24.19)

Which insurance company?
¿Cuál compañía de seguro? (Audio 24.20)

Do you have the insurance card with you today?
¿Tiene la tarjeta del seguro con usted hoy? (Audio 24.21)

Is the insurance in your name? If not, whose name is it in?
¿Está el seguro a su nombre? Si no, ¿a nombre de quién está?
(Audio 24.22)

What is the relationship of the subscriber to you? (See Box 24.1)
¿Cuál es la relación del (abonado/subscriptor) con usted? (Vea el Cuadro 24.1) (Audio 24.23)

Are you covered by any other insurance? If so, which one?
¿Está cubierto(a) por algún otro seguro? Si es así, ¿por cuál? (Audio 24.24)

Do you have the insurance identification card with you?
¿Tiene la tarjeta de identificación del seguro con usted? (Audio 24.25)

Who is the subscriber's employer?
¿Quién es el empleador del (abonado/suscriptor)? (Audio 24.26)

Do you work?
¿Usted trabaja? (Audio 24.27)

Who is your employer?
¿Quién es su empleador? (Audio 24.28)

What is your phone number at work?
¿Cuál es el número de teléfono de su trabajo? (Audio 24.29)

What is your address at work?
¿Cuál es la dirección de su trabajo? (Audio 24.30)

Box 24.1
Persons who may carry insurance for a dental patient (Audio 24.48)

- Husband (Audio 24.49)
- Wife (Audio 24.50)
- Father (Audio 24.51)
- Mother (Audio 24.52)
- Self (Audio 24.53)

Cuadro 24.1
Personas que pueden tener seguro para un paciente dental (Audio 24.47)

- Esposo (Audio 24.49)
- Esposa (Audio 24.50)
- Padre/papa (Audio 24.51)
- Madre/mama (Audio 24.52)
- Uno(a) mismo(a)/yo (Audio 24.53)

I need to have you sign this form. I have recorded all the information that you just gave me on this form.

Necesito que firme este formulario. He anotado toda la información que me acaba de dar en este formulario. (Audio 24.31)

INFORMED CONSENT
CONSENTIMIENTO INFORMADO (AUDIO 24.32)

We have examined your mouth and explained to you the dental problems that you have.
Le hemos examinado la boca y le hemos explicado los problemas dentales que tiene. (Audio 24.33)

Do you understand what your dental problems are?
¿Entiende cuáles son sus problemas dentales? (Audio 24.34)

Based on our clinical and radiographic findings, we have suggested several different treatment options to you.
De acuerdo con nuestros resultados clínicos y radiográficos, le hemos sugerido varias opciones de tratamiento. (Audio 24.35)

Do you have any questions about the treatment options?
¿Tiene preguntas sobre las opciones de tratamiento? (Audio 24.36)

Do you understand all of the consequences of treatment as explained in the paper I gave you to read?
¿Entiende todas las consecuencias del tratamiento según lo explicado en el papel que le di para que leyera? (Audio 24.37)

Please sign and date the treatment consent form.
Por favor, firme y escriba la fecha en el formulario de consentimiento del tratamiento. (Audio 24.38)

The doctor and designated staff will be providing the treatment you need.
El/La doctor(a) y el personal designado le proporcionarán el tratamiento que usted necesita. (Audio 24.39)

If something unexpected happens and we need to change the treatment plan we discussed, we will let you know immediately.

Si sucede algo inesperado y necesitamos cambiar el plan de tratamiento que discutimos, se lo informaremos de inmediato. (Audio 24.40)

What would you like us to do?
¿Qué le gustaría que hiciéramos? (Audio 24.41)

Do you understand the financial arrangements and your obligations for payment for treatment?
¿Entiende los acuerdos financieros y sus obligaciones para el pago del tratamiento? (Audio 24.42)

You will be given a copy of the treatment plan and a list of all the associated fees.
Se le entregará una copia del plan de tratamiento y una lista de todos los costos asociados. (Audio 24.43)

Once you agree to proceed, please sign the copy of the financial arrangements, and treatment can begin.
Cuando decida proceder, por favor firme la copia de los acuerdos financieros y el tratamiento podrá comenzar. (Audio 24.44)

If you have questions at any time about your treatment or finances, please let us know immediately.
Si tiene preguntas en cualquier momento sobre su tratamiento o finanzas, por favor háganos saber inmediatamente. (Audio 24.45)

Do you understand the proposed plan?
¿Entiendes el plan propuesto? (Audio 24.46)

Are you comfortable with the plan that we have presented you?
¿Está cómodo(a) con el plan que le hemos presentado? (Audio 24.47)

Chapter 25
Fees, Billing, and Insurance

Capítulo 25
Tarifas, Facturación y Seguro (Audio 25.1)

Good (morning/afternoon/evening).
Buenos(as) (días/tardes/noches). (Audio 25.2)
It is good to see you.
Qué bueno verle. (Audio 25.3)
I am _____, the office manager.
Yo soy _____, el/la encargado(a) de la oficina. (Audio 25.4)
Has your address changed since your last appointment?
¿Ha cambiado su dirección desde su última cita? (Audio 25.5)
Has your insurance changed since your last appointment?
¿Ha cambiado su seguro desde su última cita? (Audio 25.6)

DISCUSSING FEES AND DENTAL INSURANCE
DISCUSIÓN DE TARIFAS Y SEGURO DENTAL
(AUDIO 25.7)

(Mr./Mrs./Miss) _____, the cost for today is _____.
(Sr./Sra./Srta.) _____, el costo por hoy es _____. (Audio 25.8)

Your insurance covers this fee.
Su seguro cubre la tarifa. (Audio 25.9)

The insurance covers _____ of the cost.
El seguro cubre _____ del costo. (Audio 25.10)

Your insurance does not cover this fee.
Su seguro no cubre el/la (honorario/tarifa). (Audio 25.11)

You need to pay the copayment, which is _____ dollars.
Usted tiene que pagar el copago, que es _____dolares. (Audio 25.12)

Our office policy requires that payment for services be made today.
Las reglas de nuestra oficina requiere que el pago de los servicios se realice hoy. (Audio 25.13)

Our office policy is that you pay the copayment for services today.
Nuestra política de oficina es que usted pague hoy el copago de sus servicios. (Audio 25.14)

We do not accept _____ insurance but will send your forms to the company.
Nosotros no aceptamos el seguro _____ pero enviaremos sus formularios a la compañía. (Audio 25.15)

You can pay the full amount today, and you will be reimbursed by the company for the amount covered by your insurance.
Usted puede pagar el costo completo hoy y la compañía le reembolsará la cantidad que le cubra su seguro. (Audio 25.16)

We do not participate in _____ insurance company.
Nosotros no participamos en el plan de seguro _____.
(Audio 25.17)

What form of payment will you be using today? We accept checks, cash, insurance, and credit cards.
¿Qué forma de pago utilizarás hoy? Aceptamos cheques, efectivo, seguro y tarjetas de crédito. (Audio 25.18)

Chapter 26
Scheduling Appointments

Capítulo 26
Programmando Citas (Audio 26.1)

MAKING APPOINTMENTS
HACER CITAS (AUDIO 26.2)

What time of day is best for you to come to the office for an appointment?
¿A qué hora del día es mejor para usted para venir a la oficina para una cita? (Audio 26.3)

I have the_____ (day of the week) _____ (month) _____ (date) at _____ (time) available.
Tengo el _____ (día de la semana) _____ (fecha) de _____ (mes) a la(s) _____ (hora) disponible. (Audio 26.4)

Will this time be (okay/convenient) for you?
¿(Está bien/Le conviene) a esta hora? (Audio 26.5)

The doctor is going to be in a meeting on that day.
El/la doctor(a) estará en una reunión ese día. (Audio 26.6)

We need to make another appointment.
Necesitamos hacer otra cita. (Audio 26.7)

You need _____ more appointments to complete your treatment.
Usted necesita _____ citas más para completar su tratamiento. (Audio 26.8)

You need to have an appointment in _____ (days/weeks/months).
Usted necesita tener una cita en _____ (días/semanas/meses). (Audio 26.9)

Here is an appointment card with our phone number on it.
Aquí tiene una tarjeta de citas con nuestro número de teléfono. (Audio 26.10)

Be certain to call us the day before if you cannot keep this appointment.
Asegúrese de llamarnos el día anterior si no puede venir a su cita. (Audio 26.11)

Did you understand what (the doctor/the hygienist/I) told you to do?
¿Entendió lo que (el/la doctor(a)/el/la higienista/yo) le dijo(e) que hiciera? (Audio 26.12)

Do you have any questions?
¿Tiene preguntas? (Audio 26.13)

_____(Name), I am sorry you are in discomfort. The doctor can see you at _____ (time) today.
_____(Nombre), lamento que estés incómodo(a). El/La doctor(a) puede verlo(a) hoy a la(s) _____ (hora). (Audio 26.14)

APPOINTMENT RECOMMENDATIONS
RECOMENDACIONES PARA CITAS (AUDIO 26.15)

You will need to _____ before dental treatment. (See Box 26.1)
Usted necesitará _____ antes del tratamiento dental. (Vea el Cuadro 26.1) (Audio 26.16)

We will need to schedule your appointment in the (morning/afternoon) due to your health.
Necesitaremos programar la hora de su cita para que sea en la (mañana/tarde) debido a su salud. (Audio 26.17)

We recommend (nitrous oxide/oxygen) during dental treatment due to your health. It will relax you and make the situation comfortable.
Le recomendamos (óxido nitroso/oxígeno) durante el tratamiento dental debido a su salud. Le ayudará a relajarse y a hacer la situación cómoda. (Audio 26.18)

Bacteria from plaque on your teeth can enter your circulatory system during dental treatment and infect your (heart/joint prosthesis).
Bacterias de la placa en sus dientes pueden ingresar al sistema circulatorio durante el tratamiento dental y infectar su (corazón/prótesis articular). (Audio 26.19)

Box 26.1
Common recommendations (Audio 26.36)

- Eat (Audio 26.37)
- Check your bleeding time (Audio 26.38)
- Check your blood glucose (Audio 26.39)
- Decrease your dosage (Audio 26.40)
- Not eat (fast) (Audio 26.41)

- Increase your dosage (Audio 26.42)
- Rest well (Audio 26.43)
- Rinse your mouth (Audio 26.44)
- Take antibiotic premedication (Audio 26.45)
- Take a sedative premedication (Audio 26.46)
- Take your medicine (Audio 26.47)

Cuadro 26.1
Recomendaciones comunes (Audio 26.36)

- Comer (Audio 26.37)
- Evaluar su tiempo de sangrado (Audio 26.38)
- Evaluar su glucosa (azucar) en la sangre (Audio 26.39)
- Reducir su dosis (Audio 26.40)
- No comer (ayunar) (Audio 26.41)

- Aumentar su dosis (Audio 26.42)
- Descansar bien (Audio 26.43)
- Enjuagarse la boca (Audio 26.44)
- Tomar premedicación antibiótica (Audio 26.45)
- Tomar una premedicación sedante (Audio 26.46)
- Tomar sus medicamentos (Audio 26.47)

Antibiotic premedication will kill the plaque bacteria that enters the circulatory system during dental treatment.
La premedicación con antibióticos matará la placa bacteriana que ingresa al sistema circulatorio durante el tratamiento dental. (Audio 26.20)

Antibiotic premedication needs to be taken 1 hour before most dental treatments.
Debe tomarse la premedicación antibiótica una hora antes de la mayoría de los tratamientos dentales. (Audio 26.21)

MAKING REFERRALS
HACIENDO REFERENCIAS (AUDIO 26.22)

_____ **(Name), we are going to need to refer you to a**
_____ **for the treatment Dr.** _____ **has outlined.**
(See Box 26.2)
_____ (Nombre), vamos a necesitar referirle a un(a) _____ para
el tratamiento que el Dr./la Dra. _____ ha establecido. (Vea el
Cuadro 26.2) (Audio 26.23)

The name of the specialist the doctor is referring you to is
Dr. _____.
El nombre del especialista al cual el/la doctor(a) le está refiriendo es
el Dr./la Dra. _____. (Audio 26.24)

Box 26.2
Types of specialists
(Audio 26.48)

- Braces specialist
  (orthodontist)
  (Audio 26.49)
- Dental specialist
  (Audio 26.50)
- General dentist
  (Audio 26.51)
- Denture specialist
  (prosthodontist)
  (Audio 26.52)
- Dermatologist (Audio 26.53)
- Gum specialist (periodontist)
  (Audio 26.54)
- Medical doctor
  (Audio 26.55)
- Oral surgeon (Audio 26.56)
- Root canal specialist
  (endodontist) (Audio 26.57)

Cuadro 26.2
Tipos de especialistas
(Audio 26.48)

- Especialista en frenillos/
  frenos/brackets
  (ortodoncista) (Audio 26.49)
- Especialista dental
  (Audio 26.50)
- Dentista general
  (Audio 26.51)
- Especialista en dentaduras
  (Prostodoncista)
  (Audio 26.52)
- Dermatólogo(a) (Audio 26.53)
- Especialista en encías
  (periodoncista) (Audio 26.54)
- Doctor(a)/médico(a)
  (Audio 26.55)
- Cirujano(a) oral (Audio 26.56)
- Especialista en (tratamientos
  de endodoncia/conductos
  radiculares) (endodoncista)
  (Audio 26.57)

(His/Her) office is located at _____. Do you know where that street is?
Su oficina está ubicada en _____ ¿Sabe dónde está esa calle?
(Audio 26.25)

We will send Dr. _____ a letter regarding your treatment.
Le enviaremos una carta al Dr./a la Dra. _____ sobre su tratamiento.
(Audio 26.26)

We will send your radiographs to Dr. _____.
Le enviaremos sus radiografías al Dr./a la Dra. _____. (Audio 26.27)

You need to call Dr. _____ at this number to make an appointment: _____.
Usted tiene que llamar al Dr./a la Dra. _____ a este número para hacer una cita: _____. (Audio 26.28)

OFFICE HOURS
HORAS DE OFICINA (AUDIO 26.29)

Our hours are _____ to _____ (hours) on _____ (days) through _____ (days).
Nuestras horas son de _____ a _____ (horas) de _____ (día) a _____ (día). (Audio 26.30)

Our office is open on _____ (days).
Nuestra oficina está abierta los _____ (días). (Audio 26.31)

Our office is closed on _____ (days).
Nuestra oficina está cerrada los _____ (días). (Audio 26.32)

Do you know where our office is located?
¿Sabe dónde está nuestra oficina? (Audio 26.33)

Our office is located at _____. It is near _____ (local street or landmark).
Nuestra oficina está en _____. Está cerca de _____ (calle local o punto de referencia). (Audio 26.34)

Our phone number is _____.
Nuestro número de teléfono es _____. (Audio 26.35)

Chapter 27
Hispanic Heritage and Culture

Capítulo 27
Herencia y Cultura Hispana (Audio 27.1)

As diverse as Hispanics are geographically, so are they culturally. The term _Hispanic_, when used to describe a person, refers to those persons whose heritage is from a Spanish-speaking country once under the authority of Spain. In practical terms, Hispanics may originate from Spain, Mexico, Central or South America, and the Greater Antilles. While there may be many variations in the Spanish language and culture from country to country, in this section, we will focus on some commonalities among those cultures.

Los hispanos son diversos, tanto geográficamente como culturalmente. El término _hispano_, cuando se utiliza para describir a una persona, se refiere a aquellas personas cuyo legado proviene de un país donde hablan español, que estuvo una vez bajo la autoridad de España. En términos prácticos, los hispanos pueden provenir de España, México, Centro o Sur América y las Antillas Mayores. Si bien puede haber muchas variaciones en el idioma español y la cultura de un país a otro, en esta sección nos centraremos en algunos puntos en común entre las culturas. (Audio 27.2)

Latino refers to a male of Latin American origin or descent.
Latino se refiere a un hombre de origen o ascendencia latinoamericana. (Audio 27.3)

Latinos are a group of men or boys of Latin American origin or descent. It is also used to describe a group of people from Latin America.
Latinos se refiere a un grupo de hombres o niños de origen o ascendencia latinoamericana. También se utiliza para describir a un grupo de personas de latinoamerica. (Audio 27.4)

Latina refers to a female of Latin American origin or descent.
Latina se refiere a una mujer de origen o ascendencia latinoamericana. (Audio 27.5)

Latinas are a group of females of Latin American origin or descent.
Latinas se refiere a un grupo de mujeres de origen o ascendencia latinoamericana. (Audio 27.6)

Latinx is a gender-neutral or nonbinary term used to describe people of Latin American origin or descent.
Latinx es un término de género neutro o no binario que se utiliza para describir a personas de origen o ascendencia latinoamericana. (Audio 27.7)

Latine is a gender-neutral or nonbinary term used to describe people of Latin American origin or descent.
Latine es un término de género neutro o no binario que se utiliza para describir a personas de origen o ascendencia latinoamericana. (Audio 27.8)

Latinx and Latine are used in the same way, but Latine is preferred by some Spanish-speaking people because it flows better with the Spanish language.
Latinx y Latine se usan de la misma manera, pero algunas personas que hablan español prefieren el termino Latine porque fluye mejor con el idioma español. (Audio 27.9)

FAMILY VALUES AND ESTABLISHING RAPPORT
VALORES FAMILIARES Y EL ESTABLECIMIENTO DE UNA BUENA RELACIÓN (AUDIO 27.10)

Hispanic families tend to have very close relationships, even with distant relatives. It is not unusual for family members to accompany their relatives when traveling, running errands, or even going to a dental appointment. This should not be viewed as a sign of fear by your patient. Often they may be accompanied by visiting relatives from out of town. Great importance is placed on celebrating special events of family members, such as birthdays, anniversaries, weddings, and quinceañeras (a young girl's coming of age at 15 years). Holidays, particularly religious holidays, are especially important times for family gatherings.

Las familias hispanas tienden a tener relaciones muy cercanas, incluso con parientes lejanos. No es raro que los miembros de la familia acompañen a sus familiares al viajar, hacer mandados o incluso a una cita con el dentista. Esto no debe ser visto como un signo de temor por parte del paciente. A veces pueden estar acompañados por familiares que visitan desde fuera de la ciudad. Se da mucha importancia a la celebración de eventos especiales de los miembros de la familia, como cumpleaños, aniversarios, bodas y "quinceañeras" (cuando una joven cumple los quince años). Los dias festivos, particularmente los religiosos, son momentos especialmente importantes para las reuniones familiares. (Audio 27.11)

Hispanic children are generally taught early in life to respect authority figures such as doctors, clergy, police officers, teachers, and the elderly, especially parents and grandparents. The word of a medical professional will rarely be questioned. However, it is important to first establish a personal relationship with them so that they may also feel respected. Self-respect is also taught early in life and often shows in their personal appearance and manner of dressing. Acknowledging them will go a long way in building a long-term relationship.

A los niños hispanos se les suele enseñar desde temprana edad a respetar a las figuras de autoridad, como a los médicos, clérigos, policías, maestros, y a los ancianos, especialmente a los padres y abuelos. La palabra de un profesional médico rara vez será cuestionada. Sin embargo, es importante establecer primero una relación personal con ellos, de modo que también ellos se sientan respetados. El respeto a sí mismos también se enseña a temprana edad y con frecuencia se muestra en la apariencia personal y forma de vestir. El reconocerlos le ayudará a construir una relación a largo plazo. (Audio 27.12)

Hello, Mr./Mrs. _____. Is this your _____? (See Box 27.1)
Hola, señor/señora _____. ¿Es este su _____? (Vea el Cuadro 27.1) (Audio 27.13)

Where is your _____ from? (See Box 27.1)
¿De dónde es su _____? (Vea el Cuadro 27.1) (Audio 27.14)

Box 27.1
Relatives (Audio 27.39)

- Brother (Audio 27.40)
- Sister (Audio 27.41)
- Son (Audio 27.42)
- Daughter (Audio 27.43)
- Father (Audio 27.44)
- Mother (Audio 27.45)
- Grandfather (Audio 27.46)
- Grandmother (Audio 27.47)
- Aunt (Audio 27.48)
- Uncle (Audio 27.49)
- Cousin (male/female) (Audio 27.50)
- Niece (Audio 27.51)
- Nephew (Audio 27.52)

Cuadro 27.1
Familiares (Audio 27.39)

- Hermano (Audio 27.40)
- Hermana (Audio 27.41)
- Hijo (Audio 27.42)
- Hija (Audio 27.43)
- Padre/papa (Audio 27.44)
- Madre/mama (Audio 27.45)
- Abuelo (Audio 27.46)
- Abuela (Audio 27.47)
- Tía (Audio 27.48)
- Tío (Audio 27.49)
- Primo/prima (Audio 27.50)
- Sobrina (Audio 27.51)
- Sobrino (Audio 27.52)

Where are you from?
¿De dónde eres? (informal)/¿De dónde es usted? (formal)
(Audio 27.15)

Are you visiting for a special occasion?
¿Está de visita para una ocasión especial? (Audio 27.16)

Have you selected a dress for your quinceañera?
¿Ya elegiste un vestido para tu quinceañera? (Audio 27.17)

Do you have plans to celebrate Easter?
¿Tiene planes para celebrar la Pascua? (Audio 27.18)

Will you be attending the festivals?
¿Va a asistir a los festivales? (Audio 27.19)

Will you have family visiting for the holidays?
¿Tendrás familiares de visita durante las vacaciones? (Audio 27.20)

I've heard that _____ is beautiful. (See Box 27.2)
He oído decir que _____ es hermoso(a). (Vea el Cuadro 27.2)
(Audio 27.21)

Box 27.2
Locations (Audio 27.53)

- Bolivia (Audio 27.54)
- Dominican Republic (Audio 27.55)
- Spain (Audio 27.56)
- Mexico (Audio 27.57)
- Puerto Rico (Audio 27.58)
- Cuba (Audio 27.59)
- Belize (Audio 27.60)
- Costa Rica (Audio 27.61)
- El Salvador (Audio 27.62)
- Guatemala (Audio 27.63)
- Honduras (Audio 27.64)
- Panama (Audio 27.65)
- Nicaragua (Audio 27.66)
- Brazil (Audio 27.67)
- Colombia (Audio 27.68)
- Peru (Audio 27.69)
- Argentina (Audio 27.70)
- Chile (Audio 27.71)
- Venezuela (Audio 27.72)
- Ecuador (Audio 27.73)
- Paraguay (Audio 27.74)
- Uruguay (Audio 27.75)

Cuadro 27.2
Lugares (Audio 27.53)

- Bolivia (Audio 27.54)
- República Dominicana (Audio 27.55)
- España (Audio 27.56)
- México (Audio 27.57)
- Puerto Rico (Audio 27.58)
- Cuba (Audio 27.59)
- Belice (Audio 27.60)
- Costa Rica (Audio 27.61)
- El Salvador (Audio 27.62)
- Guatemala (Audio 27.63)
- Honduras (Audio 27.64)
- Panamá (Audio 27.65)
- Nicaragua (Audio 27.66)
- Brasil (Audio 27.67)
- Colombia (Audio 27.68)
- Perú (Audio 27.69)
- Argentina (Audio 27.70)
- Chile (Audio 27.71)
- Venezuela (Audio 27.72)
- Ecuador (Audio 27.73)
- Paraguay (Audio 27.74)
- Uruguay (Audio 27.75)

You have a very nice smile!
¡Tiene una sonrisa muy agradable! (Audio 27.22)

That is a beautiful dress.
Qué vestido tan bonito. (Audio 27.23)

I like your _____. (See Box 27.3)
Me gusta su _____. (Vea el Cuadro 27.3) (Audio 27.24)

Your skin is so beautiful!
¡Tiene muy linda piel! (Audio 27.25)

Box 27.3
Clothes (Audio 27.76)

- Suit (Audio 27.77)
- Dress (Audio 27.78)
- Shirt (Audio 27.79)
- Blouse (Audio 27.80)
- Tie (Audio 27.81)
- Pants (Audio 27.82)
- Shoes (Audio 27.83)
- Boots (Audio 27.84)
- Hat (Audio 27.85)
- Gloves (Audio 27.86)

Cuadro 27.3
Ropa (Audio 27.76)

- Traje (Audio 27.77)
- Vestido (Audio 27.78)
- Camisa (Audio 27.79)
- Blusa (Audio 27.80)
- Corbata (Audio 27.81)
- Pantalones (Audio 27.82)
- Zapatos (Audio 27.83)
- Botas (Audio 27.84)
- Sombrero (Audio 27.85)
- Guantes (Audio 27.86)

DIETARY HABITS
LOS HÁBITOS ALIMENTARIOS (AUDIO 27.26)

In many Hispanic countries, lunch is the largest meal of the day and is often followed by a short midday nap. Dinner is traditionally much later in the evening, generally at 9 or 10 p.m. Of course, most Hispanics living in the United States will adopt the traditional times for eating that most other Americans do. Regardless of the mealtimes, family presence is still an important part of eating.

En muchos países hispanos, el almuerzo es la comida principal del día, y a menudo le sigue una breve siesta de mediodía. La cena es tradicionalmente mucho más tarde en la noche, en general, a las nueve o diez. Por supuesto, la mayoría de los hispanos que viven en los Estados Unidos adoptará los horarios tradicionales para comer como la mayoría de los estadounidenses. Independientemente de la hora de la comida, la presencia de la familia sigue siendo una parte importante de ella. (Audio 27.27)

Hispanic diets are as varied as the individual countries from which they originate. Yet most rely on rice, beans, and fresh fruits as staples. In the United States, many Hispanics' diets also include flour and corn tortillas, whole milk, tomatoes, and beef. From a dental perspective, the large fruit

consumption may contribute to enamel demineralization from both citric acids and fermentable carbohydrates.
Las dietas hispanas son tan variadas como los países individuales de las que proceden. Sin embargo, la mayoría consisten de arroz, frijoles y frutas frescas como componentes principales. En los Estados Unidos, las dietas de muchos hispanos también incluyen tortillas de harina y de maíz, leche entera, tomate y carne de res. Desde una perspectiva dental, el gran consumo de fruta puede contribuir a la desmineralización del esmalte por los ácidos cítricos y los carbohidratos fermentables. (Audio 27.28)

Do you eat dinner late in the evening?
¿Cenas tarde? (Audio 27.29)

At what time do you typically eat your last meal for the day?
¿A qué hora suele comer su última comida del día? (Audio 27.30)

Do you eat citrus fruits often?
¿Comes frutas cítricas frequentemente? (Audio 27.31)

Do you frequently eat lemons or limes?
¿Acostumbra a comer los limones o limas? (Audio 27.32)

The acids from citrus fruits can wear down the enamel on your teeth.
Los ácidos de frutas cítricas pueden desgastar el esmalte de sus dientes. (Audio 27.33)

You should try to rinse your mouth with water after eating to minimize the effects of acids.
Usted debe tratar de enjuagarse la boca con agua después de comer para minimizar los efectos de los ácidos. (Audio 27.34)

What is your favorite restaurant?
¿Cuál es su restaurante favorito? (Audio 27.35)

Do you like to cook?
¿Le gusta cocinar? (Audio 27.36)

What is your favorite food to cook?
¿Cuál es su comida favorita para cocinar? (Audio 27.37)

What are the ingredients for that dish? (See Box 27.4)
¿Cuáles son los ingredientes para ese plato? (Vea el Cuadro 27.4) (Audio 27.38)

Box 27.4
Recipe ingredients
(Audio 27.87)

- Salt (Audio 27.88)
- Pepper (Audio 27.89)
- Onions (Audio 27.90)

- Tomatoes (Audio 27.91)
- Potatoes (Audio 27.92)
- Cilantro (Audio 27.93)
- Eggs (Audio 27.94)
- Fish (Audio 27.95)
- Pork (Audio 27.96)

- Chicken (Audio 27.97)
- Beef (Audio 27.98)
- Broth (Audio 27.99)
- Beef broth (Audio 27.100)
- Limes (Audio 27.101)
- Lemon (Audio 27.102)
- Tomatillo (Audio 27.103)
- Flour (Audio 27.104)
- Corn (Audio 27.105)
- Cheese (Audio 27.106)
- Goat cheese (Audio 27.107)

- Lard (Audio 27.108)
- Olive oil (Audio 27.109)
- Vegetable oil (Audio 27.110)
- Bread (Audio 27.111)
- Rice (Audio 27.112)
- Beans (Audio 27.113)
- Black beans (Audio 27.114)
- Milk (Audio 27.115)
- Sugar (Audio 27.116)
- Gourd (Audio 27.117)
- Wine (Audio 27.118)
- Beer (Audio 27.119)
- Tongue (Audio 27.120)

Cuadro 27.4
Ingredientes de la
receta (Audio 27.87)

- Sal (Audio 27.88)
- Pimienta (Audio 27.89)
- Cebollas (Audio 27.90)

- Tomates (Audio 27.91)
- Patatas/papas (Audio 27.92)
- Cilantro (Audio 27.93)
- Huevos (Audio 27.94)
- Pescado (Audio 27.95)
- Carne de cerdo (puerco) (Audio 27.96)

- Pollo (Audio 27.97)
- Carne de res (Audio 27.98)
- Caldo (Audio 27.99)
- Caldo de res (Audio 27.100)
- Limas (Audio 27.101)
- Limón (Audio 27.102)
- Tomatillo (Audio 27.103)
- Harina (Audio 27.104)
- Maíz (Audio 27.105)
- Queso (Audio 27.106)
- Queso de cabra (Audio 27.107)

- Manteca (Audio 27.108)
- Aceite de oliva (Audio 27.109)
- Aceite vegetal (Audio 27.110)
- Pan (Audio 27.111)
- Arroz (Audio 27.112)
- Frijoles (Audio 27.113)
- Frijoles negros (Audio 27.114)
- Leche (Audio 27.115)
- Azúcar (Audio 27.116)
- Calabaza (Audio 27.117)
- Vino (Audio 27.118)
- Cerveza (Audio 27.119)
- Lengua (Audio 27.120)

Appendix A
Accents and Pronunciations* (Audio apxa0001)

Apéndice A
Acentos y Pronunciónes

The acute accent is the only mark of its kind in Spanish. It is a small oblique line **(á)** that is drawn from right to left and specifies a syllable that has a stronger sound when pronouncing it. Accents are used generally to distinguish words written alike and identical in form with other parts of speech, but with a different meaning. For example, **papá** (*father*), **papa** (*vegetable*); **monté** (*mounted*), **monte** (*large hill*). Accents are sometimes omitted from capital letters and used to assist pronunciation.

El acento es la mayor intensidad con que se marca determinada sílaba al pronunciar una palabra. Es una rayita oblicua (á) que se escribe de derecha a izquierda y se coloca en ciertos casos sobre la vocal de la sílaba en que se carga la pronunciación. En español es necesario acentuar las palabras para darles el significado correcto que llevan. Por ejemplo, papá (padre), papa (vegetal); monté (verbo), monte (terreno elevado). A veces los acentos se omiten de las letras escritas en mayúscula y sirven para ayudar en la pronunciación. (Audio apxa0002)

ACCENTS
ACENTOS (AUDIO APXA0003)

I love	amó(AH-moh) (Audio apxa0004)
he loved	él amó(el ah-MOH) (Audio apxa0005)
road	el camino(el kah-MEE-noh) (Audio apxa0006)
he walked	él caminó(el kah-mee-NOH) (Audio apxa0007)
copper	cobre(KOH-breh) (Audio apxa0008)
I charged	yo cobré(yoh koh-BREH) (Audio apxa0009)
volumes	volúmenes(boh-LOO-meh-nes) (Audio apxa0010)
never	jamás(hah-MAHS) (Audio apxa0011)
pencil	lápiz(LAH-pees) (Audio apxa0012)

---

*From Joyce EV, Villanueva ME: *Say It in Spanish*, ed 2, Saunders, Philadelphia, 2000.

PRONUNCIATION[†]
PRONUNCIACIÓN (AUDIO APXA0013)

A sounds like *a* in *father* and is pronounced like a clipped *ah*. (Audio apxa0014)

ayudar	to help (Audio apxa0015)
el abdomen	abdomen (Audio apxa0016)
la amígdala	tonsil (Audio apxa0017)
la cama	bed (Audio apxa0018)
la bata	bathrobe (Audio apxa0019)

B has the sound of *b* in *book* when it begins a sentence and when it follows *m* or *n*. (Audio apxa0020)

el bol	basin (Audio apxa0021)
bañar	to bathe (Audio apxa0022)
el brazo	arm (Audio apxa0023)
el hombre	man (Audio apxa0024)
la boca	mouth (Audio apxa0025)

The sound of **B** becomes softened when it is located between vowels. (Audio apxa0026)

la cabeza	head (Audio apxa0027)
el rebozo	shawl (Audio apxa0028)

The Spanish **B** and **V** have the same sound. (Audio apxa0029)

C has a hard sound, as in *come* when it occurs before *a, o, u*, or before a consonant. (Audio apxa0030)

la cama	bed (Audio apxa0031)
la cuna	cradle (Audio apxa0032)
el cuello	neck (Audio apxa0033)
la cara	face (Audio apxa0034)

C before an *e* or *i* has an *s* sound. (Audio apxa0035)

la medicina	medicine (Audio apxa0036)
ciego	blind (Audio apxa0037)
la receta	prescription (Audio apxa0038)
la cintura	waist (Audio apxa0039)
el cerebro	brain (Audio apxa0040)

[†] From Chou B: *Practical Spanish in Eyecare*, Butterworth-Heinemann, Boston, 2001.

CH has the sound of *ch* in *child*. (Audio apxa0041)

el muchacho	boy (Audio apxa0042)
chupar	to suck (Audio apxa0043)
la noche	night (Audio apxa0044)
la chaqueta	jacket (Audio apxa0045)
la chica	girl (Audio apxa0046)
el chupete	pacifier (Audio apxa0047)

D is a hard dental sound at the beginning of a word. (Audio apxa0048)

la debilidad	weakness (Audio apxa0049)
los dientes	teeth (Audio apxa0050)
el doctor	doctor (Audio apxa0051)
mandar	to order (Audio apxa0052)
el dolor	pain (Audio apxa0053)

D has a *th* sound as in *them* between vowels. (Audio apxa0054)

el lado	side (Audio apxa0055)
el médico	doctor (Audio apxa0056)
el dedo	finger(Audio apxa0057)
el cuidado	care (Audio apxa0058)
el codo	elbow (Audio apxa0059)
mojado	wet (Audio apxa0060

E sounds like the English e in the word *eight*. (Audio apxa0061)

el pecho	chest (Audio apxa0062)
el pelo	hair (Audio apxa0063)
la enfermedad	illness (Audio apxa0064)
la espalda baja	lower back (Audio apxa0065)
eructar	to belch (Audio apxa0066)
el bebé	baby (Audio apxa0067)
la espalda	back (Audio apxa0068)
el papel	paper (Audio apxa0069)
el equilibrio	equilibrium (Audio apxa0070)
la mesa	table (Audio apxa0071)
estornudar	to sneeze (Audio apxa0072)
el estómago	stomach (Audio apxa0073)
empujar	to push (Audio apxa0074)

F has the same sound as in English. (Audio apxa0075)

la fiebre	fever (Audio apxa0076)
frío	cold temperature (Audio apxa0077)
la fecha	date on the calendar (Audio apxa0078)
fumar	to smoke (Audio apxa0079)
flaco	skinny (Audio apxa0080)

G before *a, o,* or *u* has a hard sound in *get.* (Audio apxa0081)

Gordo	fat (Audio apxa0082)
las gafas	eyeglasses (Audio apxa0083)
el gargajo	phlegm (Audio apxa0084)
el gato	cat (Audio apxa0085)

G before an *e* or *i* has a guttural *h* sound as in the German *ach.* (Audio apxa0086)

la gente	people (Audio apxa0087)
las alergias	allergies (Audio apxa0088)
las gemelas	twins (Audio apxa0089)

Occasionally a silent *u* will precede the *e* or *i* to indicate that the **G** is hard, as in *go.* (Audio apxa0090)

pagué	paid (Audio apxa0091)
el hormigueo	tingling sensation or "pins and needles" (Audio apxa0092)

To keep the *u* sound in the *-gue* or *-gui* combination, a dieresis (¨) is placed over the *u* as in: (Audio apxa0093)

la vergüenza	shame (Audio apxa0094)
el ungüento	ointment (Audio apxa0095)

H is a silent letter. (Audio apxa0096)

humano	human (Audio apxa0097)
hinchar	to swell (Audio apxa0098)
las hormonas	hormones (Audio apxa0099)
el hueso	bone (Audio apxa0100)
el hígado	liver (Audio apxa0101)
el huevo	egg (Audio apxa0102)

I sounds like *ee* in English, as in *keen.* (Audio apxa0103)

irritable	irritable (Audio apxa0104)
la incisión	incision (Audio apxa0105)
el instrumento	instrument (Audio apxa0106)
incómodo	uncomfortable (Audio apxa0107)
mi	my (Audio apxa0108)

J sounds like a hard English *h* but with a more guttural *h* sound as in the German *ach*. (Audio apxa0109)

la jeringa	syringe (Audio apxa0110)
las orejas	ears (Audio apxa0111)
el juanete	bunion (Audio apxa0112)
los ojos	eyes (Audio apxa0113)
la aguja	needle (Audio apxa0114)
trabajar	to work (Audio apxa0115)

K is not part of the Spanish alphabet. It is used only in words of foreign origin, and it has the same pronunciation as in English. (Audio apxa0116)

el kilo	kilogram (Audio apxa0117)
el kilómetro	kilometer (Audio apxa0118)

L is the same as in English. (Audio apxa0119)

la lengua	tongue (Audio apxa0120)
la píldora	pill (Audio apxa0121)
el líquido	liquid (Audio apxa0122)
las lágrimas	tears (Audio apxa0123)
los labios	lips (Audio apxa0124)
la luz	light (Audio apxa0125)

LL sounds like *y* in the word *yes*. (Audio apxa0126)

los tobillos	ankles (Audio apxa0127)
llorar	to cry (Audio apxa0128)
la cuchillada	gash (Audio apxa0129)
las costillas	ribs (Audio apxa0130)
las espaldilla	shoulder blade (Audio apxa0131)
la mejilla	cheek (Audio apxa0132)

M is the same as in English. (Audio apxa0133)

morir	to die (Audio apxa0134)
las manos	hands (Audio apxa0135)
la médula	marrow (Audio apxa0136)
el músculo	muscle (Audio apxa0137)

N is pronounced like *m* before *b, f, p, m,* and *v*. (Audio apxa0138)

enfermo	sick (Audio apxa0139)
la enfermera	nurse (Audio apxa0140)
un brazo	arm (Audio apxa0141)
un viejo	old man (Audio apxa0142)
un pulmón	lung (Audio apxa0143)

N otherwise sounds the same as in English. (Audio apxa0144)

la náusea	nausea (Audio apxa0145 new)
nervioso	nervous (Audio apxa0146)
la nariz	nose (Audio apxa0147)
nacer	to be born (Audio apxa0148)

Ñ has the English sound of *ny* as in *canyon* or *ni* as in *onion*. (Audio apxa0149)

los riñones	kidneys (Audio apxa0150)
el puño	fist (Audio apxa0151)
estreñido	constipated (Audio apxa0152)
el sueño	dream, sleep (Audio apxa0153)
el señor	Mr., the gentleman, sir (Audio apxa0154)
la muñeca	wrist (Audio apxa0155)

O sounds like the *o* in *born*. (Audio apxa0156)

la obesidad	obesity (Audio apxa0157)
la oreja	ear (Audio apxa0158)
emocional	emotional (Audio apxa0159)
el muslo	thigh (Audio apxa0160)
no	no (Audio apxa0161)
el pelo	hair (Audio apxa0162)

O followed by a consonant sounds like the English *o* in *or*. (Audio apxa0163)

orinar	to urinate (Audio apxa0164)
el ombligo	navel (Audio apxa0165)
el órgano	organ (Audio apxa0166)

P has the same sound as in English. (Audio apxa0167)

la parálisis	paralysis (Audio apxa0168)
el pañal	diaper (Audio apxa0169)
poco	little, referring to quantity (Audio apxa0170)
el paciente	patient (Audio apxa0171)
la pulmonía	pneumonia (Audio apxa0172)
el papá	dad (Audio apxa0173)
puje	bear down (Audio apxa0174)

There are several silent **P**s, as in: (Audio apxa0175)

la psicología	psychology (Audio apxa0176)
la psiquiatra	psychiatrist (Audio apxa0177)
la psicoterapia	psychotherapy (Audio apxa0178)

Q appears only before *ue* or *ui*. The *u* is always silent, and the Q has a *k* sound. (Audio apxa0179)

quejar	to complain (Audio apxa0180)
tranquilo	tranquil (Audio apxa0181)
la quijada	jaw (Audio apxa0182)
la izquierda	left (Audio apxa0183)
los bronquios	bronchial tubes (Audio apxa0184)
el queso	cheese (Audio apxa0185)

R is trilled at the beginning of a word. (Audio apxa0186)

la roncha	rash (Audio apxa0187)
el reumatismo	rheumatism (Audio apxa0188)
las rodillas	knees (Audio apxa0189)
el resfriado, el resfrío	cold in the nose (Audio apxa0190)

R is slightly trilled in the middle of a word. (Audio apxa0191)

primo	cousin (Audio apxa0192)
la varicela	chicken pox (Audio apxa0193)
la hernia	hernia (Audio apxa0194)
operar	o operate (Audio apxa0195)
la nariz	nose (Audio apxa0196)

RR is strongly trilled. (Audio apxa0197)

el carro	car (Audio apxa0198)
el catarro	cold in the head (Audio apxa0199)
el perro	dog (Audio apxa0200)

S has the *ess* sound in English. (Audio apxa0201)

la saliva	saliva (Audio apxa0202)
toser	to cough (Audio apxa0203)
el sarampión	measles (Audio apxa0204)
la causa	cause (Audio apxa0205)
el sudor	sweat (Audio apxa0206)
la sangre	blood (Audio apxa0207)
la vista	sight, vision (Audio apxa0208)

S before *b, d, g, l, m, n*, and *v* has the *z* sound as in *toys*. (Audio apxa0209)

el asma	asthma (Audio apxa0210)
los dientes	teeth (Audio apxa0211)
la desgana	loss of appetite (Audio apxa0212)

T is similar to English. (Audio apxa0213)

el té	tea (Audio apxa0214)
tragar	to swallow (Audio apxa0215)
las tijeras	scissors (Audio apxa0216)
el teléfono	telephone (Audio apxa0217)
tranquilo	tranquil (Audio apxa0218)
este	this (Audio apxa0219)

U sounds like the English *u* in *rule*. (Audio apxa0220)

último	last in a series (Audio apxa0221)
usar	to use (Audio apxa0222)
la unión	union (Audio apxa0223)
único	only (Audio apxa0224)

V has the same sound as *b* in Castilian Spanish, spoken in Spain. In most Latin countries *v* sounds like *v*. (Audio apxa0225)

el vértigo	dizziness (Audio apxa0226)
vestirse	to get dressed (Audio apxa0227)
la verruga	wart (Audio apxa0228)
el vientre	belly (Audio apxa0229)
aliviarse	to get well (Audio apxa0230)

W is not part of the Spanish alphabet. It is used only in foreign words and is pronounced as it is in English. (Audio apxa0231)

Washington	Washington (Audio apxa0232)

X has the sound of English *x* before a consonant. (Audio apxa0233)

explicar	to explain (Audio apxa0234)
la extensión	extensión (Audio apxa0235)
excelente	excellent (Audio apxa0236)
el extranjero	foreigner (Audio apxa0237)

When it stands between vowels, **X** has a *gs* sound as in *eggs*. (Audio apxa0238)

el examen	exam (Audio apxa0239)
el oxígeno	oxygen (Audio apxa0240)

Y sounds like the English *y* in *yes*. (Audio apxa0241)

yo	I (Audio apxa0242)
el yodo	iodine (Audio apxa0243)
yeso	cast (Audio apxa0244)
el yerno	son-in-law (Audio apxa0245)

When **Y** follows *n*, it has the sound of the English *j* as in *judge*. (Audio apxa0246)

la inyección	injection (Audio apxa0247 new)
inyectar	to inject (Audio apxa0248 new)

When **Y** stands alone, it sounds like the Spanish *i*. (Audio apxa0249)

y	and (Audio apxa0250)

Z has the s sound in most Latin American dialects. However, the letter z is pronounced like the letter z in English in some areas of Spain. (Audio apxa0251)

el zumbido	buzzing (Audio apxa0252)
embarazada	pregnant (Audio apxa0253)
el corazón	heart (Audio apxa0254)
izquierda	left (Audio apxa0255 new)
el brazo	arm (Audio apxa0256)
zurdo	left-handed (Audio apxa0257)
el zapato	shoe (Audio apxa0258)
la matriz	womb (Audio apxa0259)

Appendix B
Gender of Nouns* (Audio apxb0001)

Apéndice B
Género de los Sustantivos

Appendix B is available in the eBook at ebooks.health.elsevier.com.
See inside cover for access details.

Appendix C
Adjectives, Pronouns, and Verbs*

Apéndice C
Adjetivos, Pronombres y Verbos (Audio apxc0001)

ADJECTIVES AND PRONOUNS
(SEE BOXES C1 AND C2)
ADJETIVOS Y PRONOMBRES
(VEA LOS CUADROS C1 Y C2)
(AUDIO AUDIO APXC0002)

Adjectives describe nouns and pronouns. In Spanish, adjectives are placed after the noun. They agree in number and gender with the noun they modify. (Audio apxc0003)

ADJECTIVES ENDING IN -O (AUDIO APXC0004)

Masculine singular:	The patient is happy.
(Audio apxc0005)	El paciente está contento.
	(Ehl pah-see-ehn-teh ehs-tah kohn-tehn-toh)
	(Audio apxc0006)
Feminine singular:	She is happy.
(Audio apxc0007)	Ella está contenta.
	(Eh-yah ehs-tah kohn-tehn-tah) (Audio apxc0008)
Masculine plural:	They are happy.
(Audio apxc0009)	Ellos están contentos.
	(Eh-yohs ehs-tahn kohn-tehn-tohs) (Audio apxc0010)
Feminine plural:	They are happy.
(Audio apxc0011)	Ellas están contentas.
	(Eh-yahs ehs-tahn kohn-tehn-tahs) (Audio apxc0012)

---

*From Joyce EV, Villaneuva ME: *Say It in Spanish*, ed 2, Saunders, Philadelphia, 2000.

ADJECTIVES ENDING IN -E (AUDIO APXC0013)

Masculine singular:	He is sad.
(Audio apxc0014)	El está triste.
	(Ehl ehs-tah trees-teh) (Audio apxc0015)
Feminine singular:	She is sad.
(Audio apxc0016)	Ella está triste.
	(Eh-yah ehs-tah trees-teh) (Audio apxc0017)
Masculine plural:	They are sad.
(Audio apxc0018)	Ellos están tristes.
	(Eh-yohs ehs-tahn trees-tehs) (Audio apxc0019)
Feminine plural:	They are sad.
(Audio apxc0020)	Ellas están tristes.
	(Eh-yahs ehs-tahn trees-tehs) (Audio apxc0021)

ADJECTIVES ENDING IN A CONSONANT (AUDIO APXC0022)

Masculine singular:	The procedure is difficult.
(Audio apxc0023)	El procedimiento es difícil.
	(Ehl proh-seh-dee-mee-ehn-toh ehs dee-fee-seel) (Audio apxc0024)
Feminine singular:	The measurement is difficult.
(Audio apxc0025)	La medida es difícil.
	(Lah meh-dee-dah ehs dee-fee-seel) (Audio apxc0026)
Masculine plural:	The exams are difficult.
(Audio apxc0027)	Los exámenes son difíciles.
	(Lohs ehx-ah-meh-nehs sohn dee-fee-see-lehs) (Audio apxc0028)
Feminine plural:	The measurements are difficult.
(Audio apxc0029)	Las medidas son difíciles.
	(Lahs meh-dee-dahs sohn dee-fee-see-lehs) (Audio apxc0030)

Demonstrative adjectives precede the nouns they modify and agree with them in number and gender. (Audio apxc0031)

this book	este libro
	(ehs-teh lee-broh) (Audio apxc0032)
these pens	estas plumas
	(ehs-tahs ploo-mahs) (Audio apxc0033)

Este (this) refers to what is near or directly concerns me. (Audio apxc0034)

Esos (those) refers to what is near or directly concerns you. (Audio apxc0035)

Aquel (that) refers to what is remote to the speaker or the person addressed. (Audio apxc0036)

This pencil is red.	Este lápiz es rojo. (Ehs-teh lah-pees ehs roh-hoh) (Audio apxc0037)
John, give me that bone.	Juan dame ese hueso. (Hoo-ahn, deh-meh ah-kehl oo-eh-soh) (Audio apxc0038)

SOME COMMON LIMITING ADJECTIVES (AUDIO APXC0039)

all, everything	todo (toh-doh) (Audio apxc0040)
bad	malo (mah-loh) (Audio apxc0041)
better	mejor (meh-hohr) (Audio apxc0042)
big (age)	grande (grahn-deh) (Audio apxc0043)
first	primero (pree-meh-roh) (Audio apxc0044)
fourth	cuarto (koo-ahr-toh) (Audio apxc0045)
good	bueno (boo-eh-noh)(Audio apxc0046)
less	menos (meh-nohs) (Audio apxc0047)
little, few	poco (poh-koh) (Audio apxc0048)
more	mucho, más (moo-choh, mahs) (Audio apxc0049)
nothing	nada (nah-dah) (Audio apxc0050)
one, a, an	un (oon) (Audio apxc0051)
small (age, fit)	pequeño/chico (peh-keh-nyoh/chee-koh) (Audio apxc0052)

POSSESSIVE PRONOUNS (AUDIO APXC0053)

	Singular	**Plural**
mine	el mío, la mía	los míos, las mías
	(ehl mee-oh, lah	(lohs mee-ohs, lahs mee-ahs)
	mee-ah)	(Audio apxc0054)
yours	el tuyo, la tuya	los tuyos, las tuyas
	(ehl too-yoh, lah too-	(lohs too-yohs, lahs too-yahs)
	yah)	(Audio apxc0055)
his, hers,	el suyo, la suya	los suyos, las suyas
theirs	(ehl soo-yoh, lah soo-	(lohs soo-yohs, lahs soo-yahs)
	yah)	(Audio apxc0056)
ours	el nuestro, la nuestra	los nuestros, las nuestras
	(ehl noo-ehs-troh, lah	(lohs noo-ehs-trohs, lahs ehs-
	noo-ehs-trah)	trahs) (Audio apxc0057)

Possessive pronouns are formed by the definite article + the long form of the possessive adjective. (Audio apxc0058)

My nose is	Mi nariz es más bonita que la tuya.
prettier than	(Mee nah-rees ehs mahs boh-nee-tah keh lah
yours.	too-yah) (Audio apxc0059)

After the verb **ser**, the article preceding the possessive pronoun is generally omitted. (Audio apxc0060)

The bones are mine.	Los huesos son míos.
	(Lohs oo-eh-sohs sohn mee-ohs) (Audio
	apxc0061)
That gown is yours.	Aquella bata es suya.
	(Ah-keh-yah bah-tah ehs soo-yah) (Audio
	apxc0062)
These books are	Estos libros son míos.
mine.	(Ehs-tohs lee-brohs sohn mee-ohs) (Audio
	apxc0063)

Possession is expressed by **de** + the possessor. This corresponds to 's or s' in English. (Audio apxc0064)

his pens and yours	sus plumas y las de usted (soos ploo-mahs ee lahs deh oos-tehd) (Audio apxc0065)
Martin's pencil	el lápiz de Martín(ehl lah-pees deh Mahr-teen) (Audio apxc0066)
my book and Louisa's	mi libro y el de Luisa (mee lee-broh ee ehl deh Loo-ee-sah) (Audio apxc0067)
our patient	nuestro paciente (noo-ehs-troh pah-see-ehn-teh) (Audio apxc0068)
her rings	sus anillos (soos ah-nee-yohs) (Audio apxc0069)
a friend of theirs	un amigo de ellos (oon ah-mee-goh deh eh-yohs) (Audio apxc0070)

WHOSE? (AUDIO APXC0071)

The interrogative pronoun whose? is expressed in Spanish by **¿de quién es?** (Audio apxc0072)

Whose pen is it?	¿De quién es la pluma? (Deh kee-ehn ehs lah ploo-mah) (Audio apxc0073)
It belongs to the doctor.	Es del doctor.(Ehs dehl dohk-tohr) (Audio apxc0074)
Whose card is it?	¿De quién es la tarjeta? (Deh kee-ehn ehs lah tahr-heh-tah) (Audio apxc0075)
Mr. García's.	Del señor García. (Dehl seh-nyohr Gahr-see-ah) (Audio apxc0076)
Whose x-rays are these?	¿De quién son estas radiografías? (Deh kee-ehn sohn ehs-tahs rah-dee-oh-grah-fee-ahs) (Audio apxc0077)
They are Mrs. Luna's.	Son de la señora Luna. (Sohn deh lah seh-nyoh-rah Loo-nah) (Audio apxc0078)

SOME COMMON PREPOSITIONS (AUDIO APXC0079)

about	acerca de
	(ah-sehr-kah deh) (Audio apxc0080)
according	según
	(seh-goon) (Audio apxc0081)
after	después de
	(dehs-poo-ehs deh) (Audio apxc0082)
against	contra
	(kohn-trah) (Audio apxc0083)
among, between	entre
	(ehn-treh) (Audio apxc0084)
around	alrededor de
	(ahl-reh-deh-dohr deh) (Audio apxc0085)
before	antes de
	(ahn-tehs deh) (Audio apxc0086)
behind	detrás de
	(deh-trahs deh) (Audio apxc0087)
beneath, under	debajo de
	(deh-bah-hoh deh) (Audio apxc0088)
beside	además de
	(ah-deh-mahs deh) (Audio apxc0089)
during	durante
	(doo-rahn-teh) (Audio apxc0090)
far	lejos de
	(leh-hohs deh) (Audio apxc0091)
for	para
	(pah-rah) (Audio apxc0092)
for, by,	por
therefore	(pohr) (Audio apxc0093)
from, of	de
	(deh) (Audio apxc0094)
in, or	en
	(ehn) (Audio apxc0095)
in front of	enfrente de
	(ehn-frehn-teh deh) (Audio apxc0096)
in front of	delante de
	(deh-lahn-teh deh) (Audio apxc0097)

near	cerca de
	(sehr-kah deh) (Audio apxc0098)
outside of	fuera de
	(foo-eh-rah deh) (Audio apxc0099)
over, above	sobre
	(soh-breh) (Audio apxc0100)
since	desde
	(dehs-deh) (Audio apxc0101)
to, at	a
	(ah)(Audio apxc0102)
toward	hacia
	(ah-see-ah) (Audio apxc0103)
until	hasta
	(ahs-tah) (Audio apxc0104)
with	con
	(kohn) (Audio apxc0105)
within	dentro de
	(dehn-troh deh) (Audio apxc0106)

Box C1 Feminine and Masculine Adjectives
Cuadro C1 Adjetivos Femeninos y Masculinos (Audio apxc0107)

Adjective	Feminine	Masculine
this	esta (ehs-tah)	este (ehs-teh) (Audio apxc0108)
these	estas (ehs-tahs)	estos (ehs-tohs) (Audio apxc0109)
that	esa (eh-sah)	ese (eh-seh) (Audio apxc0110)
those	esas (eh-sahs)	esos (eh-sohs) (Audio apxc0111)
that	aquella (ah-keh-yah)	aquel (ah-kehl) (Audio apxc0112)
those	aquellas (ah-keh-yahs)	aquellos (ah-keh-yohs) (Audio apxc0113)

Box C2
Personal Pronouns

Cuadro C2
Pronombres Personales
(Audio apxc0114)

Singular	Plural
I	we (masculine)
yo	nosotros
(yoh)(Audio apxc0115)	(noh-soh-trohs) (Audio apxc0116)
	we (feminine)
	nosotras
	(noh-soh-trahs) (Audio apxc0117)
you (familiar)	you
tú	vosotros/as
(too)(Audio apxc0118)	(boh-soh-trohs/ahs) (Audio apxc0119)
you (formal)	you
ustedes	(oos-tehd) (Audio apxc0120)
(oos-tehd)	(oos-teh-dehs) (Audio apxc0121)
he	they (masculine)
él	ellos
(ehl) (Audio apxc0122)	(eh-yohs) (Audio apxc0123)
she	they (feminine)
ella	ellas
(eh-yah) (Audio apxc0124)	(eh-yahs) (Audio apxc0125)

VERBS
VERBOS (AUDIO APXC0126)

Verbs are to a sentence what the spinal cord is to the body. Verbs give structure to a sentence because they tell us what is being done and when it is being done: for example, I *talk* to the nurse (present), I *talked* to the nurse (past), I *will talk* to the nurse (future).

Los verbos son para una oración lo que la espina dorsal es para el cuerpo. Los verbos dan estructura a una oración al indicar qué es lo que se está haciendo y cuándo se está haciendo, por ejemplo: Yo *hablo* **con la enfermera (presente), Yo** *hablé* **con la enfermera (pasado), Yo** *hablaré* **con la enfermera (futuro)**. (Audio apxc0127)

Regular verbs end in **-ar**, **-er**, or **-ir** in Spanish. They are easy to conjugate because you usually take the stem of the verb and add the endings: **o**, **as**, **a**, **amos**, **an**. (See Box C3)

Los verbos regulares tienen la terminación *-ar, -er,* **o** *-ir* **en español. Son fáciles de conjugar ya que usualmente se toma la raíz del verbo y se le agrega la terminación:** *o, as, a, amos, -an.* (**Vea el Cuadro C3**) (Audio apxc0128)

to auscultate	auscultar
	(ah-oos-kool-tahr) (Audio apxc0129)
to be born	nacer
	(nah-sehr) (Audio apxc0130)
to become ill	enfermarse
	(ehn-fehr-mahr-seh) (Audio apxc0131)
to bring near	acercar
	(ah-sehr-kahr) (Audio apxc0132)
to call	llamar
	(yah-mahr) (Audio apxc0133)
to die	morir
	(moh-reer) (Audio apxc0134)
to eat	comer
	(koh-mehr) (Audio apxc0135)
to examine	examiner
	(ehx-ah-mee-nahr) (Audio apxc0136)
to get better	mejorar
	(meh-hoh-rahr) (Audio apxc0137)
to heal	sanar
	(sah-nahr) (Audio apxc0138)
to hear	oír
	(oh-eer) (Audio apxc0139)
to hurt	doler
	(doh-lehr) (Audio apxc0140)

to leave (behind)	dejar
	(deh-hahr) (Audio apxc0141)
to listen	escuchar
	(ehs-koo-chahr) (Audio apxc0142)
to live	vivir
	(bee-beer) (Audio apxc0143)
to name	nombrar
	(nohm-brahr) (Audio apxc0144)
to operate	operar
	(oh-peh-rahr) (Audio apxc0145)
to palpate	palpar
	(pahl-pahr) (Audio apxc0146)
to revise	revisar
	(reh-bee-sahr) (Audio apxc0147)
to see	ver
	(behr) (Audio apxc0148)
to vomit	vomitar
	(boh-mee-tahr) (Audio apxc0149)
to agree	acordar
	(ah-kohr-dahr) (Audio apxc0150)
to bore	aburrir
	(ah-boo-reer) (Audio apxc0151)
to come	venir
	(beh-neer) (Audio apxc0152)
to deserve	merecer
	(meh-reh-sehr) (Audio apxc0153)
to finish	acabar
	(ah-kah-bahr) (Audio apxc0154)
to go out	salir
	(sah-leer) (Audio apxc0155)
to let go	soltar
	(sohl-tahr) (Audio apxc0156)
to need	necesitar
	(neh-seh-see-tahr) (Audio apxc0157)
to reach	alcanzar
	(ahl-kahn-sahr) (Audio apxc0158)
to remain	quedar
	(keh-dahr) (Audio apxc0159)
to stop	parar
	(pah-rahr) (Audio apxc0160)

to take out	sacar
	(sah-kahr) (Audio apxc0161)
to walk	caminar
	(kah-mee-nahr) (Audio apxc0162)

Personal pronouns designate who is performing the action. Many times it is not necessary to include personal pronouns when conjugating a verb or using it in a sentence.

Los pronombres personales designan a las personas que hacen la acción. Muchas veces no es necesario incluir los pronombres personales al conjugar verbos o al usarlos en una oración. (Audio apxc0163)

PERSONAL PRONOUNS (AUDIO APXC0164)

I	yo
	(yoh) (Audio apxc0165)
you (informal)	tú
	(too) (Audio apxc0166)
he/she/you (formal)	él/ella/usted
	(ehl/eh-yah/oos-tehd) (Audio apxc0167)
we	nosotros
	(noh-soh-trohs) (Audio apxc0168)
they/you (plural)	ellos/ellas/ustedes
	(eh-yohs/eh-yahs/oos-teh-dehs) (Audio apxc0169)
To Feel	**Sentir**
	(Sehn-Teer) (Audio apxc0170)
I feel	**siento**
	(see-ehn-toh) (Audio apxc0171)
you feel	**sientes**
	(see-ehn-tehs) (Audio apxc0172)
he/she feels; you feel	**siente**
	(see-ehn-teh) (Audio apxc0173)
we feel	**sentimos**
	(sehn-tee-mohs) (Audio apxc0174)
they feel	**sienten**
	(see-ehn-tehn) (Audio apxc0175)

To Sit Down	**Sentarse**
	(Sehn-Tahr-Seh) (Audio apxc0176)
I sit	**me siento**
	(meh see-ehn-toh) (Audio apxc0177)
you sit	**te sientas**
	(teh see-ehn-tahs) (Audio apxc0178)
he/she sits; you sit	**se sienta**
	(seh see-ehn-tah) (Audio apxc0179)
we sit	**nos sentamos**
	(nohs sehn-tah-mohs) (Audio apxc0180)
they sit	**se sientan**
	(seh see-ehn-tahn) (Audio apxc0181)

REFLEXIVE PRONOUNS (AUDIO APXC0182)

The reflexive pronouns change the verb's action.
Los pronombres reflexivos cambian la acción del verbo.
(Audio apxc0183)
Mover (To Move) (Audio apxc0184)

Action on Self	Action on Object (Audio apxc0185)
yo me muevo	yo muevo
(yoh meh moo-eh-boh) (Audio apxc0185)	(yoh moo-eh-boh) (Audio apxc0190)
tú te mueves	tú mueves
(too teh moo-eh-behs) (Audio apxc0186)	(too moo-eh-behs) (Audio apxc0191)
él/ella se mueve	él/ella mueve
(ehl/eh-yah seh moo-eh-beh) (Audio apxc0187)	(ehl/eh-yah moo-eh-beh) (Audio apxc0192)
nosotros nos movemos	nosotros movemos
(noh-soh-trohs nohs moh-beh-mohs) (Audio apxc0188)	(noh-soh-trohs moh-beh-mohs) (Audio apxc0193)
ellos/ellas se mueven	ellos/ellas mueven
(eh-yohs/eh-yahs seh moo-eh-behn) (Audio apxc0189)	(eh-yohs/eh-yahs moo-eh-behn) (Audio apxc0194)

to advise	aconsejar
	(ah-kohn-seh-hahr) (Audio apxc0195)
to ask	preguntar
	(preh-goon-tahr) (Audio apxc0196)
to bathe	bañar
	(bah-nyahr) (Audio apxc0197)
to be afraid	temer
	(teh-mehr) (Audio apxc0198)
to believe	creer
	(kreh-ehr) (Audio apxc0199)
to boil	hervir
	(ehr-beer) (Audio apxc0200)
to break	romper
	(rohm-pehr) (Audio apxc0201)
to build	construer
	(kohns-troo-eer) (Audio apxc0202)
to carry	llevar
	(yeh-bahr) (Audio apxc0203)
to change	cambiar
	(kahm-bee-ahr) (Audio apxc0204)
to clean	limpiar
	(leem-pee-ahr) (Audio apxc0205)
to communicate	comunicar
	(koh-moo-nee-kahr) (Audio apxc0206)
to complain	quejar
	(keh-hahr) (Audio apxc0207)
to conduct	conducer
	(kohn-doo-seer) (Audio apxc0208)
to confuse	confundir
	(kohn-foon-deer) (Audio apxc0209)
to cook	cocinar
	(koh-see-nahr) (Audio apxc0210)
to cover	cubrir
	(koo-breer) (Audio apxc0211)
to cry	llorar
	(yoh-rahr) (Audio apxc0212)
to cut	cortar
	(kohr-tahr) (Audio apxc0213)

to deny	negar
	(neh-gahr) (Audio apxc0214)
to destroy	destruir
	(dehs-troo-eer) (Audio apxc0215)
to disappear	desaparecer
	(deh-sah-pah-reh-sehr) (Audio apxc0216)
to discover, find	descubrir
	(dehs-koo-breer) (Audio apxc0217)
to do/make	hacer
	(ah-sehr) (Audio apxc0218)
to drink	beber
	(beh-behr) (Audio apxc0219)
to eat breakfast	desayunar
	(deh-sah-yoo-nahr) (Audio apxc0220)
to embrace	abrazar
	(ah-brah-sahr) (Audio apxc0221)
to employ	emplear
	(ehm-pleh-ahr) (Audio apxc0222)
to feel	sentir
	(sehn-teer) (Audio apxc0223)
to fill	llenar
	(yeh-nahr) (Audio apxc0224)
to find	hallar
	(ah-yahr) (Audio apxc0225)
to fix	componer
	(kohm-poh-nehr) (Audio apxc0226)
to fly	volar
	(boh-lahr) (Audio apxc0227)
to get up, raise	levanter
	(leh-bahn-tahr) (Audio apxc0228)
to give	dar
	(dahr) (Audio apxc0229)
to go	ir
	(eer) (Audio apxc0230)
to go to bed, lie down	acostarse
	(ah-kohs-tahr-seh) (Audio apxc0231)
to have	haber
	(ah-behr) (Audio apxc0232)

to hunt	cazar
	(kah-sahr) (Audio apxc0233)
to joke, kid	bromear
	(broh-meh-ahr) (Audio apxc0234)
to jump	saltar
	(sahl-tahr) (Audio apxc0235)
to kiss	besar
	(beh-sahr) (Audio apxc0236)
to know	conocer
	(koh-noh-sehr) (Audio apxc0237)
to lose	perder
	(pehr-dehr) (Audio apxc0238)
to marry	casar
	(kah-sahr) (Audio apxc0239)
to paint	pintar
	(peen-tahr) (Audio apxc0240)
to point	señalar
	(seh-nyah-lahr) (Audio apxc0241)
to promise	prometer
	(proh-meh-tehr) (Audio apxc0242)
to receive	recibir
	(reh-see-beer) (Audio apxc0243)
to recognize	reconocer(reh-koh-noh-sehr) (Audio apxc0244)
to remember	recorder
	(reh-kohr-dahr) (Audio apxc0245)
to respond	responder
	(rehs-pohn-dehr) (Audio apxc0246)
to return	regresar/Volver
	(reh-greh-sahr/bohl-behr) (Audio apxc0247)
to scream	gritar
	(gree-tahr) (Audio apxc0248)
to see	ver
	(behr) (Audio apxc0249)
to sell	vender
	(behn-dehr) (Audio apxc0250)
to serve	servir
	(sehr-beer) (Audio apxc0251)

to shake	temblar
	(tehm-blahr) (Audio apxc0252)
to sit	sentar
	(sehn-tahr) (Audio apxc0253)
to sleep	dormir
	(dohr-meer) (Audio apxc0254)
to speak	hablar
	(ah-blahr) (Audio apxc0255)
to start	comenzar
	(koh-mehn-sahr) (Audio apxc0256)
to step	pisar
	(pee-sahr) (Audio apxc0257)
to suffer	sufrir
	(soo-freer) (Audio apxc0258)
to take	tomar
	(toh-mahr) (Audio apxc0259)
to thank for	agradecer
	(ah-grah-deh-sehr) (Audio apxc0260)
to try	tratar
	(trah-tahr) (Audio apxc0261)
to turn	voltear
	(bohl-teh-ahr) (Audio apxc0262)
to turn off	apagar
	(ah-pah-gahr) (Audio apxc0263)
to want	querer
	(keh-rehr) (Audio apxc0264)
to wash	lavar
	(lah-bahr) (Audio apxc0265)
to wish	desear
	(deh-seh-ahr) (Audio apxc0266)
to work	trabajar
	(trah-bah-hahr) (Audio apxc0267)
to accept	aceptar
	(ah-sehp-tahr) (Audio apxc0268)
to activate	activar
	(ahk-tee-bahr) (Audio apxc0269)
to administer	administrar
	(ahd-mee-nees-trahr)(Audio apxc0270)

to authorize	autorizar
	(ah-oo-toh-ree-sahr) (Audio apxc0271)
to beat, knock	golpear
	(gohl-peh-ahr) (Audio apxc0272)
to bleed	sangrar
	(sahn-grahr) (Audio apxc0273)
to conserve	conserver
	(kohn-sehr-bahr) (Audio apxc0274)
to control	controlar
	(kohn-troh-lahr) (Audio apxc0275)
to evaluate	evaluar
to hit	pegar
	(peh-gahr) (Audio apxc0277)
to inform	informar
	(een-fohr-mahr) (Audio apxc0278)
to interpret	interpreter
	(een-tehr-preh-tahr) (Audio apxc0279)
to present	presentar
	(preh-sehn-tahr) (Audio apxc0280)
to protect	proteger
	(proh-teh-hehr) (Audio apxc0281)
to provoke	provocar
	(proh-boh-kahr) (Audio apxc0282)
to reduce	reducer
	(reh-doo-seer) (Audio apxc0283)
to revise	revisar
	(reh-bee-sahr) (Audio apxc0284)
to select	seleccionar
	(seh-lehk-see-oh-nahr) (Audio apxc0285)
to separate	separar
	(seh-pah-rahr) (Audio apxc0286)
to suspend	suspender
	(soos-pehn-dehr) (Audio apxc0287)
to write	escribir
	(ehs-kree-beer) (Audio apxc0288)

The verbs **ser** and **estar** both translate in English as to be, but they are not interchangeable. Both are irregular in the present and the past tense. (See Boxes C4 and C5)

Los verbos ser y estar se traducen al inglés **to be**, pero no son intercambiables. Los dos verbos son irregulares en el tiempo presente y en el pasado. (Vea los Cuadros C4 y C5) (Audio apxc0289)

	SER	**ESTAR**
I am	yo soy (yo soh-ee)	yo estoy (yoh ehs-tohy) (Audio apxc0290)
you are	usted es/tú eres (oos-tehd ehs-too eh-rehs)	usted está/tú estás (oos-tehd ehs-tah/too ehs-tahs) (Audio apxc0291)
he/she/it is	él/ella/eso es (ehl/eh-yah/eh-soh ehs)	él/ella/eso está (ehl/eh-yah/eh-soh ehs-tah) (Audio apxc0292)
we are	nosotros somos (noh-soh-trohs soh-mohs)	nosotros estamos (noh-soh-trohs ehs-tah-mohs) (Audio apxc0293)
they are	ellos/ellas son (eh-yohs/eh-yahs sohn)	ellos/ellas están (eh-yohs/eh-yahs ehs-tahn) (Audio apxc0294))

USES OF SER (Audio apxc0295)

Ser *expresses a relatively permanent quality. (Audio apxc0296)*

age:	You are old.	Usted es viejo. (Audio apxc0297)
characteristic:	Snow is cold.	nieve es fría. (Audio apxc0298)
color:	Urine is yellow.	orina es amarilla. (Audio apxc0299)
shape:	The glass is round.	El vaso es redondo. (Audio apxc0300)
size:	You are tall.	Usted es alto. (Audio apxc0301)
possession:	The pencil is mine.	El lápiz es mío. (Audio apxc0302)
wealth:	The man is rich.	El hombre es rico. (Audio apxc0303)

Ser *is used with predicate nouns, pronouns, or adjectives. (Audio apxc0304)*

He is a dentist.	El es dentista (Audio apxc0305)
Who am I?	¿Quién soy yo? (Audio apxc0306)
We are Protestant.	Nosotros somos protestantes. (Audio apxc0307)

Ser *indicates material, origin, or ownership. (Audio apxc0308)*

material:	The needle is metal.	La aguja es de metal. (Audio apxc0309)
origin:	The doctor is from Texas.	El doctor es de Tejas. (Audio apxc0310)
ownership:	The dentures are mine.	Las dentaduras son mías. (Audio apxc0311)

Ser *tells time. (Audio apxc0312)*

It is one o'clock.	Es la una. (Audio apxc0313)
It is 10 o'clock.	Son las diez. (Audio apxc0314)

USES OF ESTAR (Audio apxc0315)

Estar *expresses location (permanent and temporary). (Audio apxc0316)*

Dallas is in Texas.	Dallas está en Tejas. (Audio apxc0317)
I am in the room.	Yo estoy en el cuarto. (Audio apxc0318)

Estar *expresses status of health. (Audio apxc0319)*

How are you?	¿Cómo está usted? (Audio apxc0320)
I am fine.	Estoy bien. (Audio apxc0321)
We are sick.	Estamos enfermos. (Audio apxc0322)

Estar *expresses a temporary characteristic or quality. (Audio apxc0323)*

He is nervous.	El está nervioso. (Audio apxc0324)
I am ready.	Estoy lista. (Audio apxc0325)
You are far away.	Usted está lejos. (Audio apxc0326)

Box C3 **Regular Verb**		**Cuadro C3** **Verbo (Audio apxc0327)**	
Regular Verb	**Stem**	**Endings**	**Persons**
to live	viv-	o	yo vivo (yoh bee-boh)
vivir (bee beer) (Audio apxc0328)	viv-	es	tú vives (too bee-behs)
	viv-	e	el/ella vive (ehl/eh-yah bee-beh)
	viv-	imos	nosotros vivimos (noh-soh-trohs bee-bee-mohs)
	viv-	en	ellos/ellas viven (eh-yohs/eh-yahs bee-behn) (Audio apxc0329)

Box C4 **Present and** **Past Tense**	**Cuadro C4** **Tiempo Presente y Pasado** **(Audio apxc0330)**	
Verb: to eat	comer	(koh-mehr) (Audio apxc0331)
Present Tense	**Tiempo Presente** (Audio apxc0332)	
I eat	yo como	(yoh koh-moh) (Audio apxc0333)
you eat	tú comes	(too koh-mehs) (Audio apxc0334)

Box C4 Present and Past Tense	**Cuadro C4 Tiempo Presente y Pasado (Audio apxc0330)**	
he/she eats	**él/ella come**	**(ehl/eh-yah koh-meh)** (Audio apxc0335)
we eat	**nosotros comemos**	**(noh-soh-trohs koh-meh-mos)** (Audio apxc0336)
they eat	**ellos/ellas comen**	**(eh-yohs/eh-yahs koh-mehn)** (Audio apxc0337)
Past Tense	**Tiempo Pasado** (Audio apxc0338)	
I ate	**yo comí**	**(yoh koh-mee)** (Audio apxc0339)
you ate	**tú comiste**	**(too koh-mees-teh)** (Audio apxc0340)
he/she ate	**él/ella comió**	**(ehl/eh-yah koh-mee-oh)** (Audio apxc0341)
we ate	**nosotros comimos**	**(noh-soh-trohs coh-mee-mohs)** (Audio apxc0342)
they ate	**ellos/ellas comieron**	**(eh-yohs/eh-yahs koh-mee-eh-rohn)** (Audio apxc0343)

Box C5 **Verb** **Tenses**	**CuadroC5** **Tiempo de los Verbos** **(Audio apxc0344)**	
Verb: to speak (Audio apxc0345)		
Present Tense	**Tiempo Presente** (Audio apxc0346)	
speak	hablar	(ah-blahr) (Audio apxc0347)
I speak	yo hablo	(yoh ah-bloh) (Audio apxc0348)
you speak	tú hablas	(too ah-blahs) (Audio apxc0349)
he/she speaks	él/ella habla	(ehl/eh-yah ah-blah) (Audio apxc0350)
we speak	nosotros hablamos	(noh-soh-trohs ah-blah-mohs) (Audio apxc0351)
they speak	ellos/ellas hablan	(eh-yohs/eh-yahs ah-blahn) (Audio apxc0352)
Past Tense	**Tiempo Pasado** (Audio apxc0353)	
I spoke	yo hablé	(yoh ah-bleh) (Audio apxc0354)
you spoke	tú hablaste	(too ah-blahs-teh) (Audio apxc0355)

Box C5 Verb Tenses	**CuadroC5 Tiempo de los Verbos (Audio apxc0344)**	
he/she spoke	él/ella habló	(ehl/eh-yah ah-bloh) (Audio apxc0356)
we spoke	nosotros hablamos	(noh-soh-trohs ah-blah-mohs) (Audio apxc0357)
they spoke	ellos/ellas hablaron	(eh-yohs/eh-yahs ah-blah-rohn) (Audio apxc0358)
Future Tense	**Tiempo Future** (Audio apxc0359)	
I will speak	yo hablaré	(yoh ah-blah-reh) (Audio apxc0360)
you will speak	tú hablarás	(too ah-blah-rahs) (Audio apxc0361)
he/she will speak	él/ella hablará	(ehl/eh-yah ah-blah-rah) (Audio apxc0362)
we will speak	nosotros hablaremos	(noh-soh-trohs ah-blah-reh-mohs) (Audio apxc0363)
they will speak	ellos/ellas hablarán	(eh-yohs/eh-yahs ah-blah-rahn) (Audio apxc0364)

Glossary* (Audio glos0001)

Glosario

DAYS OF THE WEEK	LOS DÍAS DE LA SEMANA (AUDIO GLOS0002)
Monday	lunes (Audio glos0003)
Tuesday	martes (Audio glos0004)
Wednesday	miércoles (Audio glos0005)
Thursday	jueves (Audio glos0006)
Friday	viernes (Audio glos0007)
Saturday	sábado (Audio glos0008)
Sunday	domingo (Audio glos0009)

MONTHS	LOS MESES (AUDIO GLOS0010)
January	enero (Audio glos0011)
February	febrero (Audio glos0012)
March	marzo (Audio glos0013)
April	abril (Audio glos0014)
May	mayo (Audio glos0015)
June	junio (Audio glos0016)
July	julio (Audio glos0017)
August	agosto (Audio glos0018)
September	septiembre (Audio glos0019)

---

*Portions of this glossary from Chou B: *Practical Spanish in Eyecare*, Butterworth-Heinemann, Boston, 2001; Wilbur CJ, Lister S: *Medical Spanish: The Instant Survivor's Guide*, ed 3, Butterworth-Heinemann, Boston, 1995.

October		octubre (Audio glos0020)
November		noviembre (Audio glos0021)
December		diciembre (Audio glos0022)

ORDINAL NUMBERS — NÚMEROS ORDINALES (AUDIO GLOS0023)

First	primero/a (Audio glos0024)
Second	segundo/a (Audio glos0025)
Third	tercero/a (Audio glos0026)
Fourth	cuarto/a (Audio glos0027)
Fifth	quinto/a (Audio glos0028)
Sixth	sexto/a (Audio glos0029)
Seventh	séptimo/a (Audio glos0030)
Eighth	octavo/a (Audio glos0031)
Ninth	noveno/a (Audio glos0032)
Tenth	décimo/a (Audio glos0033)

CARDINAL NUMBERS — NÚMEROS CARDINALES (AUDIO GLOS0034)

0	**Zero**	cero (Audio glos0035)
1	**One**	uno/a (Audio glos0036)
2	**Two**	dos (Audio glos0037)
3	**Three**	tres (Audio glos0038)
4	**Four**	cuatro (Audio glos0039)
5	**Five**	cinco (Audio glos0040)
6	**Six**	seis (Audio glos0041)
7	**Seven**	siete (Audio glos0042)
8	**Eight**	ocho (Audio glos0043)
9	**Nine**	nueve (Audio glos0044)

10	**Ten**	diez (Audio glos0045)
11	**Eleven**	once (Audio glos0046)
12	**Twelve**	doce (Audio glos0047)
13	**Thirteen**	trece (Audio glos0048)
14	**Fourteen**	catorce (Audio glos0049)
15	**Fifteen**	quince (Audio glos0050)
16	**Sixteen**	dieciséis (Audio glos0051)
17	**Seventeen**	diecisiete (Audio glos0052)
18	**Eighteen**	dieciocho (Audio glos0053)
19	**Nineteen**	diecinueve (Audio glos0054)
20	**Twenty**	veinte (Audio glos0055)
21	**Twenty-One**	veintiuno (Audio glos0056)
22	**Twenty-Two**	veintidós (Audio glos0057)
23	**Twenty-Three**	veintitrés (Audio glos0058)
24	**Twenty-Four**	veinticuatro (Audio glos0059)
25	**Twenty-Five**	veinticinco (Audio glos0060)
26	**Twenty-Six**	veintiséis (Audio glos0061)
27	**Twenty-Seven**	veintisiete (Audio glos0062)
28	**Twenty-Eight**	veintiocho (Audio glos0063)
29	**Twenty-Nine**	veintinueve (Audio glos0064)
30	**Thirty**	treinta (Audio glos0065)
40	**Forty**	cuarenta (Audio glos0066)
50	**Fifty**	cincuenta (Audio glos0067)
60	**Sixty**	sesenta (Audio glos0068)
70	**Seventy**	setenta (Audio glos0069)
80	**Eighty**	ochenta (Audio glos0070)
90	**Ninety**	noventa (Audio glos0071)
100	**One Hundred**	cien (ciento) (Audio glos0072)
101	**One Hundred One**	ciento uno (Audio glos0073)

102	**One Hundred Two**	ciento dos (Audio glos0074)
103	**One Hundred Three**	ciento tres (Audio glos0075)
104	**One Hundred Four**	ciento cuatro (Audio glos0076)
105	**One Hundred Five**	ciento cinco (Audio glos0077)
106	**One Hundred Six**	ciento seis (Audio glos0078)
107	**One Hundred Seven**	ciento siete (Audio glos0079)
108	**One Hundred Eight**	ciento ocho (Audio glos0080)
109	**One Hundred Nine**	ciento nueve (Audio glos0081)
110	**One Hundred Ten**	ciento diez (Audio glos0082)
200	**Two Hundred**	doscientos (Audio glos0083)
300	**Three Hundred**	trescientos (Audio glos0084)
400	**Four Hundred**	cuatrocientos (Audio glos0085)
500	**Five Hundred**	quinientos (Audio glos0086)
600	**Six Hundred**	seiscientos (Audio glos0087)
700	**Seven Hundred**	setecientos (Audio glos0088)
800	**Eight Hundred**	ochocientos (Audio glos0089)
900	**Nine Hundred**	novecientos (Audio glos0090)
1000	**One Thousand**	mil (Audio glos00891)
1991	**One Thousand Nine Hundred Ninety-One**	mil novecientos noventa y uno (Audio glos0092)
2001	**Two Thousand One**	dos mil uno (Audio glos0093)

INTERROGATIVES

PALABRAS INTERROGATIVAS (AUDIO GLOS0094)

How?	¿Cómo? (Audio glos0095)
How far?	¿A qué distancia? (Audio glos0096)
How often?	¿Con qué frecuencia? (Audio glos0097)
How much?	¿Cuánto? (Audio glos0098)
How many?	¿Cuántos? (Audio glos0099)
How long?	¿Cuánto tiempo? (Audio glos0100)
How many times?	¿Cuántas veces? (Audio glos0101)
What?	¿Qué? (Audio glos0102)
What else?	¿Qué más? (Audio glos0103)
What for?	¿Para qué? (Audio glos0104)
When?	¿Cuándo? (Audio glos0105)
Where?	¿Dónde? (Audio glos0106)
From where?	¿De dónde? (Audio glos0107)
To where?	¿Adónde? (Audio glos0108)
Which?	¿Cuál? (Audio glos0109)
Which (ones)?	¿Cuáles? (Audio glos0110)_
Who?	¿Quién? (Audio glos0111)
To whom?	¿A quién? (Audio glos0112)
Whose?	¿De quién? (Audio glos0113)
Why?	¿Por qué? (Audio glos0114)

EXPRESSIONS OF TIME

EXPRESIONES DE TIEMPO (AUDIO GLOS0115)

year	el año (Audio glos0116)
month	el mes (Audio glos0117)
week	la semana (Audio glos0118)

day	el día (Audio glos0119)
hour	la hora (Audio glos0120)
minute	el minuto (Audio glos0121)
second	el segundo (Audio glos0122)
today	hoy (Audio glos0123)
tomorrow	mañana (Audio glos0124)
day after tomorrow	pasado mañana (Audio glos0125)
yesterday	ayer (Audio glos0126)
day before yesterday	anteayer (Audio glos0127)
tonight	esta noche (Audio glos0128)
last night	anoche (Audio glos0129)
tomorrow morning	mañana por la mañana (Audio glos0130)
tomorrow afternoon	mañana por la tarde (Audio glos0131)
tomorrow evening	mañana por la noche (Audio glos0132)
every morning	cada mañana, todas las mañanas (Audio glos0133)
every afternoon	cada tarde, todas las tardes (Audio glos0134)
every evening	cada noche, todas las noches (Audio glos0135)
every night	cada noche (Audio glos0136)
in the morning	por la mañana (Audio glos0137)
in the afternoon	por la tarde (Audio glos0138)
in the evening	por la noche (Audio glos0139)
at night	en la noche (Audio glos0140)
all morning	toda la mañana (Audio glos0141)
all afternoon	toda la tarde (Audio glos0142)
all night	toda la noche (Audio glos0143)

2 days ago	hace dos días (Audio glos0144)
3 weeks ago	hace tres semanas (Audio glos0145)
6 years ago	hace seis años (Audio glos0146)
always	siempre (Audio glos0147)
never	nunca (Audio glos0148)
sometimes	algunas veces (Audio glos0149)
from time to time	de vez en cuando (Audio glos0150)
now	ahora (Audio glos0151)
right now	ahora mismo (Audio glos0152)
before	antes (Audio glos0153)
after	después (Audio glos0154)
later	más tarde (Audio glos0155)
next week	la semana próxima (Audio glos0156)
until	hasta (Audio glos0157)

CLOTHING

LA ROPA
(AUDIO GLOS0158)

bathing suit	el traje de baño (Audio glos0159)
bathrobe	la bata (de baño) (Audio glos0160)
belt	el cinturón (Audio glos0161)
blouse	la blusa (Audio glos0162)
blue jeans	los vaqueros (Audio glos0163)
boot	la bota (Audio glos0164)
brassiere	el sostén (Audio glos0165)
button	el botón (Audio glos0166)
cap	la gorra (Audio glos0167)
coat	el abrigo (Audio glos0168)
collar	el cuello (Audio glos0169)
corset	el corsé (Audio glos0170)

diaper	el pañal (Audio glos0171)
dress	el vestido (Audio glos0172)
hat	el sombrero (Audio glos0173)
heel	el tacón (Audio glos0174)
(low) heels	los tacones bajos (Audio glos0175)
high heels	los tacones altos (Audio glos0176)
hose	las medias (Audio glos0177)
hospital gown	el camisón (Audio glos0178)
jacket	la chaqueta (Audio glos0179)
lightweight (light clothes)	ligero (la ropa ligera) (Audio glos0180)
nightgown	el camisón de dormir (Audio glos0181)
oxfords	los zapatos bajos (Audio glos0182)
pajamas	las pijamas (Audio glos0183)
panties	las pantaletas (Audio glos0184)
pants	los pantalones (Audio glos0185)
rubber pants	los pantalones de goma (Audio glos0186)
sandals	las sandalias (Audio glos0187)
scarf	la bufanda (Audio glos0188)
shirt	la camisa (Audio glos0189)
(under)shirt	la camiseta (Audio glos0190)
t-shirt	la camiseta (Audio glos0191)
shoe	el zapato (Audio glos0192)
shorts (men's)	los calzoncillos (Audio glos0193)
skirt	la falda, la pollera (Audio glos0194)
sleeve	la manga (Audio glos0195)
long	larga (Audio glos0196)

short	corta (Audio glos0197)
slipper	la zapatilla, la chancleta (Audio glos0198)
sneakers	los zapatos de goma (Audio glos0199)
sock(s)	el calcetín, los calcetines (Audio glos0200)
stockings	las medias (Audio glos0201)
suit	el traje (Audio glos0202)
sweater	el suéter (Audio glos0203)
tie	la corbata (Audio glos0204)
trousers	los pantalones (Audio glos0205)
underwear	la ropa interior (Audio glos0206)
vest	el chaleco (Audio glos0207)

FAMILY MEMBERS (RELATIVES)
MIEMBROS DE LA FAMILIA (PARIENTES) (AUDIO GLOS0208)

aunt	la tía (Audio glos0209)
brother	el hermano (Audio glos0210)
brother-in-law	el cuñado (Audio glos0211)
children	los hijos, los niños (Audio glos0212)
cousin	el/la primo/a (Audio glos0213)
daughter	la hija (Audio glos0214)
daughter-in-law	la nuera (Audio glos0215)
father	el padre, el papá (Audio glos216)
father-in-law	el suegro (Audio glos0217)
grandfather	el abuelo (Audio glos0218)
grandmother	la abuela (Audio glos0219)
husband	el esposo, el marido, "el viejo" (slang) (Audio glos0220)

in-laws	los suegros (Audio glos0221)
mother	la madre, la mamá (Audio glos0222)
mother-in-law	la suegra (Audio glos0223)
nephew	el sobrino (Audio glos0224)
niece	la sobrina (Audio glos0225)
parents	los padres (Audio glos0226)
sister	la hermana (Audio glos0227)
sister-in-law	la cuñada (Audio glos0228)
son	el hijo (Audio glos0229)
son-in-law	el yerno (Audio glos0230)
uncle	el tío (Audio glos0231)
wife	la esposa, la mujer, "la vieja" (slang) (Audio glos0232)

TIME ON THE CLOCK (AUDIO GLOS0233)

To tell the time in Spanish, use the verb *ser* + *la(s)* and the number. (Audio glos0234)

What time is it?
¿Qué hora es? (Audio glos0235)

It is seven o'clock.
Son las siete. (Audio glos0236)

It is one o'clock.
Es la una. (Audio glos0237)

It is eight o'clock.
Son las ocho. (Audio glos0238)

It is two o'clock.
Son las dos. (Audio glos0239)

It is nine o'clock.
Son las nueve. (Audio glos0240)

It is three o'clock.
Son las tres. (Audio glos0241)

It is ten o'clock.
Son las diez. (Audio glos0242)

It is four o'clock.
Son las cuatro. (Audio glos0243)

It is eleven o'clock.
Son las once. (Audio glos0244)

It is five o'clock.
Son las cinco. (Audio glos0245)

It is twelve o'clock.
Son las doce. (Audio glos0246)

It is six o'clock.
Son las seis. (Audio glos0247)
Use *media* for "30" or half past the hour. (Audio glos0248)

It is 3:30.
Son las tres y media. (Audio glos0249)

A.M. = de la mañana (Audio glos0250)

P.M. = de la tarde (until 6 o'clock) (Audio glos0251)

P.M. = de la noche (from 6 until midnight) (Audio glos0252)
On the right side of the clock use *y* when expressing minutes.
(Audio glos0253)

It is ten after one.
Es la una y diez. (Audio glos0254)

It is two fifteen.
Son las dos y cuarto. (Audio glos0255)

It is three fifteen.
Son las tres y quince. (Audio glos0256)

It is three thirty.
Son las tres y media. (Audio glos0257)
On the left side of the clock use *menos* or *falta(n)*.
(Audio glos0258)

It is twenty to two.
Son las dos menos veinte. (Audio glos0259)

It is five to eight.
Son las ocho menos cinco. (Audio glos0260)

It is twenty to two.
Faltan veinte para las dos. (Audio glos0261)

It is five to eight.
Faltan cinco para las ocho. (Audio glos0262)

TIME EXPRESSIONS (AUDIO GLOS0263)

At what time?
¿A qué hora? (Audio glos0264)

At eight o'clock
A las ocho (Audio glos0265)

At noon
Al mediodía (Audio glos0266)

At midnight
A la medianoche (Audio glos0267)

early
temprano (Audio glos0268)

late
tarde (Audio glos0269)

on time
a tiempo (Audio glos0270)

COLORS — LOS COLORES (AUDIO GLOS0271)

black	negro/a (Audio glos0272)
blue	azul (Audio glos0273)
bluish	azulado/a (Audio glos0274)
brown	café (Audio glos0275)
clear, light (in colortone)	claro/a (Audio glos0276)
dark	oscuro/a (Audio glos0277)

gold	dorado/a (Audio glos0278)
green	verde (Audio glos0279)
gray	gris (Audio glos0280)
orange	anaranjado/a (Audio glos0281)
pale	pálido/a (Audio glos0282)
pink	rosa (Audio glos0283)
purple	púrpura, morado/a (Audio glos0284)
red	rojo/a, colorado/a (Audio glos0285)
reddish	rojizo/a (Audio glos0286)
silver	plateado/a (Audio glos0287)
transparent	transparente (Audio glos0288)
white	blanco/a (Audio glos0289)
yellow	amarillo/a (Audio glos0290)
yellowish	amarillento (Audio glos0291)

THE OFFICE

LA OFICINA
(AUDIO GLOS0292)

administration	la administración (Audio glos0293)
assistant	el/la asistente (Audio glos0294)
bathroom	el baño, el servicio (Audio glos0295)
cashier	el/la cajero/a (Audio glos0296)
chair	la silla (Audio glos0297)
dental office	el consultorio dental (Audio glos0297.1)
dental chair	La silla dental (Audio glos0297.2)
door/doorway	la puerta/la entrada (Audio glos0298) e-mail el correo electrónico (Audio glos0299)
entrance	la entrada (Audio glos0300)
exam room	el (salón/cuarto) de examen (Audio glos0301)

exam record	el expediente (Audio glos0302)
exit	la salida (Audio glos0303)
fax	el fax (Audio glos0304)
front desk	el mostrador (Audio glos0305)
hallway	el pasillo (Audio glos0306)
insurance	el seguro (Audio glos307)
insurance company	la compañía de seguro (Audio glos308)
insurance form	el formulario del seguro (Audio glos309)
laboratory	el laboratorio (Audio glos0310)
mail	el correo (Audio glos0311)
paperwork	el papeleo (Audio glos0312)
public phone	el teléfono público (Audio glos0313)
receptionist	el/la recepcionista (Audio glos0314)
specialist	el/la especialista (Audio glos0315)
telephone	el teléfono (Audio glos0316)
reception room	la sala de espera (Audio glos0317)
treatment room	el cuarto de tratamiento (Audio glos0318)

GENERAL HEALTH — LA SALUD GENERAL (AUDIO GLOS0319)

AIDS	SIDA (Audio glos0319.1)
allergy	la alergia (Audio glos0320)
asthma	el asma (Audio glos0321)
arthritis	la artritis (Audio glos0322)
blood sugar	el azúcar en la sangre (Audio glos0323)
breathing problems	los problemas respiratorios (Audio glos0324)

bruise	el moretón, la hematoma (Audio glos0325)
cancer	el cáncer (Audio glos0326)
cold	el catarro, el resfriado, la gripe (Audio glos0327)
contagious	contagioso/a (Audio glos0328)
diabetes	la diabetes (Audio glos0329)
drug sensitivity	la sensibilidad al medicamento (Audio glos0330)
fever	la fiebre (Audio glos0331)
freckle	la peca (Audio glos0332)
flu	la gripe (Audio glos0333)
headache	el dolor de cabeza (Audio glos0334)
heart attack	ataque al corazón (Audio glos0334.1)
heart murmur	murmullo/soplo del corazón (Audio glos0334.2)
heart problems	los problemas cardíacos (Audio glos0335)
HIV positive	VIH positivo (Audio glos336)
high blood pressure	la presión arterial alta (Audio glos0337)
joint replacement	el reemplazo de la articulación (Audio glos0338)
measles	el sarampión (Audio glos0339)
pacemaker	marcapasos (Audio glos0339.1)
pregnant	embarazada, esperando familia, en estado (Audio glos0340)
rheumatic fever	la fiebre reumática (Audio glos0341)
scarlet fever	la fiebre escarlatina (Audio glos0342)
thyroid problem	los problemas de la tiroides (Audio glos0343)
wart	la verruga (Audio glos0344)

DISEASES/ CONDITIONS

ENFERMEDADES/ CONDICIONES (AUDIO GLOS0345)

abrasion	**la abrasión (Audio glos0346)**
blindness	la ceguera (Audio glos0347)
burn	la quemadura (Audio glos0348)
cut	la cortadura (Audio glos0349)
infection	la infección (Audio glos0350)
inflammation	la inflamación (Audio glos0351)
injury	la lesión (Audio glos0352)
mucous (adj.)	mucoso (Audio glos0353)
mucus (n.)	la mucosidad (Audio glos0354)
scar	la cicatriz (Audio glos0355)
stitches	los puntos (Audio glos0356)
surgery	la cirugía (Audio glos0357)
trauma	el golpe (Audio glos0358)
wound	la herida (Audio glos0359)

SYMPTOMS

LOS SÍNTOMAS (AUDIO GLOS0360)

ache (v.)	**duele (Audio glos0361)**
burn (v.)	quema (Audio glos0362)
congested	congestionado/a (Audio glos0363)
cough	la tos (Audio glos0364)
distortion	la distorsión (Audio glos0365)
dizzy	mareado/a (Audio glos0366)
earache	el dolor de oído (Audio glos0367)
mouth dryness	la sequedad de boca (Audio glos0368)
fluctuate	fluctuar (Audio glos0369)
gradual	gradual (Audio glos0370)

irritation	la irritación (Audio glos0371)
itch	la comezón (Audio glos0372)
pain	el dolor (Audio glos0373)
redness	el enrojecimiento (Audio glos0374)
sensitive to light	sensible a a la luz (Audio glos0375)
sharp pain	el dolor agudo (Audio glos0376)
sinus pain	el dolor nasal (Audio glos0377)
sudden	repentino/a, súbito (Audio glos0378)
swelling	la hinchazón (Audio glos0379)
tired	cansado/a (Audio glos0380)

MEDICATIONS

MEDICAMENTOS
(AUDIO GLOS0381)

antibiotic	el antibiótico (Audio glos0382)
capsules	las cápsulas (Audio glos0383)
daily	diariamente (Audio glos0384)
drops	las gotas (Audio glos0385)
by mouth	por boca (Audio glos0386)
ointment	la pomada (Audio glos0387)
pharmacy	la farmacia (Audio glos0388)
pills	las pastillas (Audio glos0389)
shake well	agite bien (Audio glos0390)
tablets	las tabletas (Audio glos0391)

DENTAL TERMS

TÉRMINOS DENTALES
(AUDIO GLOS0392)

abfraction	la abfracción (Audio glos0393)
abrasive	el abrasivo (Audio glos0394)
abrasion of teeth	la abrasión de los dientes (Audio glos0395)

abscess	el absceso (Audio glos0396)
abutment	el estribo (Audio glos0397)
acid	el ácido (Audio glos0398)
acidulated phosphate fluoride	el fluoruro de fosfato acidulado (Audio glos0399)
acrylic appliance	el aparato de acrílico (Audio glos0400)
active caries	las caries activas (Audio glos0401)
active periodontal therapy	la terapia periodontal activa (Audio glos0402)
adhesive	el adhesivo (Audio glos0403)
adverse drug reaction	la reacción adversa al medicamento (Audio glos404)
air-abrasive machine	la máquina de aire abrasivo (Audio glos405)
air-powder polishing	pulir con aire y polvo (Audio glos0406)
air-water syringe	la jeringuilla de aire-agua (Audio glos0407)
alginate	el alginato (Audio glos0408)
allergy	la alergia (Audio glos409)
alloy	la aleación (Audio glos410)
amalgam	la amalgama (Audio glos411)
amalgam tattoo	el tatuaje de amalgama (Audio glos412)
American Dental Association	Asociación Dental Americana (Audio glos413)
American Dental Hygienists' Association	Asociación Dental Americana de Higienistas (Audio glos414)
American Heart Association	Asociación Americana del Corazón (Audio glos415)
anatomical charting	la hoja clínica anatómica (Audio glos416)
anesthetic	el anestésico (Audio glos417)

ankylosed	anquilosado/a (Audio glos418)
anterior	anterior (Audio glos419)
anticoagulant	el anticoagulante (Audio glos420)
antimicrobial	el antimicrobiano (Audio glos421)
apex	el ápice (Audio glos422)
apical	apical (Audio glos423)
appliance	el aparato (Audio glos424)
area specific	específico/a al área (Audio glos425)
arrested caries	las caries inactivas (Audio glos426)
artificial	artificial/postizo (Audio glos426.1)
aspiration	la aspiración (Audio glos427)
asprin	Aspirina (Audio glos427.1)
assessment	la evaluación (Audio glos428)
assistant	el/la ayudante, el/la asistente (Audio glos429)
attached gingiva	la encía adherida (Audio glos430)
attrition	la atrición (Audio glos431)
baby-bottle decay	caries del biberón (Audio glos432)
baby tooth	diente de (leche/bebe) (Audio glos432.1)
bacteria	las bacterias (Audio glos433)
bacterial endocarditis	la endocarditis bacteriana (Audio glos434)
bacterial infection	la infección bacteriana (Audio glos435)
bad breath	el mal aliento (Audio glos436)
baking soda	el bicarbonato de soda (Audio glos437)
bicuspid	el bicúspide (Audio glos438)
bifurcation	la bifurcación (Audio glos439)

bilateral	bilateral (Audio glos440)
biopsy	biopsia (Audio glos440.1)
bite	la mordedura/mordida (Audio glos441)
bite (v.)	muerda (Audio glos441.1)
bitewing radiograph	la radiografía interproximal (Audio glos442)
black hairy tongue	la lengua negra peluda (Audio glos443)
bleach	el blanqueador (Audio glos444)
bleaching	el blanqueo (Audio glos445)
bleeding	el sangrado (Audio glos446)
blood	la sangre (Audio glos447)
blood disorder	el desorden sanguíneo (Audio glos448)
blood glucose	la glucosa en la sangre (Audio glos449)
blood pressure	la presión arterial (Audio glos450)
bond	la ligadura (Audio glos451)
bonded	ligado/a (Audio glos452)
bonded crown	la corona consolidada (Audio glos453)
bonding agent	el agente para unir (Audio glos454)
bone	el hueso (Audio glos455)
braces	los frenillos/frenos/brackets (Audio glos456)
breath (v.)	respire/e (Audio glos456.1)
bridge	el puente (Audio glos457)
brush	el cepillo (Audio glos458)
bruxism	el bruxismo (Audio glos459)
buccal	bucal (Audio glos460)
buccal mucosa	la mucosa bucal (Audio glos461)
buccal tissue	el tejido bucal (Audio glos462)
burning mouth syndrome	el síndrome de boca ardiente (Audio glos463)

burnish	pulir, bruñir (Audio glos464)
calcification	la calcificación (Audio glos465)
calculus	el cálculo/el sarro (Audio glos466)
cancer	el cáncer (Audio glos467)
canine	el (colmillo/canino) (Audio glos467.1)
camera	la cámara (Audio glos468)
cap	la corona (Audio glos469)
carbamide peroxide	el peróxido de carbamida (Audio glos470)
caries	las caries (Audio glos471)
caries charting	la hoja clínica de las caries (Audio glos472)
caries detection	el descubrimiento de las caries (Audio glos473)
caries management	el tratamiento de las caries (Audio glos474)
caries prevention	la prevención de las caries (Audio glos475)
cementum	el cemento (Audio glos476)
cheek	el cachete/la mejilla (Audio glos477)
chin	la barbilla (Audio glos477.1)
chronic	crónico (Audio glos477.2)
cleft	la hendidura (Audio glos478)
cleft lip	el labio leporino (Audio glos479)
cleft palate	el paladar hendido (Audio glos480)
close	cerrar/cierre (Audio glos481)
cold	frio (Audio glos481.1)
complete denture	la dentadura completa (Audio glos482)
composite	el compuesto/la resina (Audio glos483)
comprehensive dental history	el historial dental exhaustivo (Audio glos484)

comprehensive medical history	el historial médico exhaustivo (Audio glos485)
computer-assisted charting	la hoja clínica computarizada (Audio glos486)
computer screen	la pantalla de la computadora (Audio glos487)
concavity	la concavidad (Audio glos488)
condyle	el cóndilo (Audio glos489)
confidentiality	la discreción (Audio glos490)
congenital disorder	el desorden congénito (Audio glos491)
congenital missing tooth	el diente ausente congénito (Audio glos492)
cosmetic dentistry	la odontología cosmética (Audio glos493)
cosmetic filling	empastadura/empaste/relleno/resina/ calza cosmética (Audio glos494)
cosmetic whitening	el blanqueador cosmético (Audio glos495)
cost of dental care	el costo de cuidado dental (Audio glos496)
cost of oral health care	el costo de cuidado de salud oral (Audio glos497)
cracked tooth	el diente fracturado (Audio glos498)
cracked tooth syndrome	el síndrome de diente fisurado (Audio glos499)
cracking	/ agrietamiento (Audio glos500)
crepitus	la crepitación (Audio glos501)
crevicular fluid	el líquido crevicular (Audio glos502)
crossbite	la mordida cruzada (Audio glos503)
cross-contamination	la contaminación cruzada (Audio glos504)
cross section	el corte transversal (Audio glos505)

crown	la corona (Audio glos506)
cure	la cura (Audio glos507)
curing	curativo/a (Audio glos508)
cusp	la cúspide (Audio glos509)
cusp fracture	la fractura de la cúspide (Audio glos510)
curet, curette	la cucharilla (Audio glos511)
curettage	el raspado (Audio glos512)
cut	la cortada (Audio glos513)
cutting edge	el filo cortante (Audio glos514)
decay	la descomposición (Audio glos515)
decayed	podrido(a)/picado(a) (Audio glos516)
delayed allergic reaction	la reacción alérgica retrasada (Audio glos517)
dental assistant	el/la asistente dental (Audio glos518)
dental emergency	la emergencia dental (Audio glos519)
dental floss	el hilo dental (Audio glos520)
dental hygienist	el/la higienista dental (Audio glos521)
dental laboratory	el laboratorio dental (Audio glos521.1)
dental insurance	el seguro dental (Audio glos522)
dental practice	(la clinica dental) (Audio glos523)
dental office	el consultorio dental (Audio glos523.1)
dental school	la facultad dental/la escuela dental (Audio glos524)
dental technician	el/la técnico(a) dental (Audio glos524.1)
dentifrice	el dentífrico (Audio glos525)
dentin	la dentina (Audio glos526)
dentist	el/la dentista/odontologo(a) (Audio glos527)

dentition	la dentición (Audio glos528)
denture	la dentadura/ placa/ dentadura postiza (Audio glos529)
desensitize	desensibilizar (Audio glos530)
desensitizing	desensibilizante (Audio glos531)
diastema	el diastema (Audio glos532)
digital imaging x-ray	la radiología digital (Audio glos533)
disclosing solution	la solución de tintura (Audio glos534)
disinfected	desinfectado/a (Audio glos535)
disinfection	la desinfección (Audio glos536)
dislocated jaw	la mandíbula dislocada (Audio glos537)
distal	distal (Audio glos538)
drill	el taladro/la piesa de mano (Audio glos539)
dry mouth	la sequedad de boca (Audio glos540)
duplication of film	la duplicación de la radiographia (Audio glos541)
edentulous	edéntulo (Audio glos542)
edentulism	el edentulismo (Audio glos543)
electric toothbrush	el cepillo eléctrico de dientes (Audio glos544)
embrasure	la embrasura (Audio glos545)
enamel	el esmalte (Audio glos546)
endodontic abscess	el absceso endodóntico (Audio glos547)
endodontist	el/la endodoncista (Audio glos548)
erosion	la erosión (Audio glos549)
esthetic	estético/a (Audio glos550)
explorer	explorador (Audio glos550.1)
exposure	la exposición (Audio glos551)

external bleaching	blanqueo externo (Audio glos552)
fiberoptic	la fibra óptica (Audio glos553)
fill	llenar (Audio glos554)
filling	la empastadura/relleno/empaste (Audio glos555)
film	el rollo negativo (Audio glos556)
fixed bridge	el puente fijo (Audio glos557)
floss	el hilo dental (Audio glos558)
fluoride	el fluoruro/fluor (Audio glos559)
fluoride rinse	el enjuague de fluoruro (Audio glos560)
fluoride tray	la bandeja para fluoruro (Audio glos561)
fracture	la fractura (Audio glos562)
frenum	el frenillo (Audio glos563)
full denture	la dentadura completa (Audio glos564)
furcation	la furcación (Audio glos565)
gauze	gasa (Audio glos565.1)
gingiva	la encía (Audio glos566)
gingival	gingival (Audio glos567)
gingivitis	la gingivitis (Audio glos568)
gloves	los guantes (Audio glos568.1)
gold crown	la corona en oro (Audio glos569)
gold inlay	el incrustacion en oro (Audio glos570)
halitosis	el mal aliento (Audio glos571)
hand scaler	la cureta manual (Audio glos572)
Hispanic Dental Association	Asociación Dental Hispana (Audio glos572.1)
hot	caliente (Audio glos572.2)

hurt	dolor (Audio glos572.3)
ice	hielo (Audio glos572.4)
illness	enfermedad (Audio glos572.5)
implant	el implante (Audio glos573)
impression	impresión (Audio glos573.1)
infected	infectado (Audio glos573.2)
injection	inyeccíon (Audio glos573.3)
injured	lastimado (Audio glos573.4)
instrument	el instrumento (Audio glos574)
internal bleaching	el blanqueo interno (Audio glos575)
intraoral examination	la examinación intrabucal (Audio glos576)
intraoral video image	la imagen de video intrabucal (Audio glos577)
jaw	la mandíbula (Audio glos578)
lateral	lateral (Audio glos579)
lead apron	delantal de plomo (Audio glos579.1)
lips	los labios (Audio glos580)
local anesthetic	anestésico local (Audio glos580.1)
lower arch	el arco inferior (Audio glos581)
mandible	la mandíbula/quijada (Audio glos582)
mask	cubreboca/mascarilla (Audio glos582.1)
maxilla	el maxilar (Audio glos583)
medicine	medicina (Audio glos583.1)
mirror	espejo (Audio glos583.2)
Miss	Señorita (Audio glos583.3)
mobility	la movilidad (Audio glos584)mouth la boca (Audio glos585)
mouthguard	el protector bucal (Audio glos586)

molar	el molar, la muela (Audio glos587)
Mr.	Señor (Audio glos587.1)
Mrs.	Señora (Audio glos587.2)
neck	cuello (Audio glos587.3)
necrotizing ulcerative periodontitis	la periodontitis necrótica ulcerativa (Audio glos588)
needle	la aguja (Audio glos589)
nerve	el nervio (Audio glos589.1)
night guard	el protector bucal de noche/guarda oclusal nocturna (Audio glos590)
occlusion	la oclusión (Audio glos591)
open(verb)	abra (Audio glos592)
operation	operacíon (Audio glos592.1)
oral cancer examination	la examinación oral para cáncer (Audio glos593)
oral condition	la condición oral (Audio glos594)
oral disease	la enfermedad oral (Audio glos595)
oral health	la salud oral (Audio glos596)
oral self-care	el cuidado oral por sí mismo (Audio glos597)
oral surgeon	el/la cirujano/a oral (Audio glos598)
orthodontist	el/la ortodoncista (Audio glos599)
oxygen	el oxígeno (Audio glos599.1)
overbite	la sobremordida (Audio glos600)
overdenture	la sobredentadura (Audio glos601)
pain	el dolor (Audio glos602)
palate	el paladar (Audio glos603)
partial denture	la dentadura (postiza) parcial (Audio glos604)

partially erupted tooth	el diente con ruptura parcial (Audio glos605)
pedodontist	odontopediatra (Audio glos606)
pericoronitis	la pericoronitis (Audio glos607)
periodontal abscess	el absceso periodontal (Audio glos608)
periodontal charting	la hoja clínica periodontal (Audio glos609)
periodontal débridement	el desbridamiento periodontal (Audio glos610)
periodontal disease	la enfermedad periodontal (Audio glos611)
periodontal dressing	la cura periodontal (Audio glos612)
periodontal ligament	el ligamento periodontal (Audio glos613)
periodontal maintenance	el mantenimiento periodontal (Audio glos614)
periodontal measurement	la medida periodontal (Audio glos615)
periodontal probe	la cánula periodontal (Audio glos616)
periodontal scaling	el raspado periodontal (Audio glos617)
periodontal surgery	la cirugía periodontal (Audio glos618)
periodontal therapy	la terapia periodontal (Audio glos619)
periodontal tissue	el tejido periodontal (Audio glos620)
periodontist	el/la periodoncista (Audio glos621)
periodontitis	la periodontitis (Audio glos622)
peroxide	el peróxido (Audio glos623)
pits and fissures	las (picaduras y aberturas/fosas y fisuras) (Audio glos624)
plaque	la placa bacteriana (Audio glos625)
polish	pulir (Audio glos626)

polishing	el pulir (Audio glos627)
pontic	el póntico (Audio glos628)
porcelain	la porcelana (Audio glos629)
powered toothbrush	el cepillo eléctrico de dientes (Audio glos630)
prophylaxis	la profilaxis (Audio glos631)
prosthodontist	el/la prostodoncista (Audio glos632)
pulp	la pulpa (Audio glos633)
pregnant	embarazada (Audio glos633.1)
pressure	presíon (Audio glos633.2)
radiation	la radiación (Audio glos634)
radiographic machine	la màquina de radiografías (Audio glos634.1)
radiographs	las radiografías (Audio glos634.2)
recession	la recesión (Audio glos635)
remove	sacar (Audio glos636)
resin	la resina (Audio glos636.1)
restroom	el baño (Audio glos636.2)
rinse	el enjuague (noun); enjuagar (verb) (Audio glos637)
rinsing	enjuagando (Audio glos638)
root	la raíz (Audio glos639)
root canal	el canal radicular(anatomy)/tratamiento de conducto (treatment)/ endodoncia (treatment) (Audio glos640)
root plane and scale	el alisado radicular y el raspado radicular/raspado y alisado radicular (Audio glos641)
rotated tooth	el diente rotado (Audio glos642)
rubber dam	la presa de goma (Audio glos643)

saliva	la saliva (Audio glos644)
salivary gland	la glándula salival (Audio glos645)
scale	raspar (Audio glos646)
scaler	la cureta, el raspador (Audio glos647)
scaling	el raspado (Audio glos648)
sealant	el sellador/sellante(Audio glos649)
sensitive	sensible (Audio glos650)
sensitivity	la sensibilidad (Audio glos651)
smile	sonrisa(n.) sonríe(v.) (Audio glos651.1)
smoke	fumar (Audio glos651.2)
soft	suave (Audio glos651.3)
soft palate	el paladar blando (Audio glos652)
sonic scaler	la cureta sónica (Audio glos653)
spit	la saliva(n.) escupe(v.) (Audio glos654)
subgingival irrigation	la irrigación subgingival (Audio glos655)
subgingival scaling	el raspado subgingival (Audio glos656)
suction	(el succionador/eyector dental) (Audio glos656.1)
sulcus	el surco (Audio glos657)
stitch	puntada (Audio glos657.1)
straighten	enderezar (Audio glos657.2)
supernumerary	super numerario (Audio glos657.3)
surgery	cirugía (Audio glos657.4)
suture	sutura(noun)/suturar(verb) (Audio glos657.5)
stitches	puntadas (Audio glos657.6)
sweets	dulces (Audio glos657.7)
swell	inflamar/hinchar (Audio glos657.8)

symptom	síntoma (Audio glos657.9)
syringe	jeringa (Audio glos657.10)
tartar	el sarro (Audio glos658)
taste bud	la papila gustativa (Audio glos659)
teeth	los dientes (Audio glos660)
temporomandibular disorder	el desorden temporomandibular (Audio glos661)
temporomandibular joint	la articulación temporomandibular (Audio glos662)
throat	la garganta (Audio glos662.1)
tissue	tejido (Audio glos662.2)
tongue	la lengua (Audio glos663)
tonsils	las amígdalas/anginas (Audio glos663.1)
tooth	el diente (Audio glos664)
toothbrush	el cepillo de dientes (Audio glos665)
toothpaste	la pasta de dientes/pasta dental/crema dental (Audio glos666)
topical anesthetic	el anestésico tópico (Audio glos667)
treatment	el tratamiento (Audio glos667.1)
ulcer	la úlcera (Audio glos667.2)
ultrasonic instrument	el instrumento ultrasónico (Audio glos668)
ultrasonic scaler	la cureta ultrasónica (Audio glos669)
unerupted	retenido/a (Audio glos670)
upper arch	el arco superior (Audio glos671)
uvula	la úvula/campanílla (Audio glos671.1)
varnish	el barniz (Audio glos672)
vesicles	vesículas (Audio glos672.1)
whitening	blanqueo (Audio glos673)

waiting area	La sala de espera (Audio glos673.1)
wisdom teeth	muelas del juicio/terceros molares/ muelas cordales (Audio glos673.2)
xerostomia	la xerostomía (Audio glos674)
x-rays	los rayos X (Audio glos675)

Spanish-English Vocabulary*
(Audio vocab0001)

Vocabulario Español-Inglés
A (Audio vocab0002)

la abfracción	abfraction (Audio vocab0003)
abierto/a	open (Audio vocab0004)
la abrasión	abrasion (Audio vocab0005)
la abrasión de los dientes	abrasion of teeth (Audio vocab0006)
abril	April (Audio vocab0007)
el absceso	abscess (Audio vocab0008)
el absceso endodóntico	endodontic abscess (Audio vocab0009)
el absceso periodontal	periodontal abscess (Audio vocab0010)
la abuela	grandmother (Audio vocab0011)
el abuelo	grandfather (Audio vocab0012)
el ácido	acid (Audio vocab0013)
el adhesivo	adhesive (Audio vocab0014)
la administración	administration (Audio vocab0015)
¿adónde?	to where? (Audio vocab0016)
el afta	canker sore (Audio vocab0016.1)
el agente para unir	bonding agent (Audio vocab0017)
agite bien	shake well (Audio vocab0018)
agosto	August (Audio vocab0019)
la aguja	needle (Audio vocab0020)
ahora	now (Audio vocab0021)
ahora mismo	right now (Audio vocab0022)
a la medianoche	at midnight (Audio vocab0023)
a las ocho	at eight o'clock (Audio vocab0024)
la aleación	alloy (Audio vocab0025)
la alergia	allergy (Audio vocab0026)
el alginato	alginate (Audio vocab0027)
algunas veces	sometimes (Audio vocab0028)
el alisado	scaling (Audio vocab0029)

---

*Modified from Chou B: *Practical Spanish in Eyecare*, Butterworth-Heinemann, Boston, 2001.

el alisado periodontal	periodontal scaling (Audio vocab0030)
el alisado subgingival	subgingival scaling (Audio vocab0031)
alisar	scale (Audio vocab0032)
al mediodía	at noon (Audio vocab0033)
la presión arterial alta	high blood pressure (Audio vocab0034)
la amalgama	amalgam (Audio vocab0035)
amarillento/a	yellowish (Audio vocab0036)
las amígdalas	tonsils (Audio vocab0036.1)
el analgésico	pain medication (Audio vocab0036.2)
el anestésico	anesthetic (Audio vocab0037)
la anestesia	anesthetic (Audio vocab0037.1)
el anestésico tópico	topical anesthetic (Audio vocab0038)
el año	year (Audio vocab0039)
anoche	last night (Audio vocab0040)
el año próximo	next year (Audio vocab0041)
anquilosado/a	ankylosed (Audio vocab0042)
anteayer	day before yesterday (Audio vocab0043)
los anteojos/las gafas	glasses (Audio vocab0044)
anterior	anterior (Audio vocab0045)
antes	before (Audio vocab0046)
el antibiótico	antibiotic (Audio vocab0047)
el anticoagulante	anticoagulant (Audio vocab0048)
el antimicrobiano	antimicrobial (Audio vocab0049)
el aparato	appliance (Audio vocab0050)
el aparato de acrílico	acrylic appliance (Audio vocab0051)
apical	apical (Audio vocab0052)
el ápice	apex (Audio vocab0053)
¿a qué distancia?	how far? (Audio vocab0054)
¿a qué hora?	at what time? (Audio vocab0055)
¿a quién?	to whom? (Audio vocab0056)
el arco inferior	lower arch (Audio vocab0057)
el arco superior	upper arch (Audio vocab0058)
la artritis	arthritis (Audio vocab0059)

el/la asistente	assistant (Audio vocab0060)
el/la asistente dental	dental assistant (Audio vocab0061)
Asociación Dental Americana	American Dental Association (Audio vocab0062)
Asociación Dental Americana de Higienistas	American Dental Hygienists' Association (Audio vocab0063)
Asociación Americana del Corazón	American Heart Association (Audio vocab0064)
la aspiración	aspiration (Audio vocab0065)
a tiempo	on time (Audio vocab0066)
la atrición	attrition (Audio vocab0067)
el aumento	power (Audio vocab0068)
ayer	yesterday (Audio vocab0069)
el/la ayudante, el/la asistente	assistant (Audio vocab0070)
el azúcar en la sangre	blood sugar (Audio vocab0071)
azul	blue (Audio vocab0072)
azulado/a	bluish (Audio vocab0073)

B (AUDIO VOCAB0074)

las bacterias	bacteria (Audio vocab0075)
la bandeja para fluoruro	fluoride tray (Audio vocab0076)
el baño	bathroom (Audio vocab0077)
el barniz	varnish (Audio vocab0078)
el bicarbonato de soda	baking soda (Audio vocab0079)
el bicúspide	bicuspid (Audio vocab0080)
la bifurcación	bifurcation (Audio vocab0081)
bilateral	bilateral (Audio vocab0082)
la biopsia	biopsy (Audio vocab0082.1)
blanco/a	white (Audio vocab0083)
el blanqueador	bleach (Audio vocab0084)
el blanqueador cosmético	cosmetic whitening (Audio vocab0085)
blanqueando	whitening (Audio vocab0086)
blanquear	bleaching (Audio vocab0087)

el blanqueo externo	external bleaching (Audio vocab0088)
el blanqueo interno	internal bleaching (Audio vocab0089)
la boca	mouth (Audio vocab0090)
bruñir	burnish (Audio vocab0091)
el bruxismo	bruxism (Audio vocab0092)
bucal	buccal (Audio vocab0093)

C (AUDIO VOCAB0094)

el cachete/la mejilla	cheek (Audio vocab0095)
cada mañana	every morning (Audio vocab0096)
cada noche	every night (Audio vocab0097)
cada tarde	every afternoon (Audio vocab0098)
café	brown (Audio vocab0099)
el/la cajero/a	cashier (Audio vocab0100)
la calcificación	calcification (Audio vocab0101)
el cálculo	calculus (Audio vocab0102)
calza dental	dental filling (Audio vocab0102.1)
la cámara	camera (Audio vocab0103)
el canal radicular	root canal (anatomy) (Audio vocab0104)
el cáncer	cancer (Audio vocab0105)
cansado/a	tired (Audio vocab0106)
la cánula periodontal	periodontal probe (Audio vocab0107)
las cápsulas	capsules (Audio vocab0108)
caries del biberón	baby-bottle tooth decay (Audio vocab0109)
las caries	caries/tooth decay (Audio vocab0110)
las caries activas	active caries (Audio vocab0111)
las caries inactivas	arrested caries (Audio vocab0112)
carilla	veneer (Audio vocab0112.1)
el catarro/la gripe	cold (Audio vocab0113)
catorce	fourteen (Audio vocab0114)
la ceguera	blindness (Audio vocab0115)
la ceja	eyebrow (Audio vocab0116)
el cemento	cementum (Audio vocab0117)
el cepillo	brush (Audio vocab0118)
el cepillo de dientes	toothbrush (Audio vocab0119)

el cepillo eléctrico de dientes	electric toothbrush, powered toothbrush (Audio vocab0120)
cero	zero (Audio vocab0121)
cerrar	close (Audio vocab0122)
la cicatriz	scar (Audio vocab0123)
cien	one hundred (Audio vocab0124)
ciento	hundred (Audio vocab0125)
ciento cinco	one hundred five (Audio vocab0126)
ciento cuatro	one hundred four (Audio vocab0127)
ciento diez	one hundred ten (Audio vocab0128)
ciento dos	one hundred two (Audio vocab0129)
ciento nueve	one hundred nine (Audio vocab0130)
ciento ocho	one hundred eight (Audio vocab0131)
ciento seis	one hundred six (Audio vocab0132)
ciento siete	one hundred seven (Audio vocab0133)
ciento tres	one hundred three (Audio vocab0134)
ciento uno	one hundred one (Audio vocab0135)
cinco	five (Audio vocab0136)
cincuenta	fifty (Audio vocab0137)
la cirugía	surgery (Audio vocab0138)
la cirugía periodontal	periodontal surgery (Audio vocab0139)
el/la cirujano/a oral	oral surgeon (Audio vocab0140)
claro/a	clear, light (in color tone) (Audio vocab0141)
colorado/a	red (Audio vocab0142)
el colmilo/canino	canine/cuspid (Audio vocab0142.2)
la comezón	itch (Audio vocab0143)
¿cómo?	how? (Audio vocab0144)
el compuesto	composite (Audio vocab0145)
la concavidad	concavity (Audio vocab0146)
la condición oral	oral condition (Audio vocab0147)
el cóndilo	condyle (Audio vocab0148)
Tratamiento de conducto	root canal treatment (Audio vocab0148.1)
congestionado/a	congested (Audio vocab0149)
¿con qué frecuencia?	how often? (Audio vocab0150)
El consultorio dental	the dental office (Audio vocab0150.1)
contagioso/a	contagious (Audio vocab0151)

la contaminación cruzada	cross-contamination (Audio vocab0152)
la corona	cap, crown (Audio vocab0153)
la corona consolidada	bonded crown (Audio vocab0154)
la corona en oro	gold crown (Audio vocab0155)
el corte	cut (Audio vocab0156)
el corte transversal	cross-section (Audio vocab0157)
el costo de cuidado de salud dental	cost of dental care (Audio vocab0158)
el costo de cuidado de salud oral	cost of oral health care (Audio vocab0159)
la articulación temporomadibular	temporomandibular joint (Audio vocab0160)
la crepitación	crepitus (Audio vocab0161)
¿cuál?	which? (Audio vocab0162)
¿cuáles?	which (ones)? (Audio vocab0163)
¿cuándo?	when? (Audio vocab0164)
¿cuántas veces?	how many times? (Audio vocab0165)
¿cuánto?	how much? (Audio vocab0166)
¿cuántos?	how many? (Audio vocab0167)
¿cuánto tiempo?	how long? (Audio vocab0168)
cuarenta	forty (Audio vocab0169)
cuarto/a	fourth (Audio vocab0170)
cuatro	four (Audio vocab0171)
cuatrocientos	four hundred (Audio vocab0172)
la cucharilla	curet, curette (Audio vocab0173)
el cuidado oral por sí mismo	oral self-care (Audio vocab0174)
la cuñada	sister-in-law (Audio vocab0175)
el cuñado	brother-in-law (Audio vocab0176)
la cura	cure (Audio vocab0177)
El **apósito periodontal** /**la cura periodontal**	periodontal dressing (Audio vocab0178)
curativo/a	curing (Audio vocab0179)
la cureta	scaler (Audio vocab0180)
la cureta manual	hand scaler (Audio vocab0181)
la cureta sónica	sonic scaler (Audio vocab0182)
la cúspide	cusp (Audio vocab0183)

D (AUDIO VOCAB0184)

décimo/a	tenth (Audio vocab0185)
¿de dónde?	from where? (Audio vocab0186)
el defecto	defect (Audio vocab0187)
de la mañana	A.M. (in the morning) (Audio vocab0188)
de la noche	P.M. (from 6 until midnight) (Audio vocab0189)
de la tarde	P.M. (until 6 o'clock) (Audio vocab0190)
la dentadura	denture (Audio vocab0191)
la dentadura completa	complete denture, full denture (Audio vocab0192)
la dentadura (postiza) parcial	partial denture (Audio vocab0193)
la dentición	dentition (Audio vocab0194)
el dentífrico	dentifrice (Audio vocab0195)
la dentina	dentin (Audio vocab0196)
el/la dentista	dentist (Audio vocab0197)
¿de quién?	whose? (Audio vocab0198)
de repente	suddenly (Audio vocab0199)
el desbridamiento periodontal	periodontal débridement (Audio vocab0200)
la descomposición	decay (Audio vocab0201)
el descubrimiento de las caries	caries detection (Audio vocab0202)
desensibilizante	desensitizing (Audio vocab0203)
desensibilizar	desensitize (Audio vocab0204)
la desinfección	disinfection (Audio vocab0205)
desinfectado/a	disinfected (Audio vocab0206)
el desorden congénito	congenital disorder (Audio vocab0207)
el desorden sanguíneo	blood disorder (Audio vocab0208)
el desorden temporomandibular	temporomandibular disorder (Audio vocab0209)
después	after (Audio vocab0210)
de vez en cuando	from time to time (Audio vocab0211)
el día	day (Audio vocab0212)
la diabetes	diabetes (Audio vocab0213)
el día de la semana	day of the week (Audio vocab0214)

diariamente	daily (Audio vocab0215)
el diastema	diastema (Audio vocab0216)——
diciembre	December (Audio vocab0217)
diecinueve	nineteen (Audio vocab0218)
dieciocho	eighteen (Audio vocab0219)
dieciséis	sixteen (Audio vocab0220)
diecisiete	seventeen (Audio vocab0221)
el diente	tooth (Audio vocab0222)
el diente ausente congénito	congenital missing tooth (Audio vocab0223)
el diente con ruptura parcial	partially erupted tooth (Audio vocab0224)
los dientes de leche	milk teeth (Audio vocab0224.1)
el diente fraccionado	cracked tooth (Audio vocab0225)
el diente rotado	rotated tooth (Audio vocab0226)
los dientes	teeth (Audio vocab0227)
diez	ten (Audio vocab0228)
la discreción	confidentiality (Audio vocab0229)
distal	distal (Audio vocab0230)
doce	twelve (Audio vocab0231)
el dolor	pain (Audio vocab0232)
el dolor de cabeza	headache (Audio vocab0233)
domingo	Sunday (Audio vocab0234)
¿dónde?	where? (Audio vocab0235)
dorado/a	gold (in color tone) (Audio vocab0236)
dos	two (Audio vocab0237)
doscientos	two hundred (Audio vocab0238)
dos mil y uno	two thousand one (Audio vocab0239)
la duplicación de rollo negativo	duplication of film (Audio vocab0240)
duele	hurt (Audio vocab0240.1)

E (AUDIO VOCAB0241)

Edéntulo/desdentada/o	edentulous (Audio vocab0242)
embarazada	pregnant (Audio vocab0243)
la embrasura	embrasure (Audio vocab0244)
la emergencia dental	dental emergency (Audio vocab0245)

la empastadura/empaste/ relleno	filling (Audio vocab0246)
la empastadura/relleno/ empaste cosmética/o	the cosmetic filling (Audio vocab0247)
el empaste en oro	gold inlay/filling (Audio vocab0248)
la encía	gums (Audio vocab0249)
la encía adherida	attached gingiva (Audio vocab0250)
el edentulismo	edentulism (Audio vocab0251)
la endocarditis bacteriana	bacterial endocarditis (Audio vocab0252)
el/la endodontcsta	endodontist (Audio vocab0253)
endodoncia	root canal (Audio vocab0253.1)
enero	January (Audio vocab0254)
la enfermedad	disease (Audio vocab0255)
la enfermedad oral	oral disease (Audio vocab0256)
la enfermedad periodontal	periodontal disease (Audio vocab0257)
enjuagando	rinsing (Audio vocab0258)
enjuagarse	rinse (Audio vocab0259)
el enjuague	rinse (Audio vocab0260)
el enjuague de fluoruro	fluoride rinse (Audio vocab0261)
la entrada	entrance (Audio vocab0262)
la erosión	erosion (Audio vocab0263)
es la una y diez	it is ten after one (Audio vocab0264)
escupe	spit(verb) (Audio vocab0264.1)
el esmalte	enamel (Audio vocab0265)
específico/a al área	area specific (Audio vocab0266)
esperando familia	pregnant/expectant family (Audio vocab0267)
la esposa	wife (Audio vocab0268)
el esposo	husband (Audio vocab0269)
esta noche	tonight (Audio vocab0270)
en estado	pregnant (Audio vocab0271)
estético/a	aesthetic (Audio vocab0272)
el estribo	abutment (Audio vocab0273)
la evaluación	assessment (Audio vocab0274)
el examen intrabucal	intraoral examination (Audio vocab0275)
el examen oral para el cáncer	oral cancer examination (Audio vocab0276)

el expediente	exam record (Audio vocab0277)
la extraccíon	extraction (Audio vocab0277.1)
extraer	to extract (Audio vocab0277.2)
la exposición	exposure (Audio vocab0278)

F (AUDIO VOCAB0279)

la facultad dental/escuela dental	dental school (Audio vocab0280)
faltan cinco para las ocho	it is five to eight (Audio vocab0281)
faltan veinte para las dos	it is twenty to two (Audio vocab0282)
la farmacia	pharmacy (Audio vocab0283)
febrero	February (Audio vocab0284)
la fibra óptica	fiberoptic (Audio vocab0285)
la fiebre	fever (Audio vocab0286)
el filo cortante	cutting edge (Audio vocab0287)
fluctuar	to fluctuate (Audio vocab0288)
el fluoruro/fluor	fluoride (Audio vocab0289)
el fluoruro de fosfato acidulado	acidulated phosphate fluoride (Audio vocab0290)
el fraccionamiento	cracking (Audio vocab0291)
la fractura	fracture (Audio vocab0292)
la fractura de la cúspide	cusp fracture (Audio vocab0293)
el frenillo	frenum (Audio vocab0294)
los frenillos/frenos/brackets	braces (Audio vocab0295)
los frenos	braces (Audio vocab0295.1)
la furcación	furcation (Audio vocab0296)

G (AUDIO VOCAB0297)

la gasa	**gauze** (Audio vocab0297.1)
gingiva	gingiva (Audio vocab0297.2)
gingival	gingival (Audio vocab0298)
la gingivitis	gingivitis (Audio vocab0299)
la glándula salival	salivary gland (Audio vocab0300)

el globo ocular/	eyeball (Audio vocab0301)
globo del ojo	
la glucosa en la sangre	blood glucose (Audio vocab0302)
el golpe/trauma	hit/trauma (Audio vocab0303)
la gorra	cap (Audio vocab0304)
gradual	gradual (Audio vocab0305)
la gripe	flu (Audio vocab0306)
gris	gray (Audio vocab0307)
los guantes	gloves (Audio vocab0307.1)
quijada	jaw (Audio vocab0307.2)

H (AUDIO VOCAB0308)

hace dos días	two days ago (Audio vocab0309)
hace seis años	six years ago (Audio vocab0310)
hace tres semanas	three weeks ago (Audio vocab0311)
hasta	until (Audio vocab0312)
la hendidura	cleft (Audio vocab0313)
la herida	wound (Audio vocab0314)
la hermana	sister (Audio vocab0315)
el hermano	brother (Audio vocab0316)
el/la higienista dental	dental hygienist (Audio vocab0317)
la hija	daughter (Audio vocab0318)
el hijo	son (Audio vocab0319)
los hijos	children (Audio vocab0320)
el hilo dental	dental floss, floss (Audio vocab0321)
el historial dental	dental history (Audio vocab0322)
el historial médico	medical history (Audio vocab0323)
la hoja clínica anatómica	anatomical charting (Audio vocab0324)
la hoja clínica computarizada	computer-assisted charting (Audio vocab0325)
la hoja clínica de las caries	caries charting (Audio vocab0326)
la hoja clínica periodontal	periodontal charting (Audio vocab0327)
la hora	hour (Audio vocab0328)
hoy	today (Audio vocab0329)
el hueso	bone (Audio vocab0330)

I (AUDIO VOCAB0331)

la imagen de video intrabucal	intraoral video image (Audio vocab0332)
el implante	implant (Audio vocab0333)
el incisivo	incisor (Audio vocab0333.1)
la infección	infection (Audio vocab0334)
la infección bacteriana	bacterial infection (Audio vocab0335)
la inflamación	inflammation (Audio vocab0336)
el instrumento	instrument (Audio vocab0337)
el instrumento ultrasónico	ultrasonic instrument (Audio vocab0338)
la inyeccíon	injection (Audio vocab0338.1)
la irrigación subgingival	subgingival irrigation (Audio vocab0339)
la irritación	irritation (Audio vocab0340)

J (AUDIO VOCAB0341)

la jeringuilla de aire-agua	air-water syringe (Audio vocab0342)
jueves	Thursday (Audio vocab0343)
julio	July (Audio vocab0344)
junio	June (Audio vocab0345)

L (AUDIO VOCAB0346)

lateral	lateral (Audio vocab0347)
el labio leporino	cleft lip (Audio vocab0348)
los labios	lips (Audio vocab0349)
el laboratorio	laboratory (Audio vocab0350)
delantal de plomo	lead apron (Audio vocab0350.1)
la lengua	tongue (Audio vocab0351)
la lengua negra peluda	black hairy tongue (Audio vocab0352)
la lesión	injury (Audio vocab0353)
ligado/a	bonded (Audio vocab0354)
la ligadura	bond (Audio vocab0355)
el ligamento periodontal	periodontal ligament (Audio vocab0356)

el líquido crevicular	crevicular fluid (Audio vocab0357)
llenar	fill (Audio vocab0358)
lunes	Monday (Audio vocab0359)

M (AUDIO VOCAB0360)

la madre	mother (Audio vocab0361)
el mal aliento, halitosis	bad breath, halitosis (Audio vocab0362)
la mamá	mother (Audio vocab0363)
mañana	tomorrow (Audio vocab0364)
mañana por la mañana	tomorrow morning (Audio vocab0365)
mañana por la noche	tomorrow evening (Audio vocab0366)
mañana por la tarde	tomorrow afternoon (Audio vocab0367)
la mandíbula	jaw, mandible (Audio vocab0368)
la mandíbula dislocada	dislocated jaw (Audio vocab0369)
el mantenimiento periodontal	periodontal maintenance (Audio vocab0370)
la máquina de aire abrasivo	air-abrasive machine (Audio vocab0371)
mareado/a	dizzy (Audio vocab0372)
el marido	husband (Audio vocab0373)
martes	Tuesday (Audio vocab0374)
marzo	March (Audio vocab375)
más tarde	later (Audio vocab0376)
masticar	to chew (Audio vocab0376.1)
el maxilar	maxilla. (Audio vocab0377)
mayo	May (Audio vocab0378)
los medicamentos	medications (Audio vocab0379)
la medida periodontal	periodontal measurement (Audio vocab0380)
el mes	month (Audio vocab0381)
miércoles	Wednesday (Audio vocab0382)
mil	one thousand (Audio vocab0383)
mil novecientos noventa y uno	one thousand nine hundred ninety-one (Audio vocab0384)

el minuto	minute (Audio vocab0385)
la mucosidad	mucous (n.) (Audio vocab0386)
el molar/la muela	molar (Audio vocab0387)
morado/a	purple (Audio vocab0388)
la mordedura/mordida	bite (noun) (Audio vocab0389)
morder/muerde	bite (verb) (Audio vocab0389.1)
la mordida cruzada	cross-bite (Audio vocab0390)
el moretón/la hematoma	bruise (Audio vocab0391)
la movilidad	mobility (Audio vocab0392)
la mucosa bucal	buccal mucosa (Audio vocab0393)
mucoso	mucous (adj.) (Audio vocab0394)
la muela del juicio/ muelas cordales	wisom tooth/wisdom teeth (Audio vocab0394.1)
la mujer	the woman (Audio vocab0395)
los músculos	muscles (Audio vocab0396)

N (AUDIO VOCAB0397)

negro/a	black (Audio vocab0398)
los niños	children (Audio vocab0399)
novecientos	nine hundred (Audio vocab0400)
noveno/a	ninth (Audio vocab0401)
noventa	ninety (Audio vocab0402)
noviembre	November (Audio vocab0403)
la nuera	daughter-in-law (Audio vocab0404)
nueve	nine (Audio vocab0405)
el número	number (Audio vocab0406)
nunca	never (Audio vocab0407)

O (AUDIO VOCAB0408)

ochenta	eighty (Audio vocab0409)
ocho	eight (Audio vocab0410)
ochocientos	eight hundred (Audio vocab0411)
la oclusión	occlusion (Audio vocab0412)
octavo/a	eighth (Audio vocab0413)
octubre	October (Audio vocab0414)

la odontología cosmética	cosmetic dentistry (Audio vocab0415)
el/la odontolog(o/a)	dentist (Audio vocab0415.1
la oficina	office (Audio vocab0416)
el ojo	eye (Audio vocab0417)
once	eleven (Audio vocab0418)
la ortodoncia	orthodontics (Audio vocab0418.1)
el/la ortodoncista	orthodontist (Audio vocab0419)
oscuro/a	dark (Audio vocab0420)
el óxido nitroso	nitrous oxide (Audio vocab0420.1)

P(AUDIO VOCAB0421)

el padre	father (Audio vocab0422)
los padres	parents (Audio vocab0423)
el paladar	palate (Audio vocab0424)
el paladar blando	soft palate (Audio vocab0425)
el paladar hendido	cleft palate (Audio vocab0426)
pálido/a	pale (in color tone) (Audio vocab0427)
el pañal	diaper (Audio vocab0428)
la pantalla de la computadora	computer screen (Audio vocab0429)
el papá	father (Audio vocab0430)
la papila gustativa	taste bud (Audio vocab0431)
¿para qué?	what for? (Audio vocab0432)
los parientes	relatives (Audio vocab0433)
pasado mañana	day after tomorrow (Audio vocab0434)
el pasillo	hallway (Audio vocab0435)
la (pasta/crema) de dientes/ pasta dental	toothpaste (Audio vocab0436)
las pastillas	pills (Audio vocab0437)
el/la pedodoncista	pedodontist (Audio vocab0438)
la rollo negativo	film (Audio vocab0439)
la pericoronitis	pericoronitis (Audio vocab0440)
el/la periodoncista	periodontist (Audio vocab0441)
la periodontitis	periodontitis (Audio vocab0442)
la periodontitis necrótica ulcerativa	necrotizing ulcerative periodontitis (Audio vocab0443)

el peróxido	peroxide (Audio vocab0444)
el peróxido de carbamida	carbamide peroxide (Audio vocab0445)
las (picaduras y aberturas/fosas y fisuras)	pits and fissures (Audio vocab0446)
picada	decayed (Audio vocab0446.1)
la piel	skin (Audio vocab0447)
placa	denture (Audio vocab0447.1)
la placa bacteriana	plaque (Audio vocab0448)
plateado/a	silver (in color tone) (Audio vocab0449)
podrido/a	decayed (Audio vocab0450)
la pomada	ointment (Audio vocab0451)
el póntico	pontic (Audio vocab0452)
por boca	by mouth (Audio vocab0453)
la porcelana	porcelain (Audio vocab0454)
por la mañana	in the morning (Audio vocab0455)
por la noche	in the evening (Audio vocab0456)
por la tarde	in the afternoon (Audio vocab0457)
¿por qué?	why? (Audio vocab0458)
la práctica dental	dental practice (Audio vocab0459)
la presa de goma	rubber dam (Audio vocab0460)
la presión arterial	blood pressure (Audio vocab0461)
la prevención de las caries	caries prevention (Audio vocab0462)
primero/a	first (Audio vocab0463)
el/la primo/a	cousin (Audio vocab0464)
los problemas cardíacos	heart problems (Audio vocab0465)
los problemas de la tiroides	thyroid problems (Audio vocab0466)
procedimiento	procedure (Audio vocab0466.1)
la profilaxis	prophylaxis (Audio vocab0467)
el/la prostodoncista	prosthodontist (Audio vocab0468)
el protector bucal	mouthguard (Audio vocab0469)
el protector bucal de noche	night guard (Audio vocab0470)
el puente	bridge (Audio vocab0471)
el puente fijo	fixed bridge (Audio vocab0472)

pulir	burnish, polish (Audio vocab0473)
puliendo	polishing (Audio vocab0474)
pulir con aire y polvo	air-powder polishing (Audio vocab0475)
la pulpa	pulp (Audio vocab0476)
la pulpectomiá	pulpectomy (Audio vocab0476.1)
púrpura/morado/a	purple (Audio vocab0477)

Q (AUDIO VOCAB0478)

¿qué?	what? (Audio vocab0479)
¿qué hora es?	what time is it? (Audio vocab0480)
la quemadura	burn (Audio vocab0481)
¿qué más?	what else? (Audio vocab0482)
¿quién?	who? (Audio vocab0483)
quince	fifteen (Audio vocab0484)
quinientos	five hundred (Audio vocab0485)
quinto/a	fifth (Audio vocab0486)

R (AUDIO VOCAB0487)

la radiación	radiation (Audio vocab0488)
la radiografía	radiograph (Audio vocab0489)
la radiología digital	digital imaging x-ray (Audio vocab0490)
la radiografía interproximal	bitewing radiograph (Audio vocab0491)
la raíz	root (Audio vocab0492)
el raspado	curettage (Audio vocab0493)
el raspado radicular y el alisado radicular	root plane and scale (Audio vocab0494)
los rayos X	the X-rays (Audio vocab0494.1)
la reacción adversa al medicamento	adverse drug reaction (Audio vocab0495)
la reacción alérgica retrasada	delayed allergic reaction (Audio vocab0496)
el/la recepcionista	receptionist (Audio vocab0497)
la recesión	recession (Audio vocab0498)
la receta	prescription (Audio vocab0499)

el relleno	filling (Audio vocab0499.1)
el resfriado	cold (Audio vocab0500)
retenido/a	unerupted (Audio vocab0501)
resina	resin (Audio vocab0501.1)
rojizo/a	reddish (Audio vocab0502)
rojo/a	red (Audio vocab0503)
la ropa	clothing (Audio vocab0504)
rosa	pink (Audio vocab0505)

S (AUDIO VOCAB0506)

sábado	Saturday (Audio vocab0507)
sacar	remove (Audio vocab0508)
la salida	exit (Audio vocab0509)
la saliva	saliva, spit (Audio vocab0510)
el (salón/cuarto) de examen	exam room (Audio vocab0511)
el (salón/sala) de espera	waiting room (Audio vocab0512)
la salud	health (Audio vocab0513)
la salud oral	oral health (Audio vocab0514)
el sangrado	bleeding (Audio vocab0515)
la sangre	blood (Audio vocab0516)
el sarro	tartar (Audio vocab0517)
el segundo	second (of time) (Audio vocab0518)
segundo/a	second (Audio vocab0519)
el seguro dental	dental insurance (Audio vocab0520)
seis	six (Audio vocab0521)
seiscientos	six hundred (Audio vocab0522)
el sellador	sealant (Audio vocab0523)
la semana	week (Audio vocab0524)
la semana próxima	next week (Audio vocab0525)
la sensibilidad	sensitivity (Audio vocab0526)
sensible	sensitive (Audio vocab0527)
septiembre	September (Audio vocab0528)
séptimo/a	seventh (Audio vocab0529)
la sequedad de boca	dry mouth (Audio vocab0530)
el servicio/baño	bathroom (Audio vocab0531)

sesenta	sixty (Audio vocab0532)
setecientos	seven hundred (Audio vocab0533)
setenta	seventy (Audio vocab0534)
sexto/a	sixth (Audio vocab0535)
siempre	always (Audio vocab0536)
siete	seven (Audio vocab0537)
la silla (dental)	chair (dental chair) (Audio vocab0538)
el síndrome de diente fraccionado	cracked-tooth syndrome (Audio vocab0539)
el síndrome de boca ardiente	burning-mouth syndrome (Audio vocab0540)
los síntomas	symptoms (Audio vocab0541)
la sobredentadura	overdenture (Audio vocab0542)
la sobremordida	overbite (Audio vocab0543)
la sobrina	niece (Audio vocab0544)
el sobrino	nephew (Audio vocab0545)
la solución de tintura	disclosing solution (Audio vocab0546)
el sombrero	hat (Audio vocab0547)
son las cinco	it is five o'clock (Audio vocab0548)
son las cuatro	it is four o'clock (Audio vocab0549)
son las diez	it is ten o'clock (Audio vocab0550)
son las doce	it is twelve o'clock (Audio vocab0551)
son las dos	it is two o'clock (Audio vocab0552)
son las dos menos veinte	it is twenty to two (Audio vocab0553)
son las dos y cuarto	it is a quarter past two (Audio vocab0554)
son las nueve	it is nine o'clock (Audio vocab0555)
son las ocho	it is eight o'clock (Audio vocab0556)
son las ocho menos cinco	it is five to eight. (Audio vocab0557)
son las once	it is eleven o'clock (Audio vocab0558)
son las seis	it is six o'clock (Audio vocab0559)
son las siete	it is seven o'clock (Audio vocab0560)
son las tres	it is three o'clock (Audio vocab0561)
son las tres y media	it is three thirty (Audio vocab0562)
son las tres y quince	it is three fifteen (Audio vocab0563)
el succionador	suction (Audio vocab0563.1)
la suegra	mother-in-law (Audio vocab0564)
el suegro	father-in-law (Audio vocab0565)

| los suegros | in-laws (Audio vocab0566) |
| el surco | sulcus (Audio vocab0567) |

T (AUDIO VOCAB0568)

las tabletas	tablets (Audio vocab0569)
el taladro	drill (Audio vocab0570)
tarde	late (Audio vocab0571)
el tatuaje de amalgama	amalgam tattoo (Audio vocab0572)
el tejido bucal	buccal tissue (Audio vocab0573)
el tejido periodontal	periodontal tissue (Audio vocab0574)
el teléfono público	public phone (Audio vocab0575)
temprano	early (Audio vocab0576)
la terapia periodontal	periodontal therapy (Audio vocab0577)
la terapia periodontal activa	active periodontal therapy (Audio vocab0578)
tercero/a	third (Audio vocab0579)
la tía	aunt (Audio vocab0580)
el tío	uncle (Audio vocab0581)
toda la mañana	all morning (Audio vocab0582)
toda la noche	all night (Audio vocab0583)
toda la tarde	all afternoon (Audio vocab0584)
todas las mañanas	every morning (Audio vocab0585)
todas las noches	every evening (Audio vocab0586)
todas las tardes	every afternoon (Audio vocab0587)
transparente	transparent (Audio vocab0588)
el tratamiento de las caries	caries management (Audio vocab0589)
trece	thirteen (Audio vocab0590)
treinta	thirty (Audio vocab0591)
tres	three (Audio vocab0592)
trescientos	three hundred (Audio vocab0593)

U (AUDIO VOCAB0594)

| uno/a | one (Audio vocab0595) |
| la úlcera | ulcer (Audio vocab0595.1) |

V (AUDIO VOCAB0596)

los vasos sanguíneos	blood vessels (Audio vocab0597)
veinte	twenty (Audio vocab0598)
veinticinco	twenty-five (Audio vocab0599)
veinticuatro	twenty-four (Audio vocab600)
veintidós	twenty-two (Audio vocab0601)
veintinueve	twenty-nine (Audio vocab0602)
veintiocho	twenty-eight (Audio vocab0603)
veintiséis	twenty-six (Audio vocab0604)
veintisiete	twenty-seven (Audio vocab0605)
veintitrés	twenty-three (Audio vocab0606)
veintiuno	twenty-one (Audio vocab0607)
verde	green (Audio vocab0608)
la verruga	wart (Audio vocab0609)
"la vieja"	wife/old lady (Audio vocab0610)
"el viejo"	husband/old man (Audio vocab0611)
viernes	Friday (Audio vocab0612)

X (AUDIO VOCAB0613)

la xerostomía	xerostomia (Audio vocab0614)

Y (AUDIO VOCAB0615)

el yerno	son-in-law (Audio vocab0616)

Informal Expressions

Expresiones Informales* (Audio inf0001)

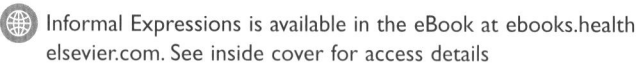 Informal Expressions is available in the eBook at ebooks.health. elsevier.com. See inside cover for access details

Index

Note: Page numbers followed *b* indicates boxes, *f* indicate figures and *t* indicate tables, and *e* indicate online content.